Mind
Matters

*Psychological Medicine
in
Holistic Practice*

J. R. MILLENSON

EASTLAND PRESS ◆ SEATTLE

Library of Congress Catalog Card Number: 94-61963
International Standard Book Number: 0-939616-21-1
Printed in the United States of America.

Library of Congress Cataloging in Publication

Millenson, John R., 1932-
    Mind matters: psychological medicine in holistic practice /
J. R. Millenson.
    p. cm.
    Includes bibliographical references and index.
    Preassigned LCCN: 94-61963
    ISBN 0-9393616-21-1

    1. Clinical health psychology.   2. Medicine, Psychosomatic.   3.
Holistic medicine—Psychological aspects.   4. Mind and body.   I.
Title.

R726.7.M55 1995   616'.0019
                                     QBI95-20248

2 4 6 8 10 9 7 5 3 1

Book design by Gary Niemeier

Table of Contents

Preface

All suffering is a call for inquiry.

—NISARGADATTA

IN NOVEMBER OF 1987 I came down with a cold. I was living in the Findhorn Community in Northern Scotland at the time, directing an educational project that combined a small herbal shop, a whole foods café and a resource center in natural medicine. I had just completed my formal qualifications as a medical herbalist and was about to expand my own naturopathic private practice.

The cold dragged on through the fall of that year, going and coming while I carried on with my duties as director of this exciting but taxing and often stress-inducing project. By Christmas of that year I found myself in bed and realized that I had been continuously ill for the longest period in my life. Moreover I felt chagrined that all the natural medicines and therapies I had tried had not succeeded in banishing a simple cold which by then had become an intractable case of influenza. My plan to go to India in the new year for my first real holiday break in many years (Findhorn is a working community, and I badly needed that vacation) was in danger of being lost, for I knew it would be foolhardy to expose myself to the unfamiliar microbes and dubious sanitation of the Indian subcontinent in my present state.

Accordingly, I bundled myself up and flew down to London on New Year's Eve of 1987 to escape the responsibilities of work and to recuperate at a friend's before my planned trip. Alas, the jet flight and the two-hour bus and train journey in bitter cold weather from the airport to my friend in suburban London was a serious new blow to my already beleaguered body and weakened immune system. I arrived very ill with some new and unrecognizable illness (later identified as mononucleosis—glandular

ix

fever, in my case without the fever and without the characteristic swollen glands) and from that moment for the next three years remained essentially bedridden. All through the winter months of that year my condition deteriorated despite the best medical attention from orthodox (allopathic) medicine and from a string of alternative practitioners and healers. The official diagnosis was post-viral debility—nothing serious to worry about, said every physician—but as the months went on and more and more symptoms developed and more and more body systems became impaired, I grew sicker and sicker, weaker and weaker, despite the good doctors' reassurances. In desperation and confusion, my thoughts began to turn to AIDS or some rare systemic cancer. My mental and emotional states had begun to deteriorate too, and by the spring of that year I had lost all interest in any aspect of life except how to get well. My IQ must have dropped 20 to 30 points. I felt desperate, despondent, terrified—in short, a complete wreck. My short-term memory was seriously impaired and I was so weak that I was only just able to care for my basic survival needs. And I felt sick, continuously ill, just as one feels with acute influenza.

It was only when I became jaundiced that I was at last able to get a clearer diagnosis, although it hardly helped dispel any mystery or relieve any of the anguish I felt. I had myalgic encephalomylitis (M.E., also known as chronic fatigue syndrome, C.F.S.), a relatively rare condition which had suddenly started appearing as if out of nowhere in the mid-1980s. I had never come across it in my medical studies, but I had recently read about it in the newspapers, and knew there was no effective treatment or cure. In looking into it I soon discovered that about 25 percent of sufferers recover significantly within two years of onset, another 25 percent more or less get over it in the next two years, and the remainder drag along indefinitely, some never recovering their normal functioning. It was an ominous prognosis, one that my stubborn and solutions-oriented personality was loath to accept. So for the next twelve months I struggled along, fighting invalidism, trying treatment after treatment, traveling from one physician and one alternative practitioner to another trying to find some glimmer of hope—either an esoteric medicine that might "work," or a different diagnosis that might have a cure.

By the summer of 1989, I reluctantly abandoned hope of finding any curative substance or therapeutic regimen. I had no option but to accept the diagnosis, and with considerable pessimism surrendered to my grim fate: I decided to live with M.E., and wait it out, hoping I would be lucky enough to fall into the first, or at worst the second, of the three statistical patient categories. After all, I rationalized, four years out of my life was considerably better than being an invalid in mind and body for the whole of the rest of it.

In that spirit I thus retired to a pleasant YMCA (preferable to a regimented nursing home or a pushy health farm) in upper Egypt where the climate—a major stressor to my sensitized, emaciated body—was mild year round, and where I could afford to live on the proceeds I received from the forced sale of my shop in Findhorn. As the months dragged on I studied Arabic just to keep occupied, even though my memory deficit meant that I rarely remembered much of what I painstakingly memorized from one day to the next, and waited . . . and waited, and waited, and waited.

Lying and sitting in my bed—and occasionally in the garden when I had the strength—I had all the time in the world to look back over my life and try to figure out why I, of all people and at exactly that moment, had been struck down by this bizarre incurable illness. For many years I had eaten a healthy low-fat vegetarian diet with an occasional piece of fresh fish, had never been a drinker or a smoker and usually retired well before midnight. At Findhorn I jogged two miles several times a week, and from May through October I swam in the frigid but invigorating waters of the North Sea. True, the Apothecary was a demanding work place, as I managed every aspect of it myself, ranging from cooking meals, doing the accounts, stocking the book section and the product line, to teaching the students who came to learn about natural medicine and the Findhorn way of working with Spirit. But although I worked six and sometimes seven days a week from 9 A.M. to after 6 P.M., and then usually took home the books to do the accounts on my personal computer, I loved the project and the community. Admittedly, there was no time for an intimate personal relationship; still, my creative life was more fulfilling than it had ever been in two prior decades as an academic at several universities in Britain and North America.

Eventually I began to see that in fact this lifestyle was perhaps not so healthy for me after all. I had plunged myself into a huge visionary project and taken on a work-load with financial responsibilities appropriate to a group. I had been working like Superman for several years, but also using my knowledge of powerful medicinal herbs to keep going under conditions well beyond the operating capacity of the human body system. In other words, I had been exceeding my own design limits for some time, hence the dire consequences I was now experiencing. I saw quite clearly that it was only my love for the work that had enabled me to go on as long as I had; and then, when my body began to warn me with relatively benign symptoms (the initial cold that progressed to flu), I kept on working.

As these insights gradually dawned upon me, I began to see medicine, health and disease in a new light. Although I knew well the theory of balanced living that is a key part of all the great ancient medical traditions—Chinese, Ayurvedic as well as our own Greek roots in the Hippocratic corpus—I obviously had not fully understood it. Now I did, first hand. Alas, perhaps too late, for I was well aware that not everyone is graced to recover from M.E. Eventually I formed a resolution: if ever I was well enough again to think logically and clearly, and to be able to write what I had learned about the complex and often hidden psychological influences in health and illness, I would endeavor to transmit this information to others. Far more subtle than realized (well-meaning but badly misguided "healers" asked me: "Why are you still holding onto this illness?"), yet also far more pervasive, I saw in my own chronic illness factors either hitherto unrecognized or insufficiently emphasized. Certainly, had I known before I fell ill the potentially lethal effects of overwork and over-commitment, and the neglect of my needs for intimacy and for simply doing nothing to balance all the activity that my work required, I would have been more careful.

My story has a happy ending, although I cannot personally take any responsibility for it. Suffice to say that in early 1991—now going into my fourth year of illness—fleeing the Gulf war, I ended up in an ashram in India (I did finally get my trip) on my deathbed. I had come to the baleful conclusion (I was by then coughing up blood) that I would at least have the dubious satisfaction of being the first person to die of chronic fatigue syndrome. At that very lowest point, just at the very moment when I completely gave up all hope and surrendered to the inevitability of my own death, help came to me. The master of that ashram took personal charge of me, assigned me a bed in his clinic, and after regressing me back to the state I had been in three years earlier when my cold/flu went to C.F.S., he instructed me exactly what to do with the simplest of natural remedies—what I should have done three years earlier, had I known—to regain health. And so it was that 17 days later, miraculously, I walked out of that ashram, weak, but clearly in a completely different state of health than when I had arrived. I was no longer sick, helpless, hopeless or despondent, but possessed with a firm sense of physical and mental well-being and a knowingness that the course of my life was back on track. I was rejoining the living.

Returning to Britain in the summer of 1991 and remembering my resolution, I set to work writing a short course module in health psychology for herbal students. That teaching module is the ancestor of this book. My formal research confirmed my experience with chronic illness, namely that psychological factors can enter into the predisposition, precipitation and perpetuation of disease in a myriad of subtle ways. Significantly, much of this material is not readily accessible to the average practitioner, being buried in scholarly journals and technical handbooks. This book, which brings together the results of that research, informed by my own experience of chronic illness, provides an introduction and overview to the major areas of interaction between psychology and medicine, and is directed particularly to the practitioner, student and aficionado of natural medicine who wishes to know more about how psychology may be of value in natural therapeutics. The tenor of the book is scientific, because that is my way. But I hope I have been able to communicate my belief that humanistic science is also an art.

Especially because much of the material in this book is science and is written in the style of science, I have wanted this preface to reflect my personal journey. I have felt it necessary to balance the personal with the abstract precisely because medicine will always remain at heart an art. Dealing in life and death, acutely aware of both the mechanical nature of the physical body and the ineffable mystery of that which informs the body, the physician stands as the symbolic link between the spirit and the body. In other times and other cultures the physician was priest, witch doctor and confessor. However sophisticated our technology becomes, this role of healer will remain and no one whose work is with sickness and death can evade it.

Many individuals helped to make this book a reality. Mary Gardner, F.R.H. was the first to offer encouragement of my initial suggestion that psychological influences in health and illness should be incorporated in the teaching of students in natural medicine, and the Secretary of the General Council and Register of Consultant Herbalists (U.K.), Kevin Embling-Evans, F.R.H., M.G.O., made it possible. Professor Debbie Allen first made me aware of the burgeoning field of modern health psychology and generously shared her knowledge with me. Leanna Standish, Ph.D., N.D. and Kay Costley-White, M.D. provided stimulation and encouragement and read portions of the manuscript, correcting numerous flaws and errors. My ever-loyal editor, Betsy Sandlin, has done the same, eliminating the most awkward instances of my prose. Even so, whatever errors and omissions that remain are my own responsibility for I am an obstinate author, set in my ways. Finally, I have to express my debt for the dubious privilege of having suffered through this long, mystifying, unwanted, but ultimately transformative, chronic illness, without which this book would never have been written.

1

Introduction:
What is Psychological Medicine?

*The history of medicine is a history of the dynamic
power of the relationship between doctor and patient.*

—W. R. HOUSTON[1]

*H*EALTH PSYCHOLOGY IS the clinical application of knowledge and methods
of the psychological and behavioral sciences to the evaluation, treatment
and prevention of disease and illness. It is thus an interdisciplinary field concerned in
part with the identification of the origins and causes of illness that lie in the psychosocial domain. And it also encompasses the clinical applications of psychotherapy
and behavioral therapy to patients with organic dysfunction wherever psychosocial
factors are known or suspected to be of significance in the illness process.

Although less than 20 years old as a distinct discipline, there are now numerous
textbooks of health psychology. Some are behaviorally oriented, others take a more
cognitive approach and a few are eclectic, but all are set in the framework of mainstream Western medicine. There the doctor is an expert authority on the diagnosis,
pathology and therapeutics of a derangement in the body, something called a disease,
which calls for treatment to be administered to a relatively passive sick person called a
patient. Diseases are believed for the most part to localize themselves in specific organs
or tissues, although some, called systemic, can ramify throughout the body. The causal agents of these diseases are invasive external agents (bacteria, viruses, parasites),
deficiencies of essential vitamins, nutrients or oxygen itself, trauma, environmental
hazards such as pollution, radiation and poisons, and defects in manufacturing called
genetic abnormalities. Disease in such a medicine denotes a malfunctioning body
part, and the physician's job is to figure out where it has gone wrong and to fix it (see
Fig. 1.1).

1

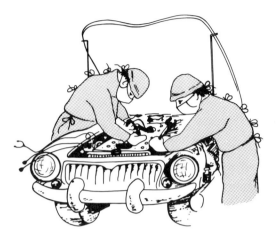

Fig. 1.1 Body Mechanics[2]

His—and this biomechanical medicine is predominantly patriarchal—primary tools are *allopathic* drugs that oppose the symptoms and pathology, and corrective surgery. If the body can't be fixed, then it can often be propped up with this medicine so that the patient can at least carry on functioning. There are of course many body systems and they vary greatly in design and function, making their complete up-to-date technical knowledge beyond the information capacity of any one human being. Medicine is thus conveniently dispensed by specialists who deal with particular body parts, e.g., the lungs, eye-ear-nose and throat, reproductive organs, brain, gut and so forth. As a set of powerful therapeutic tools amongst many, allopathy is of unquestionable value especially in infectious diseases and medical emergencies. But allopathy has become ideology, a putative synonym for all that medicine is and can be.

In this medicine the influences on people's health of how they think, feel and act do not go completely unrecognized. Indeed they are the province of another group of specialists. Clinical pychologists offer counseling to prepare the individual for medical stresses since patients are often terrified of invasive techniques, in particular surgery under general anesthesia. Hospitals in general are stressful environments as they put the individual in a dependent, relatively helpless, depersonalized role. Specialists in what has come to be called behavioral medicine also help instill skills and attitudes that enable people with chronic illnesses to cope better with unanticipated and possibly progressive disabilities. In illness we are faced with the limits of our own personal control and reminded forcibly of our mortality. So there is a place for supportive psychotherapy for those who have reacted to their disease with depression, anxiety or even panic.

But psychology touches deep aspects of illness that are not easily localized in a specialized branch of medicine. When the same treatment that proves effective for one patient with a particular disease fails with a second patient with the same disorder, biomechanical medicine has no easy answer. Something about patients, above and beyond their physical robustness—perhaps their character or their attitudes towards sickness or health, or even their will to live—seems to play a role in treatment efficacy. Certainly, from time immemorial physicians have recognized that the unexpected stresses and chronic strains of living—the slings and arrows of outrageous fortune—do influence one's susceptibility to disease. The characteristic ways a person copes with these—one's personality, in effect—has been a factor in Western medical philosophy since at least the second century when Galen incorporated the four Hippocratic humors into diagnosis and treatment. Indeed it was only relatively recently that the great successes of the germ theory of disease and modern surgery seemed to marginalize such influences. Around the middle of this century physicians who continued to work with psychological and emotional factors in illness etiology became compartmentalized in a special clinical division called *psychosomatic medicine* that dealt with a few anomalous diseases that remained refractory to biomedicine.

For all its successes in "conquering" disease and increasing longevity, allopathic medicine is faltering as it approaches the twenty-first century. Our modern health care institutions are overcrowded, our health bill is enormous and growing, new diseases have replaced the vanquished ones, and the incidence of others like cancer and heart disease have increased dramatically. On average we do not seem any healthier than our grandparents. In hindsight the limitations of allopathy might have been foreseen. Once infectious disease, deficiency disease and trauma have been brought under control with drugs, asepsis, sanitation and hygiene, average lifespan increases markedly. Then the impact of chronic disease, which was always lurking in the background, takes center stage. In the developed world, coronary heart disease, stroke, cancers and autoimmune diseases have replaced tuberculosis, influenza, polio, diphtheria and smallpox as the principal diseases of morbidity. Moreover, new chronic diseases such as AIDS, chronic fatigue syndrome and a host of environmental allergies and sensitivities have appeared, some of which may be related to modern petrochemical pollution, and others to multiple co-infection with numerous viruses that, until now, the human body has never had to deal with simultaneously. It seems that for every disease "conquered" by allopathy a new one arises to take its place.

This discouraging state of affairs serves to underline the limitations inherent in the medical philosophy of allopathy. The many-headed hydra of disease keeps growing new heads, feeding on our lack of clarity about the fundamental nature of disease. Does disease result from fortuitous contact with infectious agents and from chance factors in our genetic make-up? Or is it in fact largely due to imbalances and disharmonies with nature—our own and our environment's—that could, if recognized, be brought under our control? A new medicine is growing out of a burgeoning awareness that we must learn to live in harmony with our planet, that science at large must become more *holistic*.[3] This new medicine does not foresee the end of disease, for so long as there is life there will be a constantly evolving process; new disharmonies with the need for new balances will inevitably arise. Yet disease in this holistic philosophy is a kind of signal that warns us of imbalance. Were we to heed its earliest signs we could indeed reduce suffering. But our myopic health consciousness is still at the stage of crisis management where we rarely do anything, personally or globally, until we are forced to. In the chronic degenerative diseases the imbalances are starkly revealed in the realm of lifestyle and behavior. Here psychological factors in the predisposition, precipitation and perpetuation of organic pathology can no longer be ignored or pushed to the side.

This book is written from the perspective of a holistic medicine that sees the individual person-patient as an integral part of a larger system embracing the social, psychological and physical environment. This *biopsychosocial* framework and the systems approach to disease and illness are now familiar enough to mainstream medicine, having been introduced by Professor George Engel in a seminal paper some 15 years ago. But medicine has been slow to incorporate fully this holistic view, reluctant to realize its full implications for theory and practice. Were medicine purely science and technology, the acceptance of the biopsychosocial view would have precipitated a paradigmatic revolution. But medicine is also an industry. It is practiced within an entrenched social institution with many vested interests which resist change. We might take some consolation in knowing that although sterile procedure for surgery was introduced in the eighteenth century, it was initially viewed as a superstition and it was over 100 years before it became an accepted procedure.

It is in the niche created by this lag between the formulation of the new conceptual framework in medicine and its actual acceptance as the working paradigm that fringe medicines flourish. These complementary and alternative practices are implicitly holistic, but they frequently carry with them dualistic assumptions about mind and body and often possess anti-intellectual biases which alienate them from the scientific mainstream. Their value thus unrecognized, they remain unregulated and so, too often, they fail to train their practitioners to an acceptable standard of knowledge and skill even within their own limited domains. Nevertheless, they are the harbingers of a medicine yet to come. In time, as more physicians work in liaison with psychiatrists, and medical students are taught basic clinical psychology, orthodox medicine will move closer to "alternative medicine"; conversely, as complementary practitioners begin to incorporate basic sciences into their training and philosophy, fringe medicines will move closer to the mainstream.

Practitioners of holistic natural medicine include naturopaths, herbalists, homeopaths, acupuncturists, polarity therapists, aromatherapists, reflexologists, flower-essence practitioners, osteopaths and chiropractors, massage therapists, spiritual healers, body therapists, psychosomatic psychotherapists, holistic nutritional counselors and others. Health psychology is the obvious term for the field of psychological influences in such a medicine, but it carries a false promise. For all our aspirations, we know much less about how to create and maintain health than about how to fall ill. Most of the work in the field that encompasses psychology, behavior and medicine is still preoccupied with psychological factors of disease, not health. Israeli medical anthropologist Aaron Antonovsky has noted that given the extraordinary upheavals, frustrations, dangers, disappointments, hazards, assaults, griefs and losses to which human beings are subject, the real mystery is how so many manage to remain healthy. True, the literature makes occasional reference to the "hardy" personality who can cope well with life stressors, Antonovsky speaks of the importance for health of a "sense of coherence," Dr. Larry Dossey reminds us that health is a state of mind not of body, Abraham Maslow has written about the healthy person who is self-actualized, and Carl Rogers urged us to see the value for health of an open, authentic feeling way of being. Yet these are little more than the sketchiest of hints for a true health psychology.

The actual emergence of health psychology itself as a distinct field is in large part due to the discovery by two cardiologists in the 1960s that a certain toxic behavioral pattern consisting of aggressive hostility, impatience, freneticism and preoccupation with time predicts coronary heart disease. The real significance of this discovery is that for the first time personality variables were shown to be as relevant to disease as smoking is to lung cancer or the bite of a protozoa-carrying mosquito is to malaria. Since that seminal discovery psychologists have been drawn into a liaison role with physicians in an increasingly wide range of roles and treatment settings. Behavioral medicine is the new field dealing with the contributions of behavior theory to the treatment and prevention of disease, and it gives more clues and a few practical tools towards a health psychology.

In preparing this text, I took as much as I could from this incipient psychology of health, but like all others this book too is mostly about the psychology of disease. Since I did not wish to pretend that this was yet health psychology, I looked for another term to denote it and found it in *psychological medicine*. Ever since Daniel Hack Tuke wrote his classic textbook of psychological medicine in 1872 this term has had some currency in psychiatry and abnormal psychology. Hack Tuke's term was based on an analogy with organic medicine. Just as there were diseases of the body that affected organic function, so for Hack Tuke there were diseases of the mind that affected intellectual and affective functioning. What better term for a medicine that was to deal with these "mental diseases" than psychological medicine? This usage had its day, but one of the last textbooks to appear with this title was Tredgold's in 1945.[4] Long before then "psychiatry" had become the preferred word for psychological medicine. Today the term cannot be found in modern dictionaries of psychology or psychiatry, although several journals with this name continue to publish articles on psychiatry, health psychology, behavioral medicine, medical psychology, clinical psychology and psychosomatics. Psychological medicine seems a very appropriate description for the aspect of medicine concerned with psychological factors in the predisposition, precipitation, perpetuation and prevention of disease.[5] The term allows for a wide range of topical discussion, favors no particular theoretical position, and puts psychological medicine on an equal footing with chemical, botanical, nutritional, homeopathic, surgical, physical and other medicines that are used by the entire spectrum of practitioners and physicians.

Because I have written this book for students and practitioners of natural medicine, as well as for the general reader, who may never have formally studied psychology, I have tried to make it stand alone by including a chapter on the four principal schools of modern psychology. I do not pretend that this chapter is a substitute for an introductory course in psychology. It serves only to introduce some basic terms and to provide an orientation so that readers can understand how the different complementary psychologies approach medicine. This overview and my own eclectic predispositions have allowed me to tap a diversity of sources: many chapters rely, as do other health psychology texts, on the contemporary scientific literature. As much as possible I have endeavored to place the findings of research in a holistic context. And I have made no attempt to cover those aspects of health psychology or behavioral medicine that are specific to allopathic practice and complementary or antagonistic to natural medicine.

As this book is intended to be a practical sourcebook for working practitioners from diverse theoretical orientations, I have taken procedures and techniques from the entire therapeutic spectrum. Even so, I have not been able to include every valuable technique in psychological medicine. The reader may note the absence of neurolinguistic programming (NLP), autogenic training, the various neo-Reichian body therapies, yogic breathing exercises and other well-known therapies which are doubtless of value. In the interests of space I had to exercise some selection criteria, and the wisest course seemed to be to limit my exposition to the techniques and therapies with which I have had personal experience, either in the role of practitioner or patient.

Psychological medicine, as I have reincarnated it, is the application of psychology to problems which are presented primarily as somatic disorders. It is thus roughly equivalent to what is nowadays termed *mind-body medicine.* Complementary but distinct from mind-body medicine are those therapeutics applied through somatic channels which strongly affect mental function and emotional states, and which may appropriately be termed *body-mind medicine.* In Chinese medicine, for instance, each meridian (channel) is related to a specific emotional state, and acupuncture points and plant medicines are selected in part on the basis of mental and emotional symptomatology. Homeopathy addresses psychological aspects of disease with oral medicines, medical herbalism has its nervines, sedatives and stress reducers, and nutritional supplements have significant influences on mental and emotional symptoms. Important as these body-mind medicines are, I have elected not to treat them in this book. Although the two medicines would naturally be integrated in holistic practice, the body-mind therapies—unlike the therapeutics derived from health psychology written from the standpoint of natural medicine—are well documented in numerous sources that are readily available to the practitioner.[6]

By referring extensively to scientific literature, and recommending it to practitioners of natural medicine, I emphasize that alternative and complementary medicine need be no less scientific than biomedicine. Indeed the close attention to the individual case so characteristic of these medicines allows them to make unique contributions to medical psychology research, which for too long has been constrained by the poor resolving power of large-scale group statistics more appropriate to agricultural trials than to clinical medicine. At the same time I have not hesitated to utilize concepts and theories from medical philosophy and etiology that go beyond the realm of current experimental science, to discuss meaning in illness, to draw inspiration from individual case histories and autobiographies, and to make appeal to the healing power of nature. Key concepts of humanistic psychology and a spiritual view of illness and health are transcientific and cannot be proven or disproven by science. They are nonetheless fundamental to the holistic view of natural medicine.

Medicine remains in part an intuitive art and, as shamans have always recognized, a bit of magic as well. The idea that a modern discipline acknowledges such mystical and irrational elements troubles our scientific sensibilities. But our own present day mass-produced factory medicine in which the doctor is a "provider" of medical goods and services to a patient "consumer," whose principal role in the therapeutic enterprise is to "comply" with what the doctor orders, is what ought to shock us. In this book I have tried to strike a balance between that extreme view and an equally unbalanced New Age view which asserts that, having created them, we are fully responsible for all our illnesses. The latter view is undoubtedly simplistic. Yet by demanding quick fixes in the form of pills and knives for illness instead of addressing and correcting the imbalances in our lives and our social institutions, we are certainly responsible for our medical system.

A book such as this one that takes its facts and theories from a variety of sources is most likely to appeal to students and practitioners who are open enough to go beyond the shibboleths of our day whatever their healing persuasion. There is little that is new here, but as Pascal observed, the organization is my own.

Project 1

Psychology as a World View: The "Mind-Body" Journal

Although there is much to be learned from books about psychological medicine in the practice of natural medicine, a prime source of knowledge comes from our own personal experience distilled into a form that is general enough to be of use to our patients. In learning for ourselves what comprises harmonious and disharmonious living, in becoming sensitive to one body's needs and rhythms, in learning how these affect our health for better or worse, and in getting to know and honor the unique personality that we are, we discover the principles of one individual's (our own) medical psychology first hand. True, our needs, values and psychological requirements will not be identical to those of any other, but the process by which we go about discovering our own health psychology is a perfectly general one. Once learned it can be transmitted to others, in particular to our patients.

However, the influences and susceptibilities that constitute our personal psychology are extraordinarily subtle, interactive and fleeting. In addition, we are constantly bombarded with new information, unique situations and novel challenges every day. How to disentangle what is relevant from what is not? How to discover the correlations, patterns and regularities that can provide the basis for prediction and control of, at least, our own health? In order to cope with the diversity and volume of information, the student of natural medicine is encouraged to establish a record-keeping system in the form of a mind-body journal. Into this journal will go the descriptions and circumstances of all diseases and illnesses (serious as well as trifling) that occur to the recorder, along with the emotional background and potential sources of stress that are present at the time, since some of these may turn out to be related to the illness. The mind-body journal is also a place to record less obvious disharmonious physical states—slight feelings of tiredness at a time of day when normally strength and vigor are experienced, the sense of feeling a bit "off," reduced energy, a puzzling lack of desire to engage in normally enjoyed activities. Such signs are often the early warning signals of an impending illness arising out of a hardly noticed disharmony in our lives. In bringing our awareness to the subtle relations between our lives and our body states, the journal becomes a device for increasing sensitivity to the events that influence and regulate our health.

In terms of the concepts to be introduced in the next chapter, the journal provides the opportunity to keep track of all the so-called biopsychosocial factors that we discover correlate with early warning signs of disease. As data collection continues and sensitivity grows, we gradually acquire the ability to see patterns and regularities in how our body responds to particular events in our environment. Keeping the journal actually becomes a valuable self-monitoring device that can serve as a preventative to disease.

Throughout this text, as techniques and practical principles are introduced for ameliorating stress, balancing our emotions and establishing a nourishing and fulfilling lifestyle, the journal becomes a useful repository for our own personal experiments with these techniques and practices. The permanent record of the results of testing small, controlled changes in lifestyle in relation to potential stressors and daily hassles can tangibly reveal the effects of different coping strategies on our health.

Into the journal too can go our significant dreams, for these often carry hints about needed changes in our lives and point to unfulfilled needs that we may not be aware of in our waking life.

The mind-body journal is thus a kind of personal, ongoing "lab report" where any new and unexpected correlations between our own health and any of the factors illustrated later in the text in Fig. 2.3 can be recorded. Inevitably, in keeping the journal, new factors not shown in that diagram will be discovered, so that in time the journal becomes the emerging record of one's own significant personal biopsychosocial field. In that way the journal and the work done in keeping it help to create a science of the individual person whose complexity and detail will eventually go well beyond the sketch of Fig. 2.3. In this ongoing and systematic collection of knowledge about the self, even the beginning student of natural therapeutics can take satisfaction in knowing that he or she is helping to extend the boundaries of current medical knowledge. Requiring no elaborate equipment or instrumentation, needing no government grants, free from dependence upon the authority of another and carried out in spare time, journaling is science-in-the-making to which we can all contribute.

▨▨ Annotated Bibliography

Information about psychological medicine comes from many sources, loosely collected under the general heading of mind-body medicine. There are numerous popular books in the field, well-known authors being Drs. Bernie Siegel, Deepak Chopra and Larry Dossey. Review articles, reports of original research, book reviews and roundtable discussions can be found in professional journals representing various scientific subdivisions.

The annotated list provided here comprises a sample of some of the prominent scholarly journals in which the clinician, wishing to keep up to date with the latest findings in the field, may find articles of merit under such topics as stress, emotional dimensions of health, disease and illness, behavioral medicine, psychosomatics and similar rubrics. Although this list of periodicals is by no means exhaustive, it can provide the clinician and interested layperson with a useful entry point to the burgeoning body of literature in psychological medicine. The practitioner of natural medicine will be pleased to note that mainstream medicine and behavioral science is increasingly reflecting the holistic perspective.

Advances: The Journal of Mind-Body Health. Published quarterly since 1984 by the John E. Fetzer Institute, Inc., 9292 West KL Ave, Kalamazoo, MI 49009-9398. The journal publishes "manuscripts on all subjects relating to the capacity of mental phenomena to affect physical health."

Alternative and Complementary Therapies. A new (since September 1994) bimonthly publication for health care practitioners published by Mary Ann Liebert, Inc., 1651 Third Ave, New York, NY 10128. Promises to include cutting-edge papers and practical information on mind-body medicine, as well as book reviews, editorials and a literature watch.

Behavior Research and Therapy. Published eight times per year since 1963 by Elsevier Science Ltd., Bampfyde St., Exeter, EX1 2AH, England. "The journal publishes scientific papers pertaining to abnormal behavior and experience and their modification, and to medical psychology."

Behavioral Medicine: An Interdisciplinary Journal of Research and Practice. Published quarterly since 1974 by Heldref Publications, 1319 Eighteenth St., NW, Washington, DC 20036-1802.

Health Psychology. Published bimonthly since 1984 by the American Psychological Association, 700 First St., NW, Washington, DC 20002-4242. "A scholarly journal devoted to furthering an understanding of scientific relationships between behavioral principles on the one hand and physical health and illness on the other."

Journal of Behavioral Medicine. Published bimonthly since 1978 by Plenum Publishing Corporation, 233 Spring Street, New York, NY 10013. This "is a broadly conceived interdisciplinary publication devoted to furthering our understanding of physical health and illness through the knowledge and techniques of behavioral science." Current research topics include health risk factors (such as smoking, obesity and alcoholism), pain studies, self-regulation therapies and biofeedback.

Journal of Clinical and Consulting Psychology. Published bimonthly since 1933 by the American Psychological Association, 700 First St., NW, Washington, DC 20002-4242. Although the majority of the articles in this journal are concerned with disordered behavior, the journal occasionally publishes original review articles in the fields of psychosomatics and behavioral medicine.

Psychological Medicine. Published quarterly since 1970 by the Cambridge University Press, 110 Midland Ave., Port Chester, NY 10573-4930. "A journal primarily for the publication of original research in clinical psychiatry and the basic sciences related to it. These comprise not only the several fields of biological enquiry traditionally associated with medicine, but also the various psychological and social sciences, the relevance of which to medicine has become increasingly apparent."

Psychosomatic Medicine. Published bimonthly since 1939 by Williams and Wilkins, 428 E. Preston St., Baltimore, MD 21202-3993. "The journal welcomes original research articles, reviews and case reports."

Psychosomatics: The Journal of Consultation and Liaison Psychiatry. Published bimonthly since 1960 by the American Psychiatric Press Inc., 1400 K. St., NW, Washington, DC 20005 for the Academy of Psychosomatic Medicine. Review articles, original research reports, perspective articles, case reports, book reviews, letters and med-psych literature abstracts.

Psychotherapy and Psychosomatics. Published eight times per year since 1952 by S. Karger AG, P.O. Box C-H-4009, Basel, Switzerland for the International Federation for Medical Psychotherapy.

2

Historical and Psychological Background of Medical Models

The cause of many diseases is unknown to the physicians of Hellas because they are ignorant of the whole. For the part can never be well unless the whole is well. This . . . is the great error of our day in the treatment of the human body.

—PLATO (c. 356 B.C.)

*T*HE GREAT ERROR of the day 2300 years ago in ancient Greece remains the great error of the day in modern Western allopathic (orthodox) medicine. Since the discovery of cell pathology in 1858 by Rudolf Virchow and the discovery of bacterial involvement in infectious disease by Louis Pasteur in the late nineteenth century, illness and disease have been viewed in the framework of what is known as the doctrine of specific etiology, or more simply, the *biomedical model*. That model consists of two major postulates: (1) illness can be categorized into specific diseases characterized by identifiable organic pathology; and (2) each such disease has a unique primary cause.[1] This conceptual model is actually a *paradigm*[2] or world view in which we see illness arising out of organic malfunction, damage or disturbance in the machinery of the body. In this medical paradigm it is the physician's job to repair that machine. With the discovery of the physiological pathways of many diseases, biochemistry has spawned a huge pharmaceutical industry which each year synthesizes thousands of chemical compounds (drugs) in order to discover those which more or less selectively affect these disease pathways.

In the first half of this century the biomedical paradigm of illness—partly as a consequence of the therapeutic application of chemical drugs, antibiotics and vaccinations—achieved striking success in overcoming an appreciable segment of infectious disease. The therapeutics arising out of the biomedical model (often just called the medical model) virtually eliminated the major lethal diseases of the previous century: pneumonia, influenza and tuberculosis. Many other once deadly diseases, such

11

as diphtheria, smallpox, yellow fever, leprosy, malaria and scarlet fever, have either been eliminated or are under control.[3]

Yet it is precisely the success of the biomedical paradigm that has brought with it new *iatrogenic*[4] health problems that are very difficult to conceptualize in its terms, much less treat. The incidence of cancer, stroke, heart disease and mental disease has increased alarmingly in the twentieth century. This increase is partly due to the decline in infectious disease that used to kill many in their twenties, thirties and forties. Today the average life expectancy in the Western (developed) world has been substantially raised so that we now reach the age when degenerative disease becomes statistically more probable. But the increase in the chronic disease rate cannot be explained completely by increased longevity; by far the most important reason lies in psychological, social and behavioral factors that remain outside the conceptual schema of the biomedical paradigm. Mainstream medicine has been slow to acknowledge the importance of these factors and to bring them into the health care system.

Our Western Medical Heritage

It has been recognized since antiquity that habits, beliefs, attitudes, how we live and our physical and social environment play significant roles in sickness and health. Many ancient systems of medicine—Chinese, Indian and Tibetan, as well as the native traditions of shamanism and witch doctors—identified at least some of these factors in their practices and philosophies.[5] Nonetheless, until very recently it has not been possible to fashion a wide-angled conceptual model encompassing many temporally and spatially remote factors, influences and conditions of sickness and health into a single consistent paradigm. Still, our own Western medical heritage, which stems from the ancient Hellenic and pre-Hellenic medical practices and philosophy enshrined in the famous Hippocratic corpus, did possess primitive holistic tendencies. Hippocrates himself was born about 460 B.C. on the island of Kos where he founded a school which became famous for healing patients by rational methods, which contrasted with the orthodox medicine of the times, namely the magical cures of the temple. Hippocrates himself is considered the author of several books of the corpus; however, a large portion of it was actually compiled later, both by his disciples and his critics. The writings thus represent several diverse schools of thought that matured during the several centuries after Hippocrates, and are one of the earliest recorded attempts to create a naturalistic or truly scientific medicine.

The Hippocratic corpus contains three fundamental premises which marked substantial advances over previous magico-religious philosophies of healing:

- All illness is due to some bodily malfunction.
- The environment of the patient must be closely studied to arrive at a satisfactory diagnosis and prognosis.
- Our own natures are the physicians of our illness.[6]

Hippocratic medicine viewed the person as a combination of four bodily humors:

black bile (feces), yellow bile (urine), blood and phlegm (mucus). The four humors were the body's representation of the four basic elements of matter: air, earth, fire and water. When the humors were in equilibrium the result was health. But when any one or more humor was either overly strong or overly weak sickness was the outcome. In keeping with this scheme, remedies and medicaments were themselves classified by the degree and composition of each of the four elements, and thus a quasi-rational basis for therapeutics was constructed. Mental passions (thoughts, feelings, emotions and behaviors) and humors interacted, and both were directly dependent on deviations from an ideal temperate life, the golden mean of the Greeks—nothing to excess. The early Greek physicians held too that the humors could be affected by climate, polluted water, over- or under-activity, lack of sunlight and other conditions of the environment. Hippocrates' principal therapy was, in fact, what we would today call naturopathic: fresh air, sun and sea bathing, rest and moderate exercise. Thus this ancient medicine was holistic in the sense that illness was regarded as the result of an imbalance in the whole person. It lacked, however, a conceptual language for the precise description and investigation of the various environmental and psychological variables of personality, beliefs, emotions, attitudes and the behavior patterns we today would call "lifestyles."

Six hundred years later, in the second century A.D., Galen, a Greek physician writing and practicing in Rome, took the humoral doctrine as a basis for a theory of temperament in which the varieties of human character were attributed to various admixtures of the four humors. Galen described four basic personality types, each of which was associated with a dominance of one of the four humors. Thus a dominance of blood led to a cheerful, sanguine and ruddy person. Too much black bile led to a tendency to depression and melancholia. Yellow bile dominance was associated with an angry, bitter personality, while overbalance of phlegm characterized the apathetic person. These personality types provided a further basis for treatment within the humoral framework of disease. The humoral theory of health and illness has come and gone, but Galen's four emotional aspects of personality—optimism, depression, hostility and apathy—remain today as key ones for understanding the relationship between health and personality. We still believe as he did that the sanguine personality has a protective quality against disease, while the other three types are each in some way associated with health risk.[7]

The humoral doctrine of Hippocratic and Galenic medicine was enormously influential for two thousand years. So long as it remained naturalistic and empirical, as it did until medieval times, it provided a conceptual basis for rational therapeutics. Yet in retrospect it can be seen that because verification of the relative composition and admixture of the humors remained hypothetical, the doctrine discouraged empirical observation. Lacking the very ingredient that might have advanced the early naturalistic therapeutics the ancient Greek model never led to a systematic collection of the observed relationships between lifestyle, thought patterns, emotions and illness. Eventually, as centuries went on without empirical measurement of the

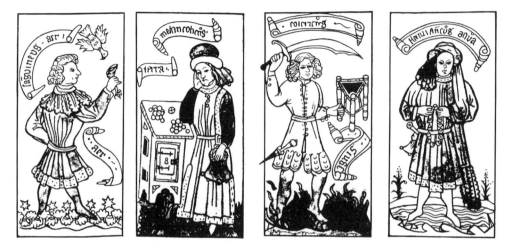

Fig 2.1 Medieval woodcuts of the four temperaments which Galen attributed to excesses of the four humors. From left to right: the man with optimistic, cheerful temperament, who has plenty of blood; the melancholy man, full of black bile; the hot-tempered man, who has a surplus of choler or yellow bile; and the sluggish man with too much phlegm.[8]

humors, the doctrine became dogmatic, and what had been an early holistic paradigm became stagnant, encouraging principally speculation on the nature and consequences of the hypothetical humors in place of the further development of knowledge and practice.

By medieval times, in what was a reversion to pre-Hippocratic medical philosophy, illness had come to be regarded as the product of demons and evil spirits, a revival in theological terms of the archaic medicines of ancient Egypt and Mesopotamia in which illness was seen as punishment from the gods. It is important to observe how the characterization of illness—what we have called the paradigm or model in which the natural phenomena of disease are viewed—occasions and justifies therapeutics. Although the ancients could not see or measure the equilibrium of the humors that they postulated as underlying sickness and health, they still could suppose that agents such as water, sunshine, rest and relaxation could affect the humors differentially, and in that sense the humoral theory was a naturalistic model. But when illness is considered to be the work of a supernatural devil which has somehow got into the body, then it becomes clearer why medieval medicine employed such techniques as bloodletting, purges, cathartics, even explicit punishment, to exorcise the evil spirits. Medical paradigms most definitely do influence the kinds of practical therapeutics that we are likely to think of as useful.

In hindsight it is very easy to criticize ancient, medieval and archaic systems of medicine in the light of twentieth century science. Yet history shows that every past and present medical system has captured some germ of truth about health and disease. The ancient Greeks knew little of anatomy and physiology, nothing about cellular pathology or infectious microorganisms, yet they had, two millennia ago, evolved a more holistic perspective on health than we have today in mainstream medicine.[9] How, a century from now, will medicine view radiation therapy, chemotherapy, electroshock therapy, surgical removal of tonsular lymph tissue, routine appendectomy and vaccination with active disease products? Will they too one day be seen as little more than superstitious, irrational "therapies" derived from a false model of illness?

And, before we scoff at the archaic and medieval ideas of illness as a punishment for sin, we should be aware that this idea too, for all its superfluous moralistic trappings, captures the grain of a very great truth that is only just beginning to be reacknowledged, namely that we ourselves are a participant in our own illness. As Dr. Edward Bach,[10] the Welsh homeopath who developed the Bach flower remedies, wrote nearly sixty years ago:

> . . . so long as our souls and personalities are in harmony all is joy and peace, happiness and health. It is when our personalities are led astray from the path laid down by the soul, either by our own worldly desires or by the persuasion of others, that a conflict arises. This conflict is the root cause of disease and unhappiness.[11]

The medieval theologians distorted this very naturalistic doctrine which they inherited from the great Master of Galilee, and added to it superfluous concepts of blame, guilt and moral condemnation, presumably because they thought it necessary to supplement the originally nonjudgmental Nazarene teachings with a dose of social punishment, just in case the flock did not heed the natural message of suffering that the body itself would give. The original meaning of the word *sin* is "to err, to miss the mark." There is no blame, no guilt, no pejorative connotation in the original Sumerian meaning. These were added long after the original use of the word to indicate that indeed we have deviated from the path of *being true to ourselves*.

Some of the newest, most hopeful programs for working with cancer and AIDS involve the patient looking very deeply into an illness and examining it in the context of his[12] own life, to discover how he participated in it and possibly helped to create the conditions which brought it about. The purpose of such analysis is far from finding fault or blame, but to give the afflicted person a very real sense of personal responsibility, which is in fact a source of control. What we helped to bring about, we can perhaps help to send away.

> Disease is in itself beneficent, and has for its object the bringing back of the personality to the divine will of the Soul; and thus we can see that it is both preventable and . . . curable. Suffering is a corrective to point out a lesson which by other means we have failed to grasp, and never can it be eradicated until that lesson is learnt.[13]

Dr. Edward Bach's Holistic Philosophy of Medicine

The ideas enunciated by homeopath and herbalist Edward Bach over half a century ago are fundamental to a holistic understanding of disease. But because they were framed in spiritual terms, because they speak of the divine soul and the lessons it must learn, the deep, fundamental truths contained in his writings have rarely reached beyond esoteric circles. Yet in fact they are quite in keeping with the most recent discoveries in modern particle physics and transpersonal psychology.

Bach's philosophy of health and disease is based on three interrelated ideas, which we shall cast in the current terminology of modern psychology:

- Disease is *often*[14] the result of a conflict between one's learned (conditioned) personality and one's basic inherited nature.
- Whenever one acts so that one's actions are in harmony with one's underlying basic nature, health and happiness will ensue. Conversely, when one acts in ways that violate one's basic nature (either because of social influences or from fears acquired in childhood), this harmony is disturbed. Failure to restore the harmony and balance increases the risks of falling ill.
- Once one has fallen ill, the only sure way to regain health is by restoring the lost harmony between one's actions and basic nature.

For the sake of completeness, Bach's three principles need to be supplemented by two other, complementary ones:

- There are various natural practices that can assist one in discovering the exact nature of the disharmony (we would today call these the psychotherapies, the counseling techniques, the psychological techniques of the "growth movement," the body therapies derived from psychoanalyst Wilhelm Reich, as well as yoga and meditation), giving us the awareness of where we erred, and thus providing the vision of what we need to do (or cease doing) to restore the balance.
- Various natural therapeutics (herbs in material doses, hydrotherapy, osteopathic adjustment, homeopathics, flower essences) will assist the body in regaining health by strengthening the healing power of nature, the vital force *(vis medicatrix naturae)*, which is nothing more than a central core of our basic nature.

We can see how different Bach's holistic model of illness is from the prevailing biomedical model when we examine how the very common (and predominantly modern) disease of hypertension (blood pressure greater than 140/90 mmHg) is dealt with by modern mainstream medicine. If we examine *MacBryde's Signs and Symptoms* (1983), a classic textbook for medical students studying pathological physiology and clinical interpretation, including treatment, we find an extensive discussion of the circulatory system, the hemodynamics of hypertension and the consequences of elevated blood pressure: untreated, hypertension increases the risk of renal damage, congestive heart failure, stroke and coronary artery disease by factors of two to six times. Although hypertension is occasionally a secondary result of a more primary pathology (diabetes, atherosclerosis, oral contraceptives), over 90 percent of cases are termed "essential hypertension," by which is meant "patients who do not have a detectable [read *organic*] cause for their blood pressure elevation."[15]

This is quite an extraordinary statement when we consider how much is known (as evidenced by the thirty-four page chapter on hypertension in *MacBryde's*) about the tissue pathology and the progress of the disease. But in fact, in the biomedical model, where could the causes be found? If they cannot be found in some infectious agent, or pathology, or mechanical organ failure prior to the appearance of the raised blood pressure, the medical model provides no appropriate place for the physician to look for them. *MacBryde's Signs and Symptoms* does mention in passing that hypertension is affected by stress, obesity, salt intake, cigarette smoking and alcohol consumption, and that it can be lowered by exercise. Aside from salt (which affects blood pressure by straightforward physiological laws of osmosis) the whole tenor of the discussion is that these factors are quite outside the purview of the physician, almost incidentals. That they lie outside the biomedical model is a fact; that it is not the doctor's job to include them in the treatment is a direct conclusion of that model. In any case, *MacBryde's* concludes, "unfortunately it is difficult to do anything about stress."[16] In this brief, dismissive sentence an entire body of psychological knowledge, built up over a half century by Hans Selye,[17] Professor of Experimental Medicine at the Université de Montréal, and his associates, concerning the nature and management of stress (which we will treat in detail in later chapters) is pronounced irrelevant for the medical student.

Holism and the Systems View of Life

In many ways the biomedical model in medicine is only a reflection of the far grander paradigm of mechanistic science which has occupied center stage in the philosophy and technology of our Western culture since the eighteenth century. Descartes in philosophy, Newton in physics and Darwin in biology created a conceptual world view in which all matter (inanimate and animate) was explained as complex bits of machinery, operating by deterministic laws in which God was reduced to chance.

The achievements in science and technology brought about by the application of the mechanistic view of the world are very familiar to us. Glance around. How many of those familiar objects which we take for granted and which are part and parcel of our daily lives would have been available even as recently as a century ago? Mechanistic biology has had no less an impact, for it has brought us an understanding of the basis of heredity and the ability to see into the cells that constitute the building blocks of our bodies.

But the very discoveries of classical science are now forcing us toward a new *systems* view of the world and ourselves. The classical scientific premise, that by analyzing the components of a system out of its context in the controlled conditions of a laboratory we could learn everything of importance about it, has broken down in modern particle physics, in biology, and now finally in medicine. The whole is not just the sum of its parts. Neither a physical nor a biological system can be reduced to a study of its components, for when the thing being studied is isolated it loses its properties. Look at Fig. 2.2, which shows a hierarchy of systems, with the focus on the *Person*. The person is simultaneously the highest level of the organismic hierarchy, and the lowest level of the social hierarchy. The person is made up of organs, and

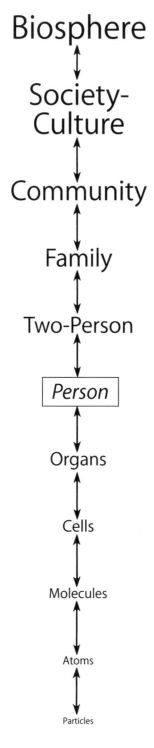

Biosphere

Society-
Culture

Community

Family

Two-Person

Person

Organs

Cells

Molecules

Atoms

Particles

Fig. 2.2
Hierarchy of Natural Systems[18]

these are made up of cells, right down to the deepest level of particulate nature that physicists have discovered to be nothing but probabilistic fields of energy.

Conversely, moving upward in the hierarchy, the person is part of a relational system whenever she is in transaction with another; she is part of a family, a culture and the biosphere, which itself displays so many characteristics of a living system that biologists have given her a name, Gaia, goddess of the earth from the Greek.

Although each particular level in Fig. 2.2 has its own laws and concepts, no level can be said to be more fundamental, for any examination of a level requires that interactions up and down the ladder be taken into account. Furthermore, although law-like relationships will be found on any given level, these will be complementary rather than subordinate to laws found on other levels. In other words, no lower level's laws will explain the phenomena of a higher level. This conceptual independence of systems in a hierarchy is radically different from classical science, which was *reductionist:* all phenomena were eventually to be reduced to physiochemical events.

One of the reasons why modern medicine has become so dehumanizing is that the physician has been operating, consciously or unconsciously, within the framework of classical Newtonian mechanistic science in identifying the patient as a diseased body. The system hierarchy expresses the fundamental idea that although persons are composed of subsystems that are in some ways machinelike, we are also part of higher order systems that cannot be explained by mechanical principles. These higher level systems make us psychosocial beings to which the relatively clocklike processes of lower systems can give no explanatory insights. There simply is no way that we, as persons, can be completely understood by the laws of physics, chemistry, molecular biology or anatomy and physiology, even though these laws are operating within us, and even though our bodies will not be violating them irrespective of what we are doing as social beings.

The systems view is not only an antidote to reductionism, it allows us to begin to understand the unique aspects of life that lie completely outside mechanistic science. Living systems are self-healing, self-renewing, homeostatic and adaptive. These are emergent phenomena simply not seen at the lowest levels of the hierarchy, and therefore their study requires a focus on the levels where they exist. Life cannot be reduced to physics.

> Systemic properties are destroyed when a system is dissected either physically or conceptually into isolated elements. Biomedical science, following Descartes, has concentrated too much on the machinelike properties of living matter and has neglected to study its organismic, or system, nature.[19]

In systems science the reality of a given level is actually created by the observer's attention or interest. We arbitrarily single out for attention the individual patient, but we are not going to be able to understand his illness until we explore him in his environment, i.e., all the systems of which he is a component. In biomedical science these are ignored, and only his subsystems are of interest.

The new systems approach to science is *holistic* science because each level is made up of whole conceptual units which cannot be dissected without loss of their identity. It is science with a wide perspective that recognizes the complexity and fundamentally probabilistic nature of its subject matter, recognizes the conceptual nature of it. Mind and matter are no longer separate. It is science which is able to see that everything is interrelated and interpenetrated, that there are no single causes, for the causal nexus is a seamless fabric, a texture of relationships running upward, outward and downward in a nested hierarchy of systems, each level with its own laws, its own conceptual reality that requires its own methods. This is a science that recognizes itself as a product of culture and tradition and our need to understand ourselves and the world of which we are a part. And it acknowledges that science itself is only one of a myriad of ways to understand. In the chapters to come we draw extensively from experimental science, in particular from one of the newest—psychological science—but we shall remain faithful to the systems view, taking what is of value to us in our humanistic perspective, discarding what is dogma, ever mindful that the mystery of life remains just beyond the boundaries of science, however much these expand.

Comparing the Holistic and Biomedical Paradigms

Consider for a moment how the holistic and the biomedical perspectives deal with the hypertensive patient discussed above. To assist with the comparison, glance at Table 2.1, which shows how the two distinctive models of illness and disease look at various aspects of the disease experience. The biomedical paradigm is very familiar to us since it denotes the prevailing medical philosophy in the West today. We want now to contrast it with the holistic approach, and in particular with what we shall be calling the *biopsychosocial*[20] model of disease and health. As the name implies, this paradigm finds the crucial factors in health and disease in *bio*logy, in *psycho*logy and in our *social* relationships with one another.

As Table 2.1 indicates, the biomedical physician's diagnostic and treatment approach to hypertension focuses on the reduction of blood pressure, which he[21] has ascertained is outside of statistically normal values. To him, the hypertension *is* the disease. Thus he concentrates on the circulatory system. He wants to detect any signs of renal impairment before irreversible damage to the kidneys occurs. He will be concerned about atherosclerosis, so he will order a salt-free diet. His treatment will be through *intervention* in the disease pathway with chemical drugs that reduce diastolic blood pressure below the accepted danger level of 100 mmHg.

	Causation Model	
	BIOPSYCHOSOCIAL	BIOMEDICAL
Emphasis	health	disease
Priority	prevention	curative
Diagnostic focus	whole person in his/her social & psychological environment	localized tissue disruption & specific pathogen
Treatment approach	support *vis medicatrix naturae;* restore balance to the whole psychosomatic system	intervention in disease pathway; symptomatic
Military metaphor for therapy	stimulate the home forces	search and destroy the invader
Patient/physician relationship	cooperative partnership; empowering	paternalistic; disempowering

Table 2.1 Comparison of the Biopsychosocial and Biomedical Paradigms of Medicine

The patient will come to him much in the manner in which you take your car to the garage to have faulty oil pressure looked at, and hopefully repaired. Similarly, the doctor's role is that of the expert body mechanic: he will treat you as your body, not expecting anything from you except that you answer his questions, which are probing for an organic cause, and once he arrives at his diagnosis, that you comply with his prescriptions. This is what Table 2.1 means by the patient/practitioner relationship being paternalistic. Some physicians will be willing to take time to explain the purpose of the medication, and some *might* even tell you the side effects, if you are brave enough to query the prescription; but because the modern practice is a very busy one indeed, you cannot count on this. Certainly the doctor will not consider such a discussion a necessary part of the therapeutics. Patients who question medicines and ask for details about their illness, and who wish to be full participants in the healing partnership, are generally not looked upon with favor by busy family practitioners, or even by many specialists/consultants. This is a key reason why people are turning more and more to alternative medicine, since holistic practitioners are not only willing to hear them out, but actually consider that the creation of a close human relationship between patient and practitioner is part of the healing process, a point we shall return to in detail in Chapter 13.[22]

Indeed, hearing them out is exactly what we want to do as biopsychosocial practitioners, because if Dr. Edward Bach's theory of the central core cause of disease is right, we are likely to have to help the patient find out what kind of a conflict or contradiction exists between his basic nature and his present habits or lifestyle. Of course, we want to be sure that this "basic nature," however complex and subtle an idea it may be, however unique for each one of us, still does not remain as vague and inscrutable as the humors of the ancient Greeks. It is actually in this detective work, where we and our patient are together searching for the causes of the loss of equilibrium and balance, that we see the depth of the new biopsychosocial paradigm. For this model requires us to treat our patient not as a machine that has developed a mechanical fault, but as a person immersed in a family, cultural and relationship *system*. Evidently it is only out of the relationship that we establish with our patient that we are going to be able to elicit the information we both, patient and practitioner, need to locate the causal nexus of the illness. And this information is critical, since the illness can only properly and lastingly be cured by eliminating its causes.

We will go into more detail in subsequent chapters about the precise ways of eliminating the cause(s), but suffice it to point out here that healing techniques as diverse as herbalism, hypnosis, surgery and even hands-on spiritual healing are all marked with relapses after apparent "cures" because, although the therapeutic technique "worked" at the time, the underlying cause (the imbalance of the Greeks, the conflict of Dr. Bach's theory, some persistent difficulty somewhere in a system level higher up than the physical body) was not eliminated. The body eventually reflects this continuing presence of imbalance in a recurrence. In a way the mechanical image has a counterpart: if you persistently drive with your foot on the clutch, your mechanic's good work of renewing the clutch will soon have to be repeated.

Different Kinds of Holistic Medicines

To give some idea of the intricate exploration into the patient's habits, experiences, sensations, beliefs, desires—in a word, psychology—that holistic practice can require, consider this examination protocol recommended by Samuel Hahnemann, the founder of homeopathic medicine:

> For example, what is the character of his stools? How does he pass his water? How is it with his day and night sleep? What is the state of his disposition, his humor, his memory? How about the thirst? What sort of taste has he in his mouth? What kinds of food and drink are most relished? What are most repugnant to him? Has each its full natural taste, or some other unusual taste? How does he feel after eating or drinking? Has he anything to tell about the head, the limbs, or the abdomen? . . . What did the patient vomit? Is the bad taste in his mouth putrid or bitter or sour, or what? Before or after eating or during the repast? At what period of the day was it worst? What is the taste of what is eructated? Does the urine only become turbid on standing, or is it

turbid when first discharged? . . . Does he start during sleep? Does he lie only on his back, or on which side? Does he cover himself well up, or can he not bear the clothes on him? Does he easily awake, or does he sleep too soundly? How does he feel immediately after waking from sleep? How often does this or that symptom occur? What is the cause that produces it each time it occurs? Does it come on whilst sitting, lying, standing, or when in motion? Only when fasting? . . . how the patient behaved during the visit—whether he was morose, quarrelsome, hasty, lachrymose, anxious, despairing, or sad, or hopeful, calm, etc. Whether he was in a drowsy state or in any way dull of comprehension; whether he spoke hoarsely or in a low tone or incoherently, or how otherwise did he talk? What was the color of his face and eyes, and of his skin generally? What degree of liveliness and power was there in his expression and eyes? What was the state of his tongue, his breathing, the smell from his mouth, and his hearing? Were his pupils dilated or contracted? How rapidly and to what extent did they alter in the dark and in the light? What was the character of the pulse? What was the condition of the skin of this or that part, or generally? Whether he lay with head thrown back with mouth half or fully open, with the arms placed above the head, on his back, or in what other position? What effort did he make to raise himself? And anything else in him that may strike the physician as being remarkable.[23]

Hahnemann's meticulous method of taking a case history reminds us that there do exist definite differences between various *holistic* medicines. Hahnemann's "taking the case" is a vivid illustration of the holism of the classical homeopath.[24] Because the homeopath is concerned to match the patient's symptom picture with the picture of a particular remedy out of many thousands of potential remedies, the practitioner must obtain as much detailed information about the patient as possible, on all fundamental levels: the physical, the mental (thoughts, beliefs, desires, intentions) and the emotional (feelings, moods, emotions). Physicist and life systems-analyst Fritjof Capra has distinguished two kinds of holistic views of health. In the first we are concerned not with a single organ or body system, but with the entire bodymind. This is the holism of homeopathy. The physical fact of hypertension, to pick a familiar example, is only one of a myriad of signs and symptoms that will make up a unique picture or reflection of the illness. In fact, the actual bodily symptom that brings the patient to the homeopathic practitioner is rarely the crucial symptom or pointer that makes the case stand out from the general background of disease, and hence rarely is the prescription (remedy) selected from what the patient regards as the most important symptom.

But Capra has distinguished a second kind of holistic medicine, a holism that goes beyond viewing a single bodymind as a unit which cannot be separated, to viewing a person in his or her environment as a holistic unit. In this holism the patient has become a *system,* which includes body, lifestyle, personality, his or her relationship to others, to family, work and culture, and even to the planet. Evidently this system, of which the person of the patient is the current focus, cannot be understood without taking into account how this person-system interacts with others, what kind of lifestyle he and his primary social groups have, how this particular identified patient's personality fosters health or how it attracts conflicts that predispose toward illness. It

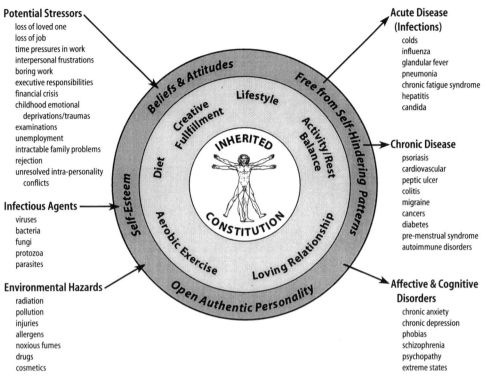

Potential Stressors
loss of loved one
loss of job
time pressures in work
interpersonal frustrations
boring work
executive responsibilities
financial crisis
childhood emotional
    deprivations/traumas
examinations
unemployment
intractable family problems
rejection
unresolved intra-personality
    conflicts

Infectious Agents
viruses
bacteria
fungi
protozoa
parasites

Environmental Hazards
radiation
pollution
injuries
allergens
noxious fumes
drugs
cosmetics

Acute Disease
(Infections)
colds
influenza
glandular fever
pneumonia
chronic fatigue syndrome
hepatitis
candida

Chronic Disease
psoriasis
cardiovascular
peptic ulcer
colitis
migraine
cancers
diabetes
pre-menstrual syndrome
autoimmune disorders

Affective & Cognitive
Disorders
chronic anxiety
chronic depression
phobias
schizophrenia
psychopathy
extreme states

Fig. 2.3 The Biopsychosocial Field of Disease

is this holism that best captures Dr. Bach's early conception of disease as arising from a conflict between our basic nature and our personality—read our systematic and particular conditioned ways of being, relating and behaving.

The Biopsychosocial Field Illustrated

In Fig. 2.3, which effectively includes and combines Capra's and Bach's holistic paradigm, the individual is seen to be influenced by three external kinds of disease-inducing agents. These are the environmental hazards, infectious agents and potential stressors shown on the diagram's left side. Typical examples of each of the three categories of causal disease-predisposing events are shown. Note that the existence of any one of the agents does not in itself produce disease. In logic we would say that these causal agents might be necessary, but not sufficient causes. In medicine we refer to them as predisposing factors or influences.

The central human figure in Fig. 2.3 is shown with three layers, which represent different facets of the whole human person. Although we shall sometimes refer to these as different "levels," there is no sense that any one facet is more fundamental than any other. You could think of these three facets esoterically as auras. The innermost core represents our inherited constitutional strengths and weaknesses. We know that many diseases tend to run in families, and a few diseases are actually inherited at birth. But like every other factor in the biopsychosocial model, the constitutional inherited component is only a predisposition; the actual manifestation of disease is multifactoral. The tendency for heart disease, diabetes, arthritis or cancer runs in families, but it may never manifest if one leads a healthy life. A constitutional disposition is a probability, and a probability whose value can be influenced up or down by many other factors, some of which—like lifestyle, exercise habits and diet—we have personal control over.

The middle (lightly shaded) layer of the human figure in Fig. 2.3 represents one aspect of what is meant by living a healthy life: this is the domain representing lifestyle. Here we include our diet, whether rest and activity are balanced in our lives, do we get sufficient aerobic exercise for our animal body, is our work creatively satisfying, do we have close intimate relationships with others, and are they fulfilling? The Hippocratic physicians were aware of these influences, but two thousand years have not been sufficient time to make their optimization for health a routine part of every twentieth century person's behavioral repertoire. Here will come one of the important uses of psychology to the practitioner, for behavioral medicine, derived from the experimental laboratory of the psychology of learning, can offer us techniques to modify unhealthy habits and to create and maintain healthy exercise regimens, diets and lifestyles.

The outer (darkly shaded) layer of our picture in Fig. 2.3 represents our personality. Here we depict the particular ways or psychological styles in which we interact with others: how open and authentic we are in relationship, how we are with authority figures, to what extent we still have (probably unconscious) childhood defensive and protective patterns developed long ago for coping with rejection and the lack of unconditional love. These patterns were useful, even crucial for childhood survival, but now are anachronistic and self-hindering for us as adults. In this personality layer, too, lie our self-esteem and our core beliefs and attitudes about ourselves and others, and significantly, how we react to potential stressors when we meet them. The personality layer also can be more or less healthy, more or less prone to predispose us to disease, not a cause of disease *per se,* but another probabilistic predisposing condition.

The effective practitioner of natural medicine is thus going to have to be able to act as a sensitive counselor for her patient. She is going to have to assist some patients to develop healthy ways of expressing and discharging the emotions of fear, resentment, shame and grief. She may sometimes have to be a teacher[25] of elementary health psychology to show a patient—delicately and gently, but firmly—how he is still retaining a childhood emotional pattern or belief system which acts against his own best interests, for these patterns are invitations to stress responses, hence constitute illness risk factors. A patient may still be holding on to feelings of guilt, despair or resentment rather than examining them to see what one part of the self is trying to tell another part, not yet claiming responsibility for his own life, still playing unconscious games.[26] Much of the material presented in the text is intended to furnish the basic conceptual tools for the practitioner to base her own work on, or in unusually difficult cases to be able to recognize when to refer a patient to an expert in psychotherapy.

Figure 2.3 is thus an attempt to portray the causal field of biopsychosocial medicine. The causes, or more accurately, the predisposing conditions, lie in the environment in three classes (potential stressors, infectious agents and environmental hazards); and they lie within the person in three other classes (constitutional strengths and weaknesses, acquired or learned lifestyles, and partly acquired, partly inherited personality traits). The actual appearance of any disease (shown on the right side of Fig. 2.3) depends on a complex interaction of all the factors on the left side. As shown, diseases themselves may be conveniently classified into three classes as well: acute disease (typically the short duration infectious diseases), chronic disease (the longer-lasting diseases that, if unresolved, become degenerative, eventually leading to death), and class three, the diseases in which the predominant or salient symptomatology is cognitive, behavioral and affective, the so-called mental diseases. The comprehensive model shown in Fig 2.3 is simply one way to organize and relate our experience of the causes and effects in illness and disease, and serves above all to remind us of the complexity of the disease process.

Alternative, Complementary and Holistic Medicines

The explicitness of the holistic picture of Fig. 2.3 is also a useful map to check uncritical uses of the trendy word "holistic," for the complete model shows us quite clearly what field of influences a treatment or technique needs to address. Merely because methods are alternative or complementary to allopathic medicine does not guarantee their holism. For instance, it is quite possible to prescribe an herbal formula for hypertension exactly as an allopathic physician would prescribe diuretics, beta blockers and vasodilators, and never inquire into the patient's life history to probe for the reasons behind the raised blood pressure. Aside from cases of first aid or for acute disease that needs immediate treatment, a holistic practitioner should address the root cause(s) of the illness, which, as Fig. 2.3 and the quotation from Hahnemann indicate, is likely to lie far from the body itself.

This is not to say that in many cases natural therapeutics alone will not be sufficient to stimulate nature's healing power, the *vis medicatrix naturae,* which in itself will be sufficient to restore the patient to health. In the final analysis, it is the patient who restores his or her own balance and harmony. Certainly natural medicines and natural therapeutics often have the ability to support us in taking the necessary actions in our life to restore the balance we temporarily lost, even help us make the changes in our ways of living and believing that are necessary. After all this is the very basis of the homeopathic philosophy and the Bach flower remedies: somehow the correct remedy brings about a psychosomatic response from within, which initiates the process that restores system harmony and health. Ultimately, it is the patient who does the curing, and the healing need not necessarily entail explicit psychological methods. To think that imbalance can only be rectified by psychology would be to go to the opposite extreme of biomedicine and elevate psychology to an unwarranted position of inflated prestige. We do not wish to replace one dogma with another. Once again, the ancient Greek ideal of the golden mean is our best guide. Psychological medicine is simply a set of valuable techniques and an orienting approach to holistic practice that effectively complement the particular therapeutics which the practitioner of natural medicine may be offering.

Project 2

Applying the Multi-Causal View to Symptoms

Go back in your own life and pick out one or two illnesses from which you have suffered. (If you have never been ill, then choose a close friend or relative.) Apply the holistic view of illness to your own symptoms, listing some of the various predisposing and causal factors. How did they interact to support a multi-causal view of illness? Were there psychogenic or iatrogenic factors? How can you understand your illness' cause and eventual resolution in terms of Dr. Edward Bach's philosophy of sickness and health as described and extended in the text?

Annotated Bibliography

Bach, Edward, and F. J. Wheeler. *The Bach Flower Remedies*. London: C. W. Daniels, 1979. Contains Bach's little treatise, "Heal Yourself," which encapsulates the holistic and modern vitalistic philosophy of medicine.

Capra, Fritjof. *The Turning Point*. New York: Simon & Schuster, 1982. Capra's chapter, "Wholeness and Health," has become a classic. But the entire book is well worth reading to see how our alternative medicines fit into the changing world view in which the Newtonian model of mechanics is giving way to the systems view.

Capra, Fritjof. *Uncommon Wisdom*. New York: Simon & Schuster, 1988. A more informal presentation than *The Turning Point*, in which Capra discusses how he arrived at his new synthesis. There are many conversations with eminent contemporary thinkers, one of the best of which is with Carl Simonton (the co-developer with Stephanie Matthews-Simonton of the use of visualizations to attack cancer cells) on his systems approach to cancer and chronic illness in general.

Cousins, Norman. *Anatomy of an Illness*. London: W. W. Norton, 1979. An extraordinary self-portrait of a man struck down by a supposedly incurable, fatal illness. The story of his recovery and indomitable will to live illustrates points from nearly all the chapters in this book.

Sobel, David S. *Ways of Health*. London: Harcourt Brace Jovanovich, 1979. A variety of chapters on holistic approaches to health, ancient systems of medicine, techniques of self-regulation and ecological views of health. The chapter on homeopathic medicine by Harris Coulter is a superb summary of the philosophy and practice of classical homeopathy.

Vithoulkas, George. *Science of Homeopathy.* New York: Grove, 1980. An excellent presentation of the theory of illness and disease by a recognized master prescriber of the twentieth century.

3

The Logics of Modern Psychology

Nasrudin was not feeling very well. He called in a doctor.

"You need a purgative," said the physician.

"I want a second opinion," said Nasrudin.

"An operation," said the second doctor.

"Send for another doctor," said Nasrudin.

"Massage is the only answer in cases like this," said the third.

"Now we have the prescription," said Nasrudin. "A third of a cut, a third of a purge, and add one-third of a massage. That should clear things up nicely!"[1]

WE COME TO the study of psychological influences in illness because we say that the mind and the body are not separate. And indeed we have seen that the field of causes and effects in medicine ranges widely from infectious agents, environmental hazards and potential stressors to personality and lifestyle risk factors. All of these causal agents—better, *predispositions*—play significant roles in the manifestation of both disease and crippling emotional/intellectual disorders.

The Concept of Mind

But what is this entity called "mind" that is able to influence and be influenced by the body in countless ways and at every level? We link the mind to the brain, no doubt because we cannot imagine thought in the absence of a brain. Yet the brain is certainly not identical to the mind, as evidenced by the fact that mental phenomena are a part of your and my everyday experience, whereas brain function is seen only by neurosurgeons and specialists in laboratories. No matter how much we discover about brain circuitry, we must still understand mental phenomena in their own right because the two systems—brain and mind—are holistic units existing at different conceptual levels (see Fig. 2.1, Chapter 2).

We speak of mind as though it were a place where our thoughts, memories, images, desires and intentions reside, as in "It came to my mind that I ought first to discuss the definition of mind." Our minds are also said to be the agents of our actions, and, as Fig. 3.1 depicts, we usually put them into our heads. Actually the mind has no location because it is *not* a thing. No doubt we are using certain parts of our brain when we think, judge, perceive, feel, reason and imagine. But so are we using our brains when we play the piano or ride a bicycle, and these activities do not go on in our heads. The examples seem to be different because while our actions take place in space, our thoughts do not.

When we are thinking, feeling, perceiving, judging, willing and desiring, we say we are "using" our mind, but perhaps our mind is using us since we aren't even aware of all our mental processes. This idea of the mind, as a kind of special private workshop where our mental processes are assembled and shipped out to awareness, ignores the developmental history of thought. We forget that thinking to ourselves is an acquired skill. The child who was admonished to "Think before you speak," and who answered, "How do I know what I think until I speak?" is a sharp reminder that as children we *first* learned to talk, and after that we learned to talk silently. Perhaps we'd do best to regard thought as *covert behavior* to emphasize its continuity with the rest of our actions.

If we turn to the dictionary for help we find that minds are places where *mental* processes take place (the workshop), *or* the processes themselves (the finished products of the workshop). When we look up "mental" for clarification, the dictionary just refers us back to "performed by or exists in the mind." We're in a circle. Another very serious problem about the concept of mind is the one inherent in Fig. 3.1. This little man (representing our mind) inside our head is supposed to be the real cause of our behavior. But if so, who or what is causing *his* actions. We seem forced to postulate an infinite regress of little people in our heads (called *homunculi*). Quite unsatisfactory. This theory, known as the "ghost-in-the-machine," is a kind of logical fiction, for it depicts our intentions and motives as though they come from a

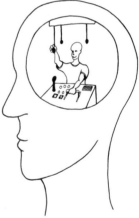

Fig. 3.1
The Ghost in the Machine

unique observational domain when actually they are concepts derived from certain characteristic aspects or qualities of our ordinary purposive behavior.

To see the spurious nature of such ghostly domains, consider an analogy from the everyday world of objects.[2] Imagine the visitor coming to a university campus for the first time. We show him around the colleges, libraries, playing fields, museums, scientific departments and administrative offices. He then says to us, "Very impressive. I have seen where the members of the colleges live, where the registrar works, where the scientists experiment and the rest. Now please show me the *university*." We then must explain to our naive visitor that the university does not constitute an additional department or institution that he has not already seen, but that in seeing the colleges, labs and offices, he has in fact seen the university. It is nothing more than the organization or sum of all the elements that he has already seen, so although it differs in level of abstraction from the elements of which it is composed, it entails no new observations.

The concept of the mind as a thing or a place on a par with another thing having a location called the body, and which houses the ghost-in-the-machine causing our actions, is a similar category mistake. It arises because we know that the laws of physics, chemistry and physiology do not suffice to explain a person's thinking, feeling and purposive doing. So we find ourselves obliged to represent these activities in ways other than, or at least in addition to, the units and dimensions of the physical and biological sciences. *Yet to admit that does not mean that we must create a fictional entity or repository for the causes of human actions.* Just as the human body represents a complex organized unit serving as a field of biomechanical causes and effects, so mind must represent another field of causes and effects. Essentially the word mind refers to the extraordinary *ways* we do what we do, the exquisitely complex *ways* we feel when we experience. Just as the university is defined by the various constituents that make it up, so too the mind is defined by the various constituents that make up our purposive behavior and everyday experience.[3]

We must therefore go beyond the everyday viewpoint which says that we act as we do because we will our actions, or because we want to do them. These statements are not wrong: they are another way of saying that we do what we do because we do it. It was once believed that we acted out of reason, and if we were ever acting in what Chapter 2 called self-hindering ways, appeal to reason would be sufficient to modify our irrational behavior. But ever since Freud we have had to abandon this simplistic rational view. We know that people go on smoking, overeating, living sedentary lives, self-destructing in all manner of ways despite the clear evidence that these habits are serious, even lethal, risk factors in health. Such discrepancies from rationality literally create the science of psychology, for they underline the task of ferreting out the causes of our feelings and actions wherever they may be found. Mind and mental phenomena can be addressed by a science that relates people's thoughts, feelings, desires and ambitions to each other, and to other independent events of the world around us. Because of the conceptual difficulties described we shall, however, rarely refer to "mind," although we certainly will be concerned with the intrinsic characteristics of thinking and emotion for the profound role they play in the biopsychosocial field of influences on health and illness.

The Spectrum of Modern Psychology

Psychology may well be the science of mind, but in practice it is the study of behavior and experience. The behavioristic critique against the introspective psychologies of the last century arose precisely out of the difficulty in creating a consistent body of knowledge from private consciousness. The critique is ongoing for it persists today in modern behavior theory where it has provided an important antidote to vague speculation, and has obliged psychologists to focus on what is verifiable and reproducible.

What we find when we examine what psychologists do (as opposed to what they say they are doing) is that they are studying how people think, learn, discriminate, judge, perceive, remember, and how and when they come to desire and fear and feel as they do, how they get and change their beliefs and attitudes, and how these in turn re-influence what they think, do and feel. Sometimes psychologists study normal people learning skills of various sorts, and sometimes they study people who are deeply emotionally disturbed. Some psychologists ask about the interrelation between people's motives and where these motives come from. That is to say, there is an ongoing examination of which aspects of behavior and experience are acquired by conditioning and learning, and which are predominantly hereditary. Another important area in psychology has to do with the measurement of complex concepts such as intelligence, personality traits and interpersonal communication. Other psychologists train animals or program computers to act intelligently, because these "simpler" systems that cannot communicate through language force their programmers to understand the principles of intelligent and purposive behavior well enough to create it.

With all these diverse activities and interests of psychologists spread over such a wide spectrum of observation, we shall hardly be surprised that there is no one grand conceptual paradigm that makes sense out of that great helter skelter of detail. On the contrary, different models, different methodologies, different schools of psychology command different areas of the terrain, and sometimes these various psychologies read like accounts from totally different planets. We are going to be obliged, like it or not, as practitioners of natural medicine, to take an eclectic position toward psychology rather like that wise fool Nasrudin took toward his doctors. Herbalists, naturopaths, osteopaths, acupuncturists and others will have to take a little bit from here and a little bit from there and be ready to use principles from any of the psychological schools.

This chapter is titled the logics of modern psychology simply because there is no one single conceptual paradigm unifying the field. This state of affairs justifies an examination of the fundamental concepts of the four current mainstream schools of psychology. We begin with Sigmund Freud because even though pure psychoanalysis itself remains today a very small enclave, every modern psychological school owes so much to the deterministic and functional viewpoint that Freud pioneered. Second, behavior theory, devoted to demonstrating that a great deal of mind is nothing but behavior, provides the basis of behavioral medicine and has spawned an impressive technology of behavior for education, therapy and self-help. We then look at a third school of thought, *cognitive* psychology, to which over 80 percent of modern psychologists claim allegiance. Influenced by the digital computer as a model of thought, cognitive psychology studies memory, perception, language and information processing in general. The cognitive treatment of the relation between beliefs, imagery and emotion will be of special interest to practitioners since these processes play such a crucial role in how we deal with life stressors, determining the degree to which we generate disease-predisposing stress responses. Finally we shall turn our attention to humanistic psychology, sometimes called "the third force" in psychology (the first two being psychoanalysis and behavior theory). Humanistic psychology provided the impetus that led to the encounter groups of the 1960s and continues to feed the present day growth movement. It is here, mixed with other "New Age" ideas derived in part from Eastern spiritual disciplines, that we shall find the most detailed attention to distinctly human motivation and to considerations of what it means to evolve a self-actualized, health-promoting personality.

The behaviorists keep us grounded in the empirical world of observation, the psychoanalysts never let us forget our darkest deepest unconscious, the cognitivists are working out the details of the black box of the rational human, and the humanists pursue the intuition that we are more than we know, more than we shall ever know, always a step beyond the pale of our own science.

Freud and Psychoanalysis

Sigmund Freud was born in 1856 in a small town in Moravia, now Czechoslovakia. He studied medicine in Vienna, which became his home until 1938 when he fled the imminent Nazi occupation to London, where he died a year later. Freud's clinical career commenced in 1885 when he went to Paris to study under the eminent professor of medicine J. M. Charcot, who was experimenting with the use of hypnosis in cases of hysteria.[4] On his return to Vienna Freud began to make use of hypnosis with patients suffering from puzzling physical symptoms (loss of limb sensation, blindness, paralysis) for which no detectable organic pathology could be found. Freud noticed that under hypnosis his patients spontaneously brought up memories and fantasies of past emotional traumas, usually in distant childhood, and usually to do with sexuality. Significantly, after re-experiencing these memories, patients' hysterical symptoms often disappeared.

Impressed as he was with this early success, Freud nonetheless found hypnosis unsatisfactory. Not all patients could be hypnotized, and cures were not invariably lasting in those who could. Freud looked for and hit upon another method, the now-classical technique of free association. The patient reclines on a couch and, unprompted, freely associates whatever thoughts arise, being instructed not to censor any of them. The therapist sits behind the patient out of eye contact, perhaps taking notes and from time to time commenting interpretatively in a nonjudgmental way. Out of this very simple situation Freud elaborated an entire system of psychology, whose basic premise is *functional*: everything a person does, says or thinks is presumed to have both meaning and motive, even though the patient might not be, and usually is not, aware of these deeper significances. Freud found that the origins of a patient's present problems invariably reside in the far distant childhood past. Remote though they are, representations of these childhood events remain incorporated in the present personality structure of the individual. Therapy consists of bringing to the light of awareness conflicting desires, suppressed painful memories and frightening thoughts, thereby allowing the appropriate emotions of fear, anger, grief, guilt and frustration—never fully discharged at the time—to be experienced in the present. The therapist's role is essentially to remain a nonjudgmental listener, occasionally suggesting or hinting at possible connections and contradictions between the past and present. The nonjudgmental climate is intended to make the treatment situation so safe that the patient can risk discharging negative emotions and expressing what might be socially unacceptable ideas. This emotional discharge (or *catharsis*), together with the patient's *insight*s about the past, are the necessary ingredients for a cure.

To make sense of his observations, Freud constructed a vast and impressive theory of personality with a threefold apparatus for representing (1) unconscious motives for lust, destruction and aggression called the *id*; (2) a partly unconscious and partly conscious system called the *ego* which deals with reality in a rational way; and (3) a part of the personality called the *superego* (conscience) containing parental and societal prohibitions. Freud found that patients consistently brought up suppressed (*repressed*) childhood sexual fantasies—and in some cases memories—of seduction, often by other family members, and these observations seemed to confirm that the core of patients' problems were sexual.

Evaluating Freud's contributions to medical psychology requires us to separate out the new and valuable findings, concepts and methods from the picturesque theory that Freud constructed to explain these findings. As an innovator, a pioneer in a land where none before him had explored, Freud was one of those who, like Copernicus and Darwin (the men with whom he compared himself), revolutionized our way of looking at ourselves and our world. These seminal contributions will endure long after his hydraulic model[5] of the mind and his psychosexual theory of personality are forgotten.

Indeed, these are but historical relics today. On the other hand, the idea that contradictions between different unconscious motives can induce conflicts that both prevent us from achieving our needs, and simultaneously induce chronic anxiety, guilt or negative self-judgment remains a lasting contribution to *psychogenesis*. A similar two-part judgment has to be made of the word "neurosis," used so casually as a cause of chronic anxiety, conflicting emotions, vacillating and self-defeating behavior. Neurosis is hardly a cause of anything. Rather it is a shorthand word summarizing the very obvious suffering and pathetic futility that characterize individuals experiencing such states. But as the term has come to acquire pejorative connotations and is clearly moving to the same judgmental pole that sin has reached over the last 2000 years, perhaps the wisest course is to dispense with it altogether. Certainly long-term depression is self-hindering, and so too is chronic anxiety, when these emotions prevent us from doing things we want to do which are not actually dangerous. Guilt too is not useful if all it does is make us feel bad without galvanizing adaptive action. The practitioner who cultivates an attitude of sympathetic, astute observation of the actual details and circumstances of a patient's negative feelings and self-defeating response patterns will find this a far more helpful healing climate than labeling patients "neurotic." Such labels always conceal the complexity of the individual person's process, and can be dehumanizing.

One of Freud's greatest contributions was to show us that our behavior is often governed by motives that we are quite out of touch with. This is really what is meant when it is said that Freud discovered the unconscious. Of course it had been known for millennia that we aren't aware of everything we do and everything we know, but the unconscious before Freud was a kind of wastebasket out of sight under our rational mind-table, with no apparent connection to anything of relevance. Freud's genius was to invest the unconscious with *motives* and to show how these motives, by conflicting and vying amongst themselves, exerted direct influence on everything we do and experience.

Freud took nothing his patients said to be chance: neither how they responded to the treatment situation, nor to the therapist, nor the content of their dreams, nor even their apparently innocuous slips of the tongue. Paralleling Darwin's functionalism in biology, Freud worked with the idea that *everything* a person does, says and feels must have a functional value, else it would not have occurred. In Chapter 12, dealing with meaning in illness, we explore how this approach provides a form of purposive or *teleological* explanation for diseases which prove difficult to locate exactly within the biopsychosocial framework. It was Freud who compiled the first great symbolic dictionary of meaning for dreams. True, he saw them primarily as expressions of repressed sexual urges, and certainly over-exaggerated the universality of the phallic symbol. Nevertheless, it was he who first attempted to bring into scientific theory the idea that *dreams speak a meaningful psychological language* which could be systematically deciphered once the therapist and the patient together discovered the keys.

The same kind of double judgment—useful to the practitioner in some ways, misleading and distorted in others—applies equally to Freud's frankly sexist developmental theory of personality. Today very few accept Freud's three stages of childhood development: the oral (age 0-18 months), the anal (age 18 months–3 years) and the phallic (age 5-6). And except for diehard psychoanalysts, the Oedipus complex (unresolved childhood sexual lust for the opposite-sex parent) is of historical interest only. But what emerges clear, strong and viable is Freud's great contribution that who we are as adults is directly related to how we compromised ourselves in childhood by building *defenses* against our own emotions to try to "buy" our parents' love. In adulthood these anachronistic childhood defenses hinder us from being open, authentic and accepting of ourselves as we are, thus preventing optimal health. These childhood defenses need to be brought to awareness and consciously rechosen or rejected as inappropriate, lest, by creating physical constrictions that lead to body armor and organ weakness, they become serious health risks. It was Freud who first taught us to see how our past lives are internalized in the present.

Even Freud's treatment situation—free association in the presence of a nonjudgmental other—so apparently simple, was a major discovery, for it represented a new way to listen, a new way to accept another's thoughts and fantasies and feelings. Modified free association is the basis for modern nondirective counseling, although counselors nowadays prefer to sit face to face with their patients (whom they generally call clients to emphasize the cooperative, nonhierarchical nature of the therapeutic enterprise), and to give simple descriptive feedback rather more neutral than traditional Freudian interpretations. The discovery, too, by Freud that patients develop a characteristic emotional relationship with the therapist, in which the patient acts toward the therapist as if the therapist were the parent, remains the basis for many therapeutic insights. This *transference* of emotion projected from childhood parent to present-day therapist is frequently seen in deep counseling and is used to demonstrate how the patient still responds as a child to the world. In this way Freud's therapeutic situation within the four walls of the practitioner's office can become a true microcosm of the patient's actual everyday life.

Freud's method was to assist (our word therapist is derived from the Greek *therapuin,* to assist) the patient to gain insight into deep conflicts. Insight plus catharsis form the basis of cure, which means freedom from domination by negative emotions arising from past hurts and early emotional wounds. As a method, psychoanalysis has not been outstandingly successful. It takes years (even when successful), is quite expensive and consequently available only to relatively few. No doubt these are important reasons why a variety of other psychotherapies now dominate the field. Nonetheless, Freud's principles of insight (increased self-awareness) and catharsis (deep, intense emotional discharge) remain central to most modern psychotherapies.

In retrospect, Freud changed and molded the character of modern psychology. His contributions will inhere throughout the field long after the specifics of his theories are forgotten. A number of Freud's most illustrious students and disciples went on to create their own systems which modified, expanded and built upon his seminal contributions. Out of the work of these men and women came two developments of abiding interest to practitioners of natural medicine. One was the formulation of psychosomatic medicine, the first systematic theory of how psychogenic factors could bring about organic disease. The second was the discovery by Wilhelm Reich that the emotional defenses erected in childhood to insure survival and to prevent rejection go beyond the personality to lodge in the very muscles and connective tissues of the body itself in the form of a kind of *body armor* which, walling us off from our own selves, can undermine our health and well-being.

Behavior Theory

Whereas Freud's work arose within the framework of European medicine, behavior theory[6] emerged out of American academic psychology as a reaction to the speculations and impracticalities inherent in the study of consciousness as introspection. John B. Watson at the University of Chicago was the first to call himself a behaviorist, and his program called for psychology to be a natural science of behavior. Mind, consciousness and experience, if these words meant anything at all, were not in themselves to be the subject of psychology. Rather, psychology was a natural science, like physics, chemistry and biology, concerned with the laws of behavior.

In 1920 about the only reproducible general set of data that resembled anything like a law in science that Watson could utilize for his program were the observations of the Nobel Prize-winning Russian physiologist, Ivan Pavlov. It was Pavlov who had demonstrated that neutral stimuli events like tones and lights, repeatedly and reliably associated with the delivery of food, caused hungry dogs to salivate. In thus demonstrating the control of physiological functioning (salivation) by an environmental factor (conditioning of stimuli), Pavlov could be said to have been an early forerunner of mind-body medicine. Watson saw in this principle of conditioning a model for association learning that he thought could be generalized to skills of all kinds, including language. Conditioning of this sort has a kind of mechanical character about it, and one might well refer to Watson's program as an attempt to create a pseudo-mechanics of behavior. The attempt failed, although Watson and his students were able to show that emotions like fear and pleasure could indeed be connected to new stimuli by Pavlov's principle.

Important as such discoveries were, they fail to throw much light upon the origin of our ordinary everyday actions. The problem really is that what we call variously purposive, voluntary and choice behaviors simply do not conform to the pattern that reflex behaviors, like salivation and innate emotional responses, do. It was not until the work of the now well-known American behaviorist B. F. Skinner, beginning in the late 1930s and extending through the next half century, that behavior theory was able to formulate a consistent model for voluntary action. From experiments conducted first in higher animals and later extended to human beings, Skinner showed that the crucial principle governing choice or purposive behavior was not Pavlov's conditioning, but a variant of Darwin's natural selection. By looking at choice behaviors as being *emitted* by an individual organism—initially for unknown reasons that exist prior to the experimental investigation—those behaviors which resulted in producing favorable or desirable environmental consequences (food, water, access to a mate) became differentially strengthened, learned and maintained in that situation. Skinner called that selection process *reinforcement* and saw it as the great principle governing purposive behavior. And because reinforcement could as well or more easily be studied in rats, pigeons and monkeys as in humans, Skinner took it as the job of behavior theory to discover the laws of reinforcement in the animal laboratory.

What he and his associates discovered of interest to psychological medicine were some very general principles of learning and behavior maintenance that apply to everyday behavior of normal human beings. This is the kind of behavior which operates on the environment, so Skinner called it *operant* behavior to avoid the murky ghost-in-the-machine issues of locating and identifying the causal agency of behavior that the terms voluntary or purposive seem to require. Operant behavior is simply behavior that can be *shaped* and maintained by reinforcement, and in its domain are actions such as talking, walking, reading—skills of every sort—in short, quite ordinary activities. In this scheme, motivation and emotion are considered two of the major classes of controls that turn such learned activities on or off and govern its strength. This is because the appearance or strength of the tendency to engage in an action depends on the current value of its reinforcer, i.e., how much the reward or reinforcement for that action is currently desired. And that in turn depends on factors traditionally placed in the fields of motivation and emotion. For instance, if you aren't hungry or if you are frightened, you aren't likely to produce any food-directed activities, even though you know how (i.e., you have learned what to do to get food). Conversely, having spent all day indoors, your motivation to go out for a walk will increase the likelihood of your doing so, and your tendency to do so will also be affected by your general emotional mood at the time. Generally speaking, in the language of behavior theory, every action, from the simplest to the most complex, involves three aspects. First there is a learned skill, having been shaped up by a reinforcement history, known or unknown. Next there must be the environmental supports for the skill to occur. And lastly the reinforcer (motive) involved must have sufficient attractive power. For instance, if you like to dance, you are most likely to do so when (1) you've learned the steps to the music, (2) you have the opportunity (a congenial partner, good music), and (3) your motive (desire) to dance is strong—i.e., the reinforcement value of dancing is high at that moment.

These principles, conceptualized by behavioral psychology, are eminently practical:

- To best maintain behavior, reinforcement should come immediately after the action is made.
- Whether the behaving person knows reinforcement is coming for a particular behavior isn't as important as the fact that in the past it actually has done so. That is to say, the action of reinforcement has an automatic quality about it.
- To create new behaviors never before made by the person, the teacher begins with an existing operant (say a low jump) and gradually makes reinforcement contingent on a progressive operant series (higher and higher jumps). This progressive *shaping* of behavior is the key to creating complex new behaviors.
- The *if-then* behavior-reinforcement relation, which can be determined by the natural structure of the environment or created artificially by society or a teacher, is called a *reinforcement contingency*. Knowing the detailed reinforcement contingencies that exist in a person's world is a way of understanding what maintains that person's behavior patterns.
- If a particular reinforcement contingency is operative only in a particular environmental condition, then the presence or absence of that environmental state will eventually come to control the behavior. So, when you find that weeding the garden is easiest after a rain, you'll wait for rain to do your weeding. And if you get sympathy from some but not from others for complaining about your back pains, your com-

plaints will pretty soon be selectively directed to those who reinforce (pay attention to) them.

- Unreinforced acts eventually decline in probability or *extinguish,* and the time it takes them to extinguish fully is governed both by their strength and by how strong their related motive happens to be.
- Another useful principle states that when you want to chain various units of behavior together, as you do when you teach a child to lace her shoe, it is better to start at the end and train backwards.
- An important principle turned up when the behavior theorists tried reinforcing only some, not every, instance of a selected behavior. They discovered that if only every 10th or every 100th or even every 1000th key peck by a hungry pigeon produced food, vast amounts of work could be evoked from the animals with very little payment.
- Behavior theorists investigated punishment too, usually in the form of nasty, brief electric shocks to the feet of their animal subjects, which were enclosed in small boxes. In general it was found that punishment, while it had suppressive effects on previously learned actions, wasn't a useful principle for learning itself. Punishment had to be maintained indefinitely to be effective in suppressing behavior, and it invariably caused emotional effects (fear and aggression) which interfered with new learning.

Beginning about the mid-twentieth century behavioral psychologists began to develop a theory of human behavior based on their findings from the animal labs. In general they saw the world as one of reinforcement contingencies, and they saw the causes of our behavior as due to our past history with these contingencies, our unique personalities built up from unique operant conditioning histories. They also saw our maladaptive habits—what we have called neurotic traits and self-hindering behaviors—as established by past social reinforcers that, while quite subtle and perhaps not verbalizable, nonetheless continue to maintain themselves in the present. Thus if a child only received its parents' attention by acting out, it could grow to adulthood still getting people's attention—albeit negative attention—by playing the role of helpless victim, by behaving aggressively, being the troublemaker, the destructive critic and so forth. In addition, because quite a few situations in everyday life, especially piecework in factories, seemed closely to resemble the conditions in laboratory experiments, behavior theory seemed a way to interpret and explain a great deal of everyday human activity in the world at large.

Behaviorists are often criticized for their lack of attention to the inherited or innate genetic structure of the individual. Actually Skinner did acknowledge the importance of biological natural selection in molding us to what we are. But because this *phylogenetic* selection lies in the very remote past of our ancestors, thus already predetermined, Skinner concluded that it could be disregarded in a practical program concerned with a *technology of behavior.* Such a program, whose aim would be to create and maintain desirable personal habits and social behaviors, would be obliged to focus on the relevant functional factors which could be currently controlled and manipulated. Those of course are located in a person's immediate environment. This pragmatic *environmentalism*, however, seems to suggest that whatever is not under our control is best ignored. Yet it would be a poor woodcarver or sculptor indeed who ignored the grain of his material simply because he had no hand in its nature and couldn't modify it.

Much of this focus on environment is derived from Skinner's view that the value of behavior theory is directly related to its power to create a technology of behavior. The principles being systematized and clarified in the animal lab must, he felt, be helpful to improve educational practices, to bear on child rearing, to carry over into psychotherapy and even to social engineering. To illustrate some of the possibilities for how reinforcement might work to create communities and ideal societies, he wrote a novel (*Walden II*) about a hypothetical intentional society where detailed reinforcement contingencies were explicitly engineered for every desired aspect of every individual's behavior. In a less extreme way, behavior theory does in fact provide valuable principles for use in medicine, as we'll see in Chapter 6 on behavioral medicine. It has also given us an objective way of looking at the side of ourselves that we do share with our friends in the animal kingdom. But very serious and legitimate concerns have been raised about the restrictiveness and hence the generalizability of the laboratory situation out of which the principles are derived. And the emphasis in behavior theory on *control* of (usually other people's) behavior can too easily serve as a justification for authoritarian and oppressive social control.

People often have one of two reactions upon first hearing about behavioral psychology. In the first place a recital of the principles seems like nothing very new. After all, every sports coach and animal trainer knows the principles of shaping and chaining; reward and punishment have been used for thousands of years, and who wants a psychology that can justify (or even make more efficient) factories based on piece work. To be fair, reinforcement is more accurately characterized as *feedback* than as reward, as the simple example of learning to throw darts with and without seeing the target proves. But people often have another very strong reaction: if these principles really are true then behavior theory is very dangerous, for it opens the door to scientific brainwashing and grim Orwellian visions of Big Brother control over every aspect of our lives.

Skinner's consistent reply to the issue of control was that it is better to know the variables of which your behavior is a function than to remain in ignorance and allow your behavior to be manipulated on the pretext that you have free will. Once in possession of the scientific principles of behavior, we are then in a position to choose to use them for benign ends: e.g., let's create a society where people are happy, productive and well-behaved (Skinner's choice of goals).

Without caricaturizing behavior theory, it is crucial to grasp what it leaves out of its picture of human nature. First of all, by concentrating on the animal model as a source of its principles, if there are any other principles of psychology that apply uniquely to the human being, this psychology is certainly not going to find them. The eminent British neuroanatomist Grey-Walter once remarked that a bowl of jelly is a good model of the brain so far as it goes (which clearly is not very far); and the same might be said of reinforcement theory. It is not that people are not influenced by reinforcers such as food, water and money; and it's not that our behavior sequences are not held together by detailed reinforcement feedback from unit to unit. But there are more things in heaven and earth than are dreamt of in this philosophy. Existential issues like meaning, death, freedom, isolation, our dreams, our human uniqueness, find no place in this scheme. And because there is a strong environmental bias as to where to look for the causes of behavior, very little can be said about an enduring concept that consistently recurs in the history of vitalistic medicine—namely, our real self, our inherited human nature, our "grain" if you like. There is an implicit assumption that everybody has the same set of innate reinforcers, the only differences between us being due to conditioning. In fact, genetically inherited individual differences might be quite fundamental. Animals observed outside the restricted conditions of Skinner's box misbehave: innate behaviors not predicted or even easily studied in the restricted situation arise and start to override reinforcement contingencies. Even animals start "becoming themselves" out of the box.

Behavior theory, then, remains a useful source of ideas and principles, a corrective toward the naïveté implicit in ghost-in-the-machine thinking. Let its principles serve as reminders that all those influences in the psychobiosocial field which influence disease and wellness—however remote in time and space—must be cast in descriptive empirical terms. If there appear places (as there surely will) when we can apply Skinner's reinforcement or Pavlov's conditioning to relieve suffering while preserving human dignity, we shall certainly not hesitate to do so. Like osmosis, gravity and oxidation, reinforcement of behavior—including illness behavior—will operate whenever and wherever it can.

Cognitive Psychology

Some 80 percent of academic psychologists describe their orientation to the field as *cognitive*. In distinct contrast to behavior theory, for which the mind is at best a simile or a category mistake, cognitive psychology cheerfully embraces the mind as its definitive subject matter. The word cognitive refers to knowledge and thought, and thus this is a psychology predominantly concerned with thinking, reasoning and problem solving. Consequently much of cognitive psychology is concerned with verbal behavior. But imagery, or thinking in pictures, is an important topic too. Cognitive visualization techniques have been developed for ameliorating pain, coping with stress, and even more remarkably, combating disease processes in cancer and AIDS.

Cognitive psychology also concerns itself with perception: how we get our knowledge, what form we represent it in, and in particular how we process information about the world to create knowledge of the world. A notable accomplishment of cognitive psychology has been to demonstrate that children do not learn chains of specific operants when they acquire their first language. Rather children learn *rules* for when to use the various parts of speech, nouns, pronouns, verbs and so forth. Acquisition of these rules—actually tendencies and probabilities to respond in certain specific ways, sometimes called behavioral *dispositions*—gives us the ability to generate an infinite variety of grammatically correct sentences.

It was the development of the digital computer that gave cognitive psychology its impetus, for prior to the advent of the computer much of the theorizing about how we process information and represent the stimuli out in the world around us remained speculative, virtually impossible to verify. But the computer provided psychologists with a concrete model on which to base their theorizing. By creating computer programs that solve problems, recognize patterns, plan and execute actions, learn about the environment and adapt to it, cognitive psychologists found themselves for the first time in a position to be able to test their theories about how people do these things. One of the very salutary effects of trying to get a computer to solve any complex problem that requires intelligence—e.g., to play chess—is that in so doing the programmer as theorist is obliged to break down the problem to its component skills and try to work out what ordinary players and grand masters do when they play the game. From such endeavors, cognitive psychologists have discovered various strategies that prove to be generalizable to many different intelligent problem solving computer programs. One such principle may be described as trial-and-error rules of thumb (called *heuristics)* that, while not guaranteeing a solution, make it more likely. These heuristics—different for each kind of problem, of course—are applied to *search trees* representing potential valuable steps to subgoals in the solution of a problem or sub-problem. Each potential step—and there may be millions in the course of determining the best move in chess—is then evaluated using variously weighted competing strategies. In the most complex programs the computer actually learns from its mistakes, creating and evaluating its own heuristics. It seems quite likely that when we solve puzzles and problems in an intelligent way, the human brain is using analogous principles.

Heuristic problem solving, complex pattern recognition and human language processing by computer are important areas in the field of *artificial intelligence,* which feeds back and forth to and from natural intelligence. The evolving digital computer with its integrated hardware and software is actually a very tantalizing model of the mind. Moreover, as computers become ever more sophisticated with faster parallel processing and vastly increased memories, as more advanced problem-oriented software is developed, and as the machinery becomes smaller and more accessible to everyone, the computer simulates more and more of the things that we do and call intelligent.[7]

The practitioner of natural medicine utilizes cognitive psychology's analysis of *attitudes and beliefs* to understand the particular ways that patients respond to emotionally charged novel situations and circumstances. Beliefs are crucial to an understanding of how we deal with potential stressors because our beliefs govern just how we respond emotionally to challenges and changes in our lives. The particular emotional response pattern known as stress (described in considerable detail in later chapters) is highly relevant to psychological medicine since, unrelieved, it forms a significant health risk. Some events that we encounter, such as extremes of temperature, noise and light, bodily insult, radiation, infection and pollution are inherently stressful. But the vast majority of our stressors have somehow *become* stressful, meaning that we learned to respond to them with stressful emotions. Actually, according to cognitive psychotherapy, it is the *beliefs* behind these stressful emotions that we learn, and which determine our emotions. That is to say, given a particular belief about an event—for instance, whether we believe that it is a threat, challenge or inconsequential—our emotions flow quite automatically. It should be apparent then, that any modifications we can make to our belief systems are going to have a direct effect on how stressful an actual event is perceived. Since the so-called "negative emotions" like anxiety, shame, guilt and depression become health risks when they become chronic and unrelieved, the importance of psychological principles that can intervene in this pathological sequence cannot be underestimated. This direct connection between belief and stress lays the basis for an important potential health-promoting principle, although it is far from new. In Roman times, Epictetus and Marcus Aurelius, the Stoics, recognized that people's unrealistic beliefs (cognitions) made them anxious and miserable, and that if their attitudes and belief systems could be changed, they could become serene and happy.

To see how belief works in emotion, consider a nasty, potentially stressful circumstance: the loss of a job, rejection by a new friend or failure at an examination. Call this circumstance the **A**ctivating event (**A**). What is the emotional consequent reaction to **A**? It might be anger, depression, anxiety or even indifference, but whatever it is, it is mediated by our attitudes or **B**eliefs about the event. This **ABC** theory of the emotions says that no matter how quickly or automatically or apparently out of our control our response is to an **A**ctivating situation, the **C**onsequent response we make is actually a product of the interpolated belief system we hold. Therefore our emotional response, **C**, is potentially under our control, since changing the **B**elief about **A** will change **C**, how we react to it.

Someone slams the door in our face and we get furious. Why? Because we believe we deserve, nay *demand,* respect. We're rejected for a job and we become despondent. Why? Because we believed that we *required* that job for our happiness. An intimate friend leaves us without warning and we respond with resentment and then depression. Why? Because we believe that we *ought* to be treated better, and we then take the rejection as confirming our belief that we are not worthwhile, not a valuable person, *not OK.*

All the words italicized in the last paragraph refer to what cognitive psychotherapy would call unrealistic or irrational beliefs, and that, more times than not, are also unconscious. Such beliefs create reactions that go beyond an adaptive healthy response to the actual situation. Cognitive psychotherapists tell us that while there are no doubt hundreds of individual unrealistic beliefs, they all fall into one of three basic categories: (1) *demandingness* (of approval, achievement, comfort), (2) *catastrophizing* (blowing up a nasty situation to make it an unbearable one), and (3) *confirming a negative self image* (what happened is just another proof that I am not good enough). These three categories of beliefs also have a way of perpetuating themselves. If they are ingrained, then the world is likely to prove them self-fulfilling, and contradictory experiences will just be perceived as exceptions that prove the rule. The bad news is that many of us—practitioners as well as patients—unconsciously hold such unrealistic beliefs; the good news is that they are amenable to change. Among the ways are the path of the Buddha, who recommended the "cultivation of a mind that clings to naught"; or the way of the great *Bhagavad Gita,* which teaches that as suffering is always a result of being attached to our desires, "Act not for the fruits of action, act for the action itself."

Just as beliefs predict emotions, their reciprocal relationship implies that emotions can reveal hidden beliefs. When we respond to an unexpected situation with surprisingly strong or painful feelings, by analyzing these negative feelings we can trace them back to strong beliefs we perhaps did not know we held. This symmetry in the reciprocity between emotions and beliefs is the basis of the old phrase, "The heart has reasons that reason can know." And is this not just another way of expressing a cardinal principle of natural medicine—that the suffering and pain of sickness are calls for inquiry and investigation?

Humanistic Psychology

Each of the three psychologies—Freudian, behavioral and cognitive—has an implicit view of human nature. We want to make their views explicit, because according to the perennial philosophy of holistic medicine, a crucial but often neglected factor in disease is the clash between our deep innate nature, our *real self,* and our acquired or conditioned personalities that evolve out of adapting to social and cultural norms.

In these terms, Freud's view of human nature can be accurately described as pessimistic. The *id,* that great reservoir of unconscious instinctual drives and motives, has been likened to a cesspool, full of antisocial impulses like aggression, unbounded lust and competition, murderous hatred and jealousy. Although the acquired *ego* and *superego* work to constrain and channel these id impulses, Freud's theory leaves little room for a person to transcend their dark nature on the one hand, and their childhood conditioning on the other. The goal of psychoanalysis was the modest one of bringing us to a better, but still uneasy compromise with the conflict between our nature and the demands of a social world.

Behavior theory holds an equally deterministic view of human nature, but about man's possibilities it can be described as optimistic, because its extreme environmentalism implies a highly plastic nature. By gaining control over the environmental variables of which behavior is a function, we can infinitely mold and shape people. At the same time, it remains unclear what, if any, unique features human behavior might have that the higher apes don't have. Moreover, behavior theory has little to say or offer to the uniquely personal and individual sides of each of us that are surely of great importance in the practitioner/patient relationship.

Cognitive psychology seems to offer no uniform view of human nature except that we are exceedingly complex information and symbol processors, and that our ability to do this processing and represent the world in language is a function of a wired-in genetic structure (a conceptual nervous system) whose properties we shall eventually be able to infer quite accurately.[8] From the observed fact that many people in therapy seem to have irrational and unrealistic beliefs underlying their negative emotions, some cognitive psychotherapists[9] have concluded that it is also our nature to build unrealistic belief systems out of very little input.

It is in humanistic psychology that we find the most well-developed benign and optimistic concept of human nature, a nature whose growth is toward health and holism. Respecting, nurturing and honoring this nature are essential parts of humanistic psychology, thus bringing explicit attention to the realm of values. There are two men—both Americans born in the first decade of this century—associated with the development of humanistic psychology: personality and motivation theorist Abraham Maslow, and psychotherapist Carl Rogers. Out of their work has been fashioned the twentieth century human potential movement, the encounter group, and a very distinctive approach to science. It attempts to reconcile the great paradox between the determinism of science and the inalienable sense of free personal choice each of us feels as part of our essence of being human.

From studies with people who were especially creative, fulfilled and optimistic—individuals he called *self-actualized*—Maslow formulated a model of human motives that has become known as Maslow's hierarchy.[10] The pyramid in Fig. 3.2 is a modified illustration of Maslow's theory.

At the base of the pyramid are the basic physiological and safety survival needs that we share with the other members of the animal kingdom. They are at the base because, according to Maslow, until they are satisfied the organism (in this case the person) is not going to be in a position to expend much energy toward achieving any motives (needs) higher up the pyramid.

Once these base needs are secured, however, we can begin to climb the pyramid. Our procreation needs will be satisfied by sex, love and intimacy. We meet our social needs by communicating, affiliating and cooperating with kith and kin. In lower levels, productive work might just be to satisfy shelter, food and procreation needs, but once those needs are secured, work has its own intrinsic creative value. Higher yet lies the existential need of finding meaning for our lives, as well as the quest to come to terms with our finiteness and essential aloneness. At the pinnacle of the hierarchy stands the ultimate goal of life, unity with the cosmos in unitary cosmic consciousness, what Maslow calls peak experiences, what the yogis call flashes of enlightenment, and what psychologists call the realm of the transpersonal.

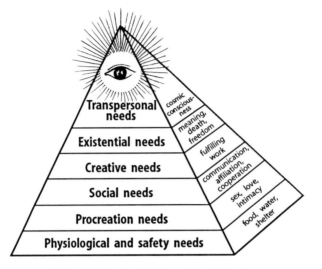

Fig. 3.2 Maslow's Hierarchy of Motives

Although the hierarchy is simplistic, it does provide an advance in sophistication over the pictures of human nature suggested by our three other psychologies. It is surely over-simplified because in its static form it seems to imply that a person struggling with poverty could not also be interested in creativity or enlightenment, clearly incompatible with the great Master traditions of India, one of the poorest nations of the world. The structure also fails to fit highly collectivized societies in which the group meets the individual's basic needs of food and safety, thus transposing on the hierarchy group needs and physiological/safety needs.

For all its defects, the pyramid of needs constitutes a valuable step in the direction of attempting to portray the complexity and intricacy of human motivation. In constructing this hierarchy Maslow studied exceptionally well-adjusted, happy, creative, healthy people. This in itself was a breakthrough for a social science that has traditionally found its material in the lab rat, the psychopath and the neurotic. Maslow referred to his subjects as *self-actualized,* by which he meant that they had become the potential self that they could be: they had satisfied, and were satisfying, the motives from many, perhaps all, levels of the pyramid.

There is no particular form for self-actualization. What is creative for one individual may not necessarily be creative for another. One could come from any walk of life, engage in any endeavor, and be actualizing one's self. This of course implies that there is some sort of *real self* that is different from some other, socially acquired conditioned self, and that part of the actualization process is a dropping away of the false persona and coming more to live in one's real self.

This concept of the real self is a very crucial one in humanistic psychology, and a core part of the vitalistic tradition in medicine as well. Appealing as it is on the surface, the "real self" is actually a very elusive concept to pin down. In humanistic psychology the human organism is conceived as a system that grows instinctively toward health just as a plant grows towards light. This is a bold and transcendent view, for it implies that each of us has the unique potential to grow toward what optimizes us as human beings. But for all the beauty in this concept it is very difficult to establish what this real self is that we are growing to, or into. One hint of it is given by an account of residents at an American yoga center:

> They report learning such things as being able to know when to rest before becoming overly tired; to eat as a response to hunger rather than social expectations or anxiety; to express love and appreciation when it is felt; to let others know when they feel friction in a relationship; to be able to induce emotional release in themselves; to detect and acknowledge when they are reacting out of fear.[11]

From his experience in psychotherapeutic relationships, Carl Rogers found that individuals grew more tolerant of stress, moved towards socialization, became more autonomous, more similar to the person they would like to be, more accepting of self and of others, more open, more expressive. People became less defensive, less rigid, increasingly discovering that their own organism is trustworthy, better able to satisfy their needs.

Maslow said about this real self:

> We have, each one of us, an essential inner nature that is instinctoid, intrinsic, given, "natural," i.e., with an appreciable hereditary determinant. . . . This inner core, even though it is biologically based and "instinctoid," is weak. . . . All that we have left are instinct-remnants. . . . Authentic selfhood can be defined in part as being able to hear these impulse-voices within oneself, i.e., to know what one really wants or doesn't want, what one is fit for and what one is not fit for.[12]

Even if there is not quite a definition here, there is a tendency, a direction, that seems to fit both Rogers' observations from psychotherapy, Maslow's exceptionally healthy people and the American yogis. We may not know exactly where the plant that is ourselves is growing, but we can at least get a glimpse of the direction.

British psychologist Michael Daniels has warned, however, that while this concept may well sensitize us to our own experience and latent talents, it also could be taken as a prescription for rampant hedonism and excessive individualism. One of the excesses of the encounter group is certainly a preoccupation with self-indulgence; and unfortunately, an uncritical reading of humanistic psychology can move one away from cooperative lifestyles, away from a concern for others and the planet. We have stressed in Chapter 2 that holistic medicine is merely a part of a broad perspective that must prevail toward all of life. The psychology we adopt must not be exempt. Our actions here affect everyone, and ultimately we are all tied up in one system where the good of the individual must become indistinguishable from the good of the whole.

Perhaps the concept of actualizing the real self ought to be viewed as a *myth*: the actualization and search for the real self is nothing less than everyman's and every-woman's search for the grail. Although a myth must not contradict empirical scientific evidence, it need not meet the strict criteria for a scientific theory, i.e., that it is testable and verifiable. We ask of a myth not whether it be true or false, but whether it is good or bad. A good myth leads to useful and valuable practical implications. The myth of self-actualization is good it if leads individuals to become more fully human, if it is capable of guiding and supporting us in our quest for healing and wholeness, and if it increases the common good by bringing us into contact with the interconnectedness of all of nature.

Self-actualization reveals the unique potential for psychological theories to become self-fulfilling prophecies. Medical psychology must be extraordinarily cautious of the portrait it paints of human nature, for people tend to become what they believe they are. The special relationship between patient and practitioner means that the latter's view of human nature can influence the patient's beliefs, including the very will to live. There is disturbing evidence[13] that behavior theory's limited view of human nature as factory nature has a tendency to become self-fulfilling. Psychology must take to heart what modern physicists are discovering: scientific theories are neither existentially true nor false, only *useful.* In the other sciences useful means useful in predicting and controlling the world around us. In psychology useful is always going to have to be referred to some value system which inevitably lies outside of the science. Useful to whom? Useful toward what goal? Whose goal? In psychological medicine useful means useful to the patient's desire for health and wholeness.

Several other noteworthy psychological schools whose views provide valuable insights for psychological medicine can be subsumed under the humanistic wing. In particular, there is the work of the Swiss analyst Carl G. Jung who split with Freud over the nature of the unconscious. Jung found with his patients what he believed were evidences of powerfully positive, uniquely human archetypes which, if explored deeply, could bring us to the very gate of cosmic consciousness. Both in dreams and in his appraisal of the unconscious Jung found the antidote to the darkness and pessimism of Freud's id. Jung's symbolisms have particularly influenced therapists interested in the meaning of illness.

Existential psychology is yet another sub-branch of psychology that is appropriately called humanistic. Here the issues of death, the meaning of life, our essential isolation and our struggle with how to use freedom to choose alternative courses of action are seen as the springs of uniquely human action and feeling. The existentialists believe that no one can achieve true health until these issues are faced and resolved; and that conversely, illness is often a symptom of the failure to achieve such resolution. In the humanistic wing too are the transpersonal psychologists who study the altered states of consciousness arising from the practice of meditative and yogic disciplines. The realization of such states and the peace, harmony and tranquility associated with them is part of the human potential, the highest rung on Maslow's pyramid, the very epitome of what it means to be healthy in body and spirit. The transpersonalists stand at the last outpost of psychology, at the very threshold of the bridge leading beyond science and medicine, to the spiritual.

Conclusion
Three perennial questions, dating from the philosophical legacy of modern psy-

chology, linger on in method and theory in each of the four major schools of psychology. The practitioner of natural medicine cannot ignore these seminal issues of psychology pertaining to the resolution of three great dichotomies: nature *vs.* nurture, mind *vs.* body, free-will *vs.* determinism. The first is the ever-present question of how much of our selves is due to our innate genetic structure, and how much is due to our socialization, our learned habits, our environmental conditioning. The second dichotomy questions whether it is possible to make a meaningful distinction between what is somatic and what is psychological. Do these poles stand for two relatively independent but interrelated aspects of nature? Are they merely two ways of looking at the same process? Or do they actually denote an illusion, a kind of conceptual double vision? The final great dichotomy represents the confusion as to how psychology can be a properly well-behaved member of the science club, which finds nothing but law-like relations among phenomena, and still be the promiscuous gadfly, allowing its subjects personal freedom to choose their lives moment to moment.

No one of the four schools can offer the definitive answer to these old chestnuts, but each one in its way provides suggestive evidence for one or another side of the dichotomy, thus expanding our knowledge base, and forcing the next generation of thinkers to pose the problem with yet greater sophistication, with yet deeper insight. In the end each individual practitioner

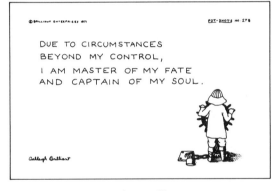

Fig. 3.3[14]

must arrive at his own existential solutions. Whatever ideas, methods and viewpoints of the several psychologies are useful and valuable he will take and use in his own practice. The highly condensed overview of this chapter can do no more than introduce fundamental problems and possibilities, illustrate different psychological dialects and point up the indeterminacies, prejudices, strengths and weaknesses of the traditions out of which the practical tools of psychological medicine are arising.

Project 3

Tracking Down the Concept of Mind

Imagine that you are a private detective hired by your appropriate professional body to track down the missing identity of an elusive secret agent who poses under the alias of "Mind." Clues to his identity come through his consistent reference to "mind" or "minds" that you can see and hear on television, in the newspapers, popular magazines, books and from fleeting but significant conversational references of your own and others that you overhear. Your job is to spy on and to compile a list of all these references, including the one best known to all practitioners and patients: "Your illness is all in your mind."

Decode each reference into simple basic English, eliminating the term "mind" from each one in the hope that if you get enough messages you can break his code. Compile your report in your mind-body journal, drawing whatever general conclusions you can about the whereabouts of this secret agent and his identity (if any).

For comparison, you might want to consider what would have happened had this project focused on his more respectable double, who goes by the name of "Body."

Annotated Bibliography

Brown, James A. C. *Freud and the Post-Freudians.* Harmondsworth: Pelican, 1961.

Daniels, Michael. "The Myth of Self-actualization." *Journal of Humanistic Psychology* 28 (1988): 7-37; **Andrew Neher,** "Maslow's Theory of Motivation: A Critique." *Journal of Humanistic Psychology* 31 (1991): 89-112; **Stephen Wilson,** "The Real Self Controversy." *Journal of Humanistic Psychology* 28 (1988): 39-65; **Willard Mittleman,** "Maslow's Study of Self-actualization." *Journal of Humanistic Psychology* 31 (1991): 114-35. These four papers flesh out Maslow's and Rogers' concepts of the real self and self-actualization, pointing out difficulties with the original concepts and making suggestions about how the concepts need to grow and evolve.

Jaynes, Julian. *The Origin of Consciousness in the Breakdown of the Bicameral Mind.* Boston: Houghton-Mifflin, 1976. The first three chapters provide a readable discussion of the nature of consciousness and the attempts of psychologists to bring it into their science.

Johnson-Laird, Phillip. *The Computer and the Mind.* Cambridge, MA: Harvard University Press, 1988; **Daniel Dennett,** *Consciousness Explained.* Boston: Little-Brown, 1991; **Roger Penrose,** *The Emperor's New Mind.* New York: Oxford University Press, 1989. Three sources for pursuing the pros and cons of computer models of the mind.

Nye, Robert D. *Three Views of Man: Perspectives from Sigmund Freud, B. F. Skinner and Carl Rogers.* Monterey, CA: Brooks Cole, 1975.

Rogers, Carl R. *On Becoming a Person.* Boston: Houghton-Mifflin, 1961. The title says it well. A fine and readable exposition of the principles of humanistic psychology from one of the founders of the school.

Schwartz, Barry. *The Battle for Human Nature.* London: W. W. Norton, 1986. A comprehensible account of modern behavior theory and the dangers arising from an extrapolation of its interpretations of human nature. The account is especially compelling because the author was trained in behavior theory and made significant contributions to it before realizing the self-fulfilling implications of its limited view of human nature.

4

The Psychobiology of Stress

Men are disturbed not by things but by the views they take of them.

—EPICTETUS

Stress can be avoided only by dying.

—HANS SELYE

A COUPLE OF MILLENNIA elapsed between the words of the two gentlemen cited above, and in the meantime, thanks in part to Hans Selye himself, our disturbances to things are now called "stress." Indeed, we would not be far off the mark to say that the stress of living constitutes the very thread out of which the cloth of psychosomatic medicine is cut. Yet the word stress did not appear in professional psychology's abstracting journal until 1944. But fashions, even in science, change quickly. Just a decade later, Selye, Professor of Endocrinology at the University of Montreal, was publishing an annual review of some 6000 articles on stress, and by the late 1970s the stress literature amounted to over 110,000 titles. Most of these were animal studies investigating physiological effects in a variety of body systems to a variety of biophysical stressors. It is safe to say that now, in the last decade of the twentieth century, stress research remains among the most popular research topics in psychophysiology, while books on stress comprise a large percentage of psychological self-help volumes.

The Development of the Stress Concept

Despite an intense interdisciplinary research effort and our strong intuitions that stress must be at the core of the mind-body interaction in the disease process, it may come as something of a surprise to learn that "after 35 years no one has formulated a definition of stress that satisfies even a majority of stress researchers."[1] It would seem that the concept is so obvious that a definition would be virtually self-evident.

51

We can all identify sources of potential stress—physical trauma, extremes of temperature, overcrowding, loud unabated noise, a disappointing love affair, a run-in with the law, strife at home or at work, unemployment—and yet any listing immediately raises the systematic question of what the various items in the list have in common. Moreover, it is quite clear that for *some* people, *some* of the time, *some* of the items might actually not act as stressors. The loud rock noise playing in my neighbors' apartment late at night is certainly a stressor for me, but evidently not for them. Not every divorce or even death of a spouse is necessarily a stressor, especially if the partner's living presence had been one.

Selye (1956) originally gave two distinctly different definitions for stress. One was "the rate of wear and tear within the body"; and the other, a rather abstract medical definition: "the state manifested by a specific syndrome which consists of all the non-specifically induced changes within a biologic system." The first definition is really more poetic than descriptive, for the body is not quite like a machine which continually wears out with use. Indeed we thrive on optimum use, and are perhaps as likely to wear out if under-used as we are if over-used. We shall be examining in the next section some of the non-specific changes referred to in the second definition, but to anticipate the conclusion, there will actually not be any single set of responses that when evoked constitutes *the* stress syndrome. Rather there are a great many neuroendocrine and behavioral-emotional components set in a highly complex network of negative feedback circuits of chemical and central nervous system events which respond in incredibly diverse ways to positively and negatively valenced[2] stimuli.

Selye's original work was carried out with mice subjected to physical restraint, extremes of temperature, overcrowded living cages, forced exercise and infectious micro-organisms. These biophysical stressors did tend to produce a particular non-specific response triad of adrenal hypertrophy, duodenal ulceration and atrophy of the thymus and lymphatics. But when investigators turned to the far more interesting and complex psychosocial stressors of human beings the picture became far cloudier than Selye's original observations might have led one to expect. It is not clear how stress differs from emotional arousal, so its definition must be so broad that it seems sometimes to include essentially anything that might happen to someone. Selye himself is partially responsible for this definitional quagmire, for although in his earliest work he spoke of stress as a response to noxious stimuli, he later widened this definition to include strong positive stimuli as well, and named the stress response triad the *General Adaptation Syndrome,* implying that it was the cluster of non-specific effects that arose whenever any demand whatsoever was placed on the organism.

The word stress goes back at least to the fourteenth century when it meant "hardship, straits, adversity, or affliction."[3] Three hundred years later physicist Robert Hooke gave the term a technical scientific meaning referring to the force per unit area acting on an object. Strain was the resultant deformation or distortion of the object due to that force. When you stretch a rubber band you are applying stress to it, and the resultant change in shape is the strain:

$$\text{STRESS} \longrightarrow \text{STRAIN}$$

But in psychobiology stress is a way that an organism responds to a stimulus, taking the form

$$\text{STRESSOR} \longrightarrow \text{STRESS}$$

So whereas in physics and engineering stress is an antecedent variable and strain is the result, in psychobiology stress is a result, not the antecedent cause. It was Selye himself who coined the word "stressor" for the antecedent causes of stress.

But exactly what are the characteristics of the antecedents of stress? In fact there does not seem to be any independent way to define a stressor except to say that it is whatever produces the characteristic response syndrome we call stress. In other words, there are no universal characteristics of stressors. Another way to say this is that despite a vast quantity of data collected in this field over half a century, there exists nothing like a unified theory of stress. Indeed, so daunting is the problem that few have even tried to produce such a theory.[4] Having laid bare serious difficulties with the concept of stress—the failure to know independently in advance what is or isn't a stressor for any given person, and the failure to find a uniform set of responses that specifically defines stress—we are better able now to appreciate the tentative, preliminary status of the present stress models of disease and illness.

Physiology of the Stress Response

The modern pre-history of the stress response really begins with Nobel Prize-winning Harvard physiologist Walter B. Cannon, who, early in the twentieth century, described the physiology of the *fight or flight* response as an organism's characteristic mode of responding to a life threat. Encountering, e.g., a predator, the individual responds with a strong *alarm* arousal involving principally the sympathetic nervous system and the endocrine system. Some of the main components of this alarm response are shown on the right side of Figure 4.1. The threat stimulus (equated to a stressor in Fig. 4.1) is received via (say) the visual channel (the eye) and transmitted up to the cerebral cortex. There it is decoded as a threat and impulses are then sent down to the limbic cortex where emotions of fear or rage are generated.

Impulses then reach the hypothalamus, the head ganglion of the sympathetic branch of the autonomic nervous system. The sympathetic branch simultaneously activates many systems, including muscles, heart, liver, lungs, digestion and peripheral circulation.

Within a few dozen milliseconds the hypothalamus signals a general alarm throughout the entire sympathetic nervous system and the body is rapidly aroused for action. The catecholamines *noradrenalin* and (mostly) *adrenalin* are released at nerve endings along the sympathetic chain, thereby resulting in pupil dilation, muscle tension, increased heart rate and stroke volume along with peripheral circulatory constriction, which results in raised blood pressure. Simultaneously the liver converts

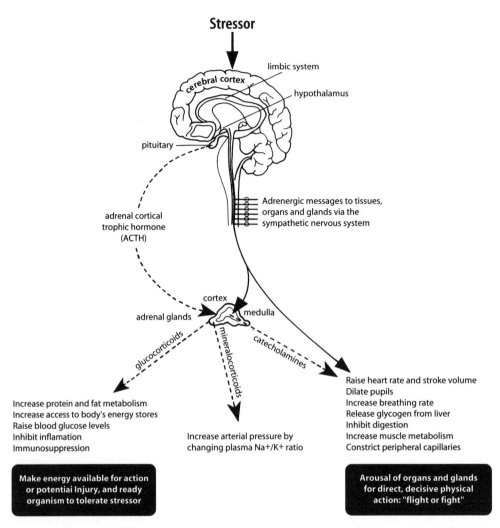

Stressor

limbic system

cerebral cortex

hypothalamus

pituitary

adrenal cortical
trophic hormone
(ACTH)

Adrenergic messages to tissues,
organs and glands via the
sympathetic nervous system

cortex

adrenal glands

medulla

glucocorticoids

mineralocorticoids

catecholamines

Increase protein and fat metabolism
Increase access to body's energy stores
Raise blood glucose levels
Inhibit inflamation
Immunosuppression

Increase arterial pressure by
changing plasma Na+/K+ ratio

Raise heart rate and stroke volume
Dilate pupils
Increase breathing rate
Release glycogen from liver
Inhibit digestion
Increase muscle metabolism
Constrict peripheral capillaries

**Make energy available for action
or potentiai Injury, and ready
organism to tolerate stressor**

**Arousal of organs and glands
for direct, decisive physical
action: "flight or fight"**

Fig. 4.1 Two axes of the stress response. Autonomic nervous pathways are shown by solid lines, hormonal bloodstream pathways by dashed lines.

glycogen to glucose and releases it into the bloodstream, digestion is inhibited, blood being diverted elsewhere to muscles and brain, and the adrenal medulla is stimulated to secrete adrenalin into the bloodstream, a profound event which amplifies and perpetrates the entire sympathetic response. All of these changes are beautifully adaptive, for they instantly arouse and energize the organism for fight or flight.

This description is an idealized pattern. In human beings it is still generally true, although there will be individual differences in patterning and emphasis. We have all felt our own fight or flight responses when something has occurred to "make our blood boil," or when involved in a serious car crash, or a near-death experience. The pumping of adrenalin in a terrifying situation is a common experience. Yet one of the anachronistic aspects of the biological fight or flight response is that in our

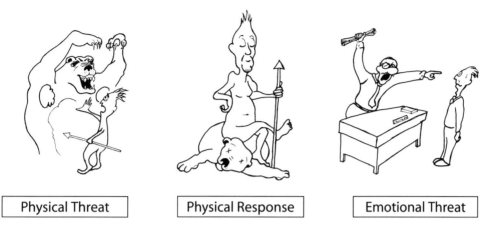

| Physical Threat | Physical Response | Emotional Threat |

Fig. 4.2 The Fight or Flight Response, in Cave-dwelling Era and Today[5]

socialized lives, fight or flight are no longer appropriate responses, as the cartoon above depicts.

What happens when our biology prepares us for one kind of response pattern but our society has come to sanction something quite different? Unless we can find ways to discharge the buildup of catecholamines (through exercise, sport, psycho-therapeutic catharsis, physical work) the state of physiological arousal and muscle tension may continue unabated, i.e., we remain in a state of stress which if prolonged is extremely detrimental to health. And indeed, experiments with rats, dogs and monkeys[6] have revealed that prolonged exposure to anxiety-generating conditions can produce gastric ulcers. Prolongation of the fight/flight syndrome apparently inhibits normal protective secretions that keep stomach tissue from being dissolved by its own hydrochloric acid milieu.

But the fight/flight response (via the sympathetic-adrenal-medulla axis) is only part of the story of the stress response. Another part is associated with the hypothala-mic-pituitary-adrenal-cortical axis (the left side of Fig. 4.1), and that is Hans Selye's story. Selye subjected mice to a number of biophysically noxious situations: extremes of temperature, forced exercise on a treadmill, physical restraint and injections of vir-ulent infectious microbes as well as poisons (formaldehyde). Selye found a triad of responses to such noxious stimulation: (1) adrenal enlargement, (2) shrinkage of the thymus and other lymphatic tissue, and (3) stress ulcers in the stomach and duode-num. These effects are mediated mainly by hormones (glucocorticoids and mineralo-corticoids) secreted by the adrenal cortex in response to adrenal-corticotrophic hor-mone (ACTH) released by the pituitary gland of the brain. ACTH is itself triggered by a neurochemical messenger from the hypothalamus called cortical releasing factor (CRF). The glucocorticoids mobilize fats into the bloodstream where they can be picked up, converted to glucose and returned to the blood for rapid transport to the tissues, which will use them for energy. Glucocorticoids also reduce inflammation and allergic responses via a suppressive action on the output of cells from the lymphatic organs. The mineralocorticoids increase blood pressure by causing salt and water retention by the kidneys and sweat glands.

Selye was struck by the *nonspecific* nature of the stress response produced by the hypothalamic-pituitary-adrenal-cortical system: the same familiar triad pattern was evoked by a wide variety of challenges to and demands made upon the organism. Indeed, it appears likely that it is evoked by virtually all noxious or aversive stimuli. The picture of the stress response to this point involves two separate though interacting physiological systems that act to create one integrated response syndrome that both prepares the organism for fight or flight and to resist threats to its integrity. This notion of resistance to a stressor adds the crucial dimension of time (see Fig. 4.3) to Selye's notion of the General Adaptation Syndrome.

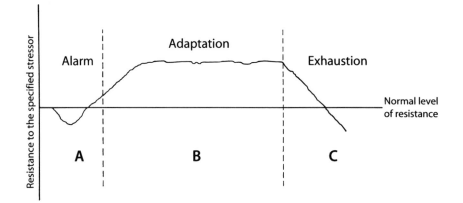

Fig. 4.3 The Three Phases of the General Adaptation Syndrome (after Selye, 1956)

Phase A of Fig. 4.3 constitutes the *alarm* response, the body's acute reaction to a stressor or a threat. At this time there is a pouring out of the hormones and neurotransmitters described previously. At the same time the individual's resistance to that stressor is temporarily diminished, and if the stressor is sufficiently strong (severe burns, extremes of temperature, great shock), death may result. Phase B is the stage of *adaptation* or *resistance* which occurs with continued exposure to the threat or stressor. The bodily signs associated with the initial alarm reaction virtually disappear, and resistance to the particular stressor rises above normal (although it will be lower for any new and different stressors concurrently encountered). Phase C is the stage of *exhaustion* that eventually results from long-term continued exposure to the stressor. As resistance to the stressor falls, the signs of the initial alarm reaction briefly reappear, but they cannot prevent the organism succumbing, for all physiological reserves have been depleted. This physiological model of stress, combining as it does Cannon's sympathetic-adrenal-medulla axis with Selye's hypothalamic-pituitary-adrenal-cortical axis, helps to explain the body's adaptation to biophysical threats. If psychosocial stressors act similarly to biophysical ones, then the three phases of the General Adaptation Syndrome could provide us with a doorway to understanding the effects of prolonged stress of any sort.

Selye's seminal investigations into the nature of the stress response were carried out principally with biophysical stimuli—extremes of temperature and noise, overcrowding, forced exercise, X-rays, mechanical trauma and bodily insult. It is an inference that psychosocial stressors, whose potential depends on cultural conditioning and an idiosyncratic learning history, display similar effects. A fifteen-year program of research examining the conditioned and behavioral aspects of stress by John Mason and collaborators at the Walter Reed Institute of Research indicates that a more comprehensive description of the stress response reveals many features which are stressor specific.[7] Mason's experiments with monkeys and humans have shown that when a variety of neuroendocrinological systems in addition to the two axes shown in Fig. 4.1 are studied concurrently, qualitatively different stressors produce highly patterned and quite different physiological response profiles. In Mason's research, hormonal activity was measured[8] to various stressors in a number of diverse systems that, aside from the adrenals, included thyroid output, insulin production, pituitary growth and sex hormones.[9] All these systems do participate in the stress response,[10] and the way they do so depends in part on the qualitative nature of the stressor, and in part on each animal or person's biochemical individuality.[11] Measuring 17-hydroxycorticosterol levels in plasma and urine, adrenalin and noradrenalin, testosterone, insulin, thyroxin and other hormonal indices, strikingly different endocrinological profiles were found for monkeys exposed to acute heat exposure, sustained exercise and fasting.[12]

How can these findings of very specific response profiles to different stressors be reconciled with Selye's generalized nonspecific GAS? Recall that all of Selye's biophysical stressors had a noxious (aversive) quality. Thus, in terms of behavior theory they all involve the presentation of unconditioned aversive stimuli—i.e., powerful biologically-negative reinforcers. As I have discussed elsewhere,[13] the presentation of both conditioned *and* unconditioned negative reinforcers elicits strong emotional disturbances. When these are life-threatening events, involving discomfort or pain, organisms—humans and animals—respond appropriately with a heightened arousal response that involves, among other things, the neuroendocrinological systems studied in stress. The nonspecific response to a stressor appears to be nothing more nor less than that generalized arousal to any aversive stimulation, regardless of its nature. Going along with that nonspecific response, however, will also be a specific adaptive pattern that differs depending on the nature of the stressor, and apparently is as different for each individual as is their fingerprint.[14] This has very important clinical implications, for it means that different people are going to respond to stressors in very different ways. Just as posture, gait, facial expression and gestures represent basic characteristics of the personality, so too does the way we each respond to stressors. Some of our differences are due to individual socialization and cultural learning, but others are doubtless derived from individual genetic predispositions.

In real life every aversive stimulus/stressor contains both a general emotional arousal factor *and* specific, finely tuned physiological and behavioral elements. To observe the specific effects in biophysical stressors, special laboratory techniques are required to minimize the threatening or anxiety-producing aspects of the stressor. Thus extremes of temperature can be introduced imperceptibly, abrupt withdrawal of food in starvation stress can be masked by feeding animals caloric-free pellets, and forced treadmill exercise can be imposed gradually over a period of time.

> When special precautions are taken . . . to minimize psychological reactions in the study of physical stimuli such as heat, fasting and moderate exercise, it now appears that the pituitary-adrenal cortical system is not stimulated in non-specific fashion by these stimuli which are generally regarded as "noxious," "demanding," or as appreciably disturbing to homeostatic equilibrium.[15]

In other terms, the nonspecific response to a stressor is almost certainly due to its *conditioned* aspect, not to its properties as a biological disturbance.[16] This is a radical conclusion because it suggests that the pressing question is not "Do psychosocial stressors behave like biophysical ones?" but rather "In nature, is a biophysical stressor ever separated from its psychological, i.e., threatening, anxiety-producing components?" In this inverted conceptual framework, *conditioned* aversive stimuli—of which psychosocial stressors are prime exemplars—constitute the necessary conditions for evoking the General Adaptation Syndrome. They do this via their ability to elicit the generalized emotional arousal—physiological, behavioral and motivational— that accompanies any abrupt unfavorable (negatively valenced) change in an organism's environment that requires considerable adaptation and adjustment, and for which effective coping behavior may not immediately be available. The emotions that go with such conditions of uncertainty are typically fear, frustration, hopelessness, despair, anxiety and rage—in a word, *distress*.

This conceptualization effectively takes the nonspecific aspect of stress out of biology and puts it squarely in psychology. Whereas a generalized nonspecific alarm response seemed puzzling at the physiological level (why should extremes of heat *and* cold produce the same physiological response?), at the behavioral level a generalized *dis*-stress response makes far more adaptive sense since in every case of a perceived threat or challenge to the organism, optimizing the body for motor behavior of some sort to cope with the challenge is likely to be of functional value. Emotional arousal has apparently developed over evolutionary time as a way of enhancing the likelihood of such effective coping with abrupt, negative environmental change.

Skeletal Muscle Stress Responses[17]

There is solid evidence that the stress response typically includes an increase in muscle tension. Actually, the very term "tension" implies both a psychological meaning (distress) as well as a muscular state (contraction). Various methods have been used to measure muscular contraction, one being lactic acid levels in the urine, since this is a breakdown product of muscle activity. However, the most common measure is muscle electrical activity picked up from surface electrodes placed on the skin above the selected muscle group. A special-purpose electronic instrument integrates these signals and provides a continuous readout known as an electromyogram (EMG). The EMG varies linearly with isometric skeletal muscle contraction over most of its range, and also correlates well with subjects' reports of their muscle tension.

Typically the EMG is set up to measure the contractions at a particular muscle site or muscle group. Thus, e.g., the EMG can record from the frontalis, trapezium, quadriceps and biceps. Although there is a small but significant tendency for tension to occur to a similar degree in muscles throughout the body, such generalized activation is limited. Just as there exist profiles and patterns of autonomic and endocrine responses to different stressors, so too there is *stimulus specificity* for muscles. In addition, individuals tend to react to stressors in a preferential fashion when several muscle groups are studied concurrently, showing maximum tension in a particular muscle group. There is thus a *response specificity* in muscles paralleling similar findings for the neuroendocrine systems in stress.[18] Moreover, this specificity coexists with a tendency for the generalized muscle tension stress response analogous to the way that hormonal profiles coexist with the GAS.[19]

Emotional stressors of essentially every kind have been demonstrated to be associated with muscle tension. Anger, frustration and especially anxiety are closely correlated with chronic muscle tension. The tendency for muscles to react in a generalized fashion is not a strong one, so that often in the laboratory experimenters have to search for a muscle group that is responsive to the stressor under study. In addition, the sensitive site will vary among individuals. In general, resting muscle tension tends to be high in disorders in which anxiety is a major concomitant, and indeed the degree of anxiety in a psychiatric patient population was highly correlated with the extent of rise in muscle tension to benign stimuli. Muscle tension is so intimately connected to anxiety that the systematic desensitization technique used in behavior therapy for anxiety disorders is based in part on muscle tension reduction. Evidently the participation of the skeletal muscle system in the stress response as muscle tension has significant clinical implications. Not only tension headaches, but such musculoskeletal disorders as rheumatism, rheumatoid arthritis and possibly Parkinson's disease may be stress-potentiated. That having been said, however, a detailed description of the pathways and mechanisms that might mediate links between chronic muscle tension and tissue pathologies remains to be worked out.

Psychoneuroimmunology

The Immune System.[20] Broadly speaking, the human immune system may be classified into those components that are *nonspecifically* directed towards a great variety of microorganisms or toxins, and those that recognize, remember and resist *specific* invaders. Nonspecific components are phylogenetically the oldest and make up *innate immunity.* Specific immunity, on the other hand, was evolved relatively recently by the vertebrates. Because it involves developing or acquiring for each particular invader a specific response which was not actually present until the invasion, it is termed *acquired immunity.*

The prominent cells of both acquired and innate immunity (see Fig. 4.4) arise as stem cells in embryonic bone marrow. Stem cells are primal undifferentiated cells that must be preprocessed before they can develop into lymphocytes. Some are preprocessed in the juvenile thymus, and others are thought to be preprocessed in the fetal liver. Preprocessed cells disperse to lymphoid tissues and organs of the body, thus providing a reservoir of lymphocytes able to develop specific functions appropriate to acquired immunity as required.

Principal innate immune components shown in Fig. 4.4 are the circulating white blood cells known as granulocytes and monocytes, and possibly the natural killer (NK) cell lymphocytes. Granulocytes and monocytes are ameboid cells that have the ability to engulf (phagocytose) and digest foreign cells. They can squeeze themselves through blood vessel pores much smaller than their own diameters, and into intercellular spaces to search and destroy viruses, parasites, bacteria and cellular debris. Monocytes typically remain only 4 to 8 hours in the bloodstream, after which they migrate to reticular endothelial tissue where they lurk in waiting for foreign

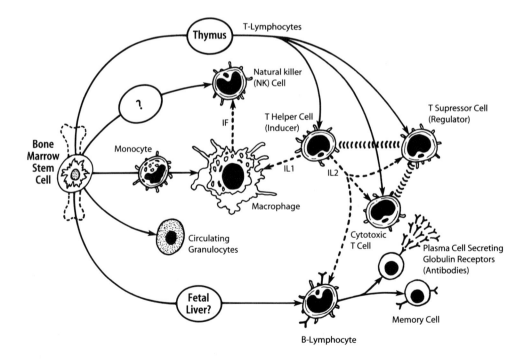

Fig. 4.4 Prominent Cells and Chemical Messengers (Cytokines: IL1, IL2, IF) of the Immune System

invaders. Once stationed there they mature into huge macrophages, swelling to four or five times their previous size. This gives them the ability to ingest as many as 100 bacteria. Macrophages can live for months performing their phagocytic function.

Natural killer (NK) cells also perform nonselective defensive functions. Like other lymphocytes they arise from bone stem cells, but where they are preprocessed remains unknown. NK cells act nonspecifically, releasing lethal chemicals against poorly differentiated cells, hence their anti-tumor function. They also participate in resistance to viral infection, acting as a first line of defense before the slower acquired immunity response has time to come into play. It is not clear how NK cells recognize their targets, but it is likely that they are sensitized to viruses through a chemical messenger known as *interferon* (IF), which is released when body cells (such as macrophages, see Fig. 4.4) are stimulated by viral, bacterial or fungal invasions.

Specific (acquired) immunity involves T and B lymphocytes in interaction with components of innate immunity, macrophages in particular. Although T and B lymphocytes cannot be distinguished under the microscope and both accumulate in lymphoid tissue (spleen, tonsils, Peyer's patches, lymph nodes), they carry out quite different functions. Each T or B lymphocyte carries receptors on its surface which, under appropriate conditions, can bind to one and only one of a vast number of possible foreign non-self molecules called *antigens* (derived from "antibody generators"). Think of this binding between lymphocyte receptor and antigen molecule as a key fitting into a lock. The power of such a system resides in its comprehensive nature: the body contains a key to unlock any foreign antigen imaginable. But there is a cost to be paid for this staggering repertoire. For the immune system to mount a concerted attack against a particular antigen recognized by a T or B cell it needs time, several days in fact, to multiply (clone) an army of identical T and B cells from the very few original progenitors possessing the appropriate receptor.

The first stage of the process is the locking on or attachment of a B lymphocyte to its matching antigen. The result of this attachment is to cause the B cell to begin to multiply rapidly, its progeny differentiating into plasma cells and memory cells (see Fig. 4.4, bottom right). Memory cells have a long life span and their function is to ensure that if its particular antigen appears in the future, a much more rapid response can be made. Memory cells are what prevent us from getting most of our childhood diseases more than once.

Plasma cells, on the other hand, begin to secrete at a rapid rate the particular receptor molecule keys (globulin molecules, now called antibodies) into blood and lymph. These antibodies are specific for the antigen, and whenever they come into contact with it throughout the body, they bind to its surface receptor. In some cases this bound antibody-antigen attachment can neutralize or destroy the antigen directly. More often, however, the attachment results (through a cascade of chemical events called the *complement* system) in attracting and sensitizing granulocytes and macrophages to engulf the antigen-antibody complex. Just as blood in the water attracts and excites sharks, so elements of the complement cascade attract and excite phagocytes.

Because secretion (of antibodies) is so central to the activity of the B lymphocytes, their role in the defense is called *humoral* immunity. But humoral immunity is only part of the picture of acquired immunity. Recall that each T lymphocyte also carries a particular one of the billion-plus possible antigen receptors on its surface. However, unless T cells are sensitized (we shall see in a moment how they become sensitized) they remain inert. There is one exception, however. T helper cells *can* bind to antigen if it is presented to them in a processed form by a macrophage who has phagocytosed an antigen-antibody complex. And once that presentation and subsequent binding takes place a dramatic process is set in motion.

It begins with the attached T helper cells emitting a chemical messenger called *interleukin2* (IL2), that (a) stimulates B lymphocytes with the crucial receptor to produce plasma and memory cells, (b) promotes multiplication and maturation of a type of T cell (cytotoxic) specialized and sensitized to fight the particular antigen, and (c) communicates its involvement to T suppressor cells, which will eventually wind down the immune response when the battle with the invader is won (see the dotted lines representing chemical communications in Fig. 4.4).

Over the next few days the titer of cytotoxic T cells bearing the critical surface receptor increases substantially. These cytotoxic T cells, sensitized by IL2 from the T helpers, are direct attack cells capable of killing microorganisms and even the body's own cells. When they encounter their antigen they bind to it and then release cytotoxic substances directly into the attacked cell. Once having destroyed a cell they move on, killing many separate cells, often without being harmed themselves. Cytotoxic T cells are particularly effective against virus particles that have invaded cells, but they also destroy cancer cells. Because this type of immune defense involves cells directly attacking antigens, it is called *cell-mediated* immunity.

Psychoimmunology. For behavioral events such as psychosocial stress to influence acquired immunity, with its intricate network of interlaced and interdependent elements, implies that the immune system must be in physical or chemical contact with the brain. Up until very recently it was believed that the immune system, serving as a surveillance and attack system against foreign invaders and wayward cancer cells, was a relatively autonomous unit. That view was challenged by the demonstration that immune responses can be conditioned by classical Pavlovian methods. A variety of agents (saccharine solutions, lights, tones), when paired repeatedly with an immunosuppressive drug, have been shown to acquire the capacity to suppress antibody reaction to antigen.[21] This is a robust finding, confirmed in many laboratories, first with animals and then extended to humans.

At what places do the immune system and the brain interface to make possible behavioral conditioning? First of all the sympathetic nervous system innervates the immune organs of thymus, bone marrow, spleen and the lymph nodes themselves. The sympathetic nerves release their catecholamines (see Fig. 4.1) in these organs, and lymphocytes residing there have receptors for receiving them.[22] Thus a pathway exists for the central nervous system to contact lymphocytes directly.

The existence of these catecholamine receptors in T and B cells means that the sympathetic-adrenal-medulla axis of the stress response can also be detected by the immune system. In addition, T and B cells also have receptors for the glucocorticoids released by the hypothalamic-pituitary-adrenal cortex axis, and indeed, corticosteroids are immunosuppressive.

These connections mean that the brain can exercise control of the immune response in the same way that it can control other organs of the body. That in fact it does so is suggested by numerous experiments in which lesions and electrical stimulation of the hypothalamus, as well as sympathetic blocks, resulted in profound changes in immune function.[23]

Stress and Immunity. Given the intimate connections between the cells of the immune system and the sympathetic nervous system, and the neurochemicals released in the stress response, it should come as no surprise to find that psychosocial stressors can modulate immunity. The list of stressors depressing one or another aspect of immune functioning (in animals) includes electric shocks, social defeat, maternal separation, cage rotation, the odor of a stressed conspecific, immersion in cold water, restraint, handling, intraperitoneal injection of saline, and loud noise. In humans the list includes academic examinations, sleep deprivation, divorce and separation, Alzheimer's caregiving, marital disruption and conjugal bereavement.[24]

In the past decade there has been an explosion of research into the stressor–immunity relationships. Yet the newness of the field means that numerous methodological and procedural pitfalls are still being worked out. Moreover, the patchwork of empirical findings and the lack of an overall integrative framework means that it is very difficult at this time to see the woods for the trees.[25] Thus, it is one thing to show that one or more quantitative aspects of the immune system is affected in psychosocial stress; it is something quite different to understand what the results might mean in terms of the overall adaptive function of this highly interactive system. How, e.g., does it serve the organism for its immune system to be depressed during stress? Is this adaptive in a way which we cannot yet see? Or is it merely an anomalous consequence of the way the immune system and the physiology of stress are constructed? I conclude that, given the current state of the art in psychoneuroimmunology, the practitioner's interest is best served through a few illustrations of the kind of experiments that are being done, noting the various measures taken, and a brief enumeration of some provocative questions for health psychology that psychoneuroimmunology raises.

In that spirit we look at a set of experiments dealing with the effects on the immune system of the common stressor of academic exams. This relatively mild and episodic stressor depresses a number of immune functions, suggesting that examination stress could be a mild health risk, especially for those individuals whose immune systems may already be compromised.

Ronald Glaser and Janet Kiecolt-Glaser, an immunologist-psychologist team at Ohio State University, have carried out a series of investigations into the effects of academic examinations on various aspects of immune functioning.[26] The subjects of their experiments have been medical students participating as volunteers in research on stress and the immune response. The medical curriculum at Ohio State University is such that students have seven or eight 3-day examination blocks spaced throughout the academic year. Since the dates are known at the beginning of the academic year it is easy to plan studies that compare the immune response at times of relatively high and low stress. Thus, blood samples were drawn for immunological assays four to six weeks prior to exams (low stress baseline) and on one of the days during the exam block (high stress period).

At the time blood was drawn the subjects were also administered a pencil and paper checklist to collect information on various physical symptoms and distress levels. Additionally, because any changes in immune response around the time of exams could be indirect products of sleep deprivation, dietary changes or increased coffee consumption, data were collected for these factors as well.

The results of these experiments can be summarized succinctly. First, the checklists confirmed that exam times are associated with higher self-reported degrees of anxiety. Second, T lymphocyte population statistics, NK cell activity, cytotoxic T cell response to mitogen[27] stimulation and latent Epstein-Barr virus, and levels of some of the critical chemical messengers by which immune cells regulate each other were all significantly altered during the examination days. Statistical tests consistently indicated that the results were independent of the changes in diet, sleep and coffee intake that are associated with exams. Thus, the relatively mild psychosocial stressor of academic exams has the ability to produce immunodeficiency in healthy young students.

Biological Significance of Stress-Induced Immunosuppression. Taken along with the results of numerous other experiments with humans and animals exploring the relation between aspects of stress and immune function, the weight of the evidence is clear. Psychosocial stressors can and do produce immunosuppression. But why? Is this merely a curious biological anomaly, perhaps due to the fact that the fight-flight alarm syndrome developed phylogenetically much earlier than the system of acquired immunity? Or is there an adaptive value to an organism if its immune response is lowered during challenge and threat?

Stephen Maier and associates at the University of Colorado have argued persuasively that it is indeed useful for an organism facing a stressor to turn down its immune response.[28] When an organism faces a threat, the alarm stress response depicted in Figure 4.3 sets off a train of neurochemical events that result in a sharp shift in the body's energy distribution as blood glucose is diverted towards muscles and brain. This energy must be taken temporarily from other body systems, such as digestion, sexual function *and* the immune system. Indeed, the immune system's various functions—the mounting of an immune response to antigen, the development of local inflammation to tissue damage, the lowering of pain thresholds that normally draw the organism's attention to infection, and the onset of the systemic changes in immunochemicals that cause fever and the feelings of malaise and sickness—are highly energy intensive.

Thus, both the fight/flight and immune systems require unusual energy mobilization. However, in each system energy must go to very different places and be ready to arouse and support very different behaviors. During a fight/flight emergency it would hardly be useful for energy to be reserved for inflammation and the malaise associated with sickness. The lowered pain thresholds of a fully competent immune response could distract an organism wounded in combat and reduce its chances of fleeing or successfully fighting. It therefore makes plausible biological sense for the immune system to be temporarily suppressed in stress, and that appears to be one of the major roles of the glucocorticoids released by the adrenal cortex.[29] Nevertheless, this shift in energy resources was apparently not designed to be a long-lasting one. Persistent chronic stress of the kind associated with modern social pressures leading to a chronic suppression of the immune system represents a new challenge for this delicately balanced distribution of energy. Stress-associated disease could well be nature's signal that she has not yet adapted these mechanisms to the high frequencies and prolonged durations characteristic of psychosocial stressors.

Health Implications. How clinically significant are the immunological changes in stress likely to be? One study in the medical students' examinations series found that there was in fact a significant increase in self-reported upper respiratory disease associated with the exam periods.[30] This is certainly a provocative finding and suggests that with patient or geriatric populations, or individuals already battling a chronic illness or a neoplasm, moderate psychosocial stress could have serious health consequences. The results of these and the many other experiments showing that the immune system is sensitive to psychosocial stressors raise basic questions toward which further research will certainly be directed:

- Does stress influence the etiology or severity of illnesses modulated by the immune system, e.g., autoimmune diseases, immunodeficient diseases, infectious disease and allergies?
- Are personality traits (such as stress hardiness, highly strung, or anger-prone) reflected in the differential susceptibility of the immune system to stress?
- Can immunocompetence be shown to be enhanced by techniques known to moderate stress, such as relaxation, biofeedback, meditation and the induction of positive emotional states?

Conclusions

The psychobiology of stress is important to the clinician because it provides the conceptual basis for an understanding of the basic pathways by which a psychosocial event (a potential stressor) can influence bodily events (organ pathology). Even though we have much to learn about how a particular stressful event such as bereavement, the repetitive monotony of a boring job, or an attack on our self-esteem can help bring about a particular physical disease, investigation of the systems described in this chapter are yielding suggestive mechanisms. As the mediators that constitute the stress response in all its behavioral and physiological complexity are clarified, the outlines of the bridge linking psychosocial stressors and disease begin to take plausible form. And in that process, much of the mystery in the age-old conundrum, "How can the mind, being non-material, influence the material body in health and illness?" is dispelled. Actually the question is poorly conceived, for it implies that threats cause emotion which causes physiological change which causes organ and tissue pathology. In fact, experience (including the emotions) and physiology are *not* separate, interconnecting events. Rather they are both part of an integrated response to threats that has both specific *and* nonspecific aspects adaptively attuned to the nature of the stimulation. One part of that integrated response entails psychoneuroendocrinological pathways. Wear and tear on organ systems via the release of catecholamines and corticosteroids in prolonged and intense stress constitutes a very real pathogenic factor. Furthermore, chronic stress-induced suppression of immunity suggests that infectious and autoimmune disease, and perhaps cancer as well, could be stress modulated. Thus, the question of how the mind influences the body in the context of stress and disease boils down to a search for the relationships between the history that gives particular events in an individual's environment significance and meaning, and the observed sequence of reactions—behavioral, physiological, neurochemical, and ultimately the tissue alterations called disease—to these events.

The tangled web of these relationships and their interactions suggest that it is best to think of stress not as a cause of illness, but as a kind of psychological "pathogen" influencing susceptibility to disease.[31] Viruses and bacteria acting through known pathways may lead to disease, yet because many other factors influence disease susceptibility, not all organisms exposed to these pathogens actually develop disease. Likewise stress reactions, propagated through the pathways described here (and those yet to be elucidated), may also have the potential to lead to disease. Whether in any given case they will actually do so depends on a variety of other susceptibility factors in the biopsychosocial field.

Project 4

Measuring Your Own Stress at Work[32]

Please fill out the questionnaire to assess your own current stressors and the particular ways that you use to cope with them.

Do you feel more stressed at work now than you did a year ago?

☐ Yes
☐ No

When you feel stress, by what *physical signs* does it manifest?

☐ Headaches
☐ Stomach/bowel problems
☐ Chest pains
☐ Frequent infections
☐ Sleep problems
☐ Weight gain or loss
☐ Loss of libido
☐ Other (please specify)

By what *psychological signs* does this stress manifest?

☐ Moodiness, irritability
☐ Tiredness
☐ Apathy
☐ Depression
☐ Anxiety
☐ Frustration
☐ Indecision
☐ Boredom
☐ Feelings of guilt
☐ Poor concentration
☐ Other (please specify)

By what *behavioral signs* does stress manifest?

☐ Being accident-prone
☐ Alcohol abuse
☐ Drug abuse
☐ Aggressiveness
☐ Relationship problems
☐ Absenteeism
☐ Other (please specify)

How does stress in your personal life affect how you feel at work?

☐ Not at all
☐ A bit
☐ Quite a lot
☐ Very much

How does stress at work affect your personal life?

☐ Not at all
☐ A bit
☐ Quite a lot
☐ Very much

What are the major causes of your stress?

☐ Excessive workload
☐ Lack of resources
☐ Problems with colleagues
☐ Problems with management
☐ Personal difficulties
☐ Worry about job security
☐ Other (please specify)

What facilities are provided at work to help you cope with stress?

	Provided	Used
Counseling services	☐	☐
Support groups	☐	☐
Recreation facilities	☐	☐
Other	☐	☐

What other strategies do you use to help you cope with stress?

☐ Relaxation/physical exercise
☐ Talking to colleagues
☐ Making sure to take breaks
☐ Don't bring home work
☐ Smoking
☐ Drinking alcohol
☐ Drinking coffee or tea
☐ Taking other drugs
☐ Other (please specify)

How do you rate your abilities to cope with stress?

☐ Poor
☐ Average
☐ Better than average
☐ Very good

How many sick days have you taken in the past 12 months?

How many of those sick days were stress-related?

Annotated Bibliography

Dobson, Clifford B. *Stress: The Hidden Adversary.* Ridgewood, NJ: Bogden & Son, 1983. A useful introduction to the field of stress as it was understood in the early 1980s. Accessible to the practitioner without a scientific background.

Henry, James P., and Patricia M. Stephens. *Stress, Health and the Social Environment.* Berlin: Springer-Verlag, 1977. The first chapter provides a very clear introduction to the history of the stress concept and its relation to disease.

Newberry, Benjamin H., et al. "Stress and Disease: An Assessment." In *Human Stress,* vol. 2, edited by James H. Humphrey. New York: AMS Press, 1987. A very readable account of the conceptual and methodological problems besetting stress research, with a useful introduction to psychoimmunology.

Rossi, Ernest L. *The Psychobiology of Mind-Body Healing.* London: W. W. Norton, 1986. All the topics of this chapter are discussed in greater depth here. In addition, hypnosis, state-dependent learning and the placebo effect are set in the same neurophysiological framework.

Selye, Hans. *The Stress of Life.* 1956. Reprint, New York: McGraw-Hill, 1990. This is the classic book by the father of stress research. Selye is at his best as he describes how medical research often proceeds serendipitously, revealing itself to be as much art as science.

Solomon, George F. "The Emerging Field of Psychoneuroimmunology, with a Special Note on AIDS." *Advances* 2 (1985): 6-19. An easily understood introduction to the newly emerging field of psychoneuroimmunology.

5

Stress and Human Disease

*T*HE PRACTITIONER'S INTEREST in the psychobiology of stress and human disease is inherently pragmatic: what kinds of stressors affect health, when, where and how? Our intuitions tell us—indeed our daily practice confirms—that stress and how patients cope with it certainly is one of the main risk factors in disease. What can behavioral scientists tell us beyond these intuitions? To answer that question we shall have to inquire into a chain of reasoning that begins with the way that behavioral scientists have measured psychosocial stress. Perhaps the practitioner can borrow some of these measuring instruments for clinical use. If there is a way (or ways) to measure stress, then perhaps there are consistent correlations between degree of measured stress and incidence (or degree) of reported sickness.

This hypothesis appears to be quite straightforward, but actually a number of methodological problems have to be surmounted to research it in human situations. These problems will lead to an examination of the kinds of *research designs* that psychologists use to try to tease out the various factors that could contribute to the relationships between personality traits, stress responses and the nature of the stressor. Once we find a relationship between stress (however measured) and illness (however defined), we then must try to create a chain of inferences about how psychological events could affect bodily ones.

The Measurement of Psychosocial Stress

We often speak very uncritically about "stress" as though it were a unitary, all-or-nothing variable. Actually stressors have many dimensions that, aside from the specific situation and its context, can include whether it is acute (time-limited) or long-term, whether it initiates a sequence of stressors each of which in turn must be adapted to, whether it is chronic ongoing and unremitting, or chronic intermittent. Some examples of different *types* of stressors are shown in Table 5.1.

Type of Stressor	Examples
Acute (time-limited)	visit to dentist to drill tooth, wasp entering car while driving on highway, woman awaiting results of breast biopsy, long jet flight
Sequential	marriage, divorce, bereavement, job loss, pregnancy, geographic move, significant financial loss or gain, aging
Chronic intermittent	examinations, unpleasant periodic meetings with disliked business associates, scheduled trips to physician or dentist for painful treatments, monthly deadlines
Chronic ongoing	debilitating illness, prolonged relationship discord, long-term exposure to environment hazards or occupational dangers, constant deadlines and unending time pressures, poverty, meaningless boring work, academic pressures such as "publish or perish," oppressive employer

Table 5.1 Types of Stressors, with Examples

In addition to the type of stressor, there are variations in the *source* of the stress. Stressors can be *biogenic,* of which there are two types: *biophysical* (hit by a car on a pedestrian crossing, a skiing accident, a severe burn) or *somatopsychic* (serious disabling or terminal illness, or loss of sensory or motor functioning). In addition, stressors can be *social* (unexpected job layoff, property value decline due to new nearby freeway construction), *interpersonal* (abrupt departure of a lover), *personal* (failure to find publisher for a book, lucrative business contract not reached), or even *spiritual* (loss of sense of purpose, burnout, "in a rut"). The great variation in the type and source of stressors needs to be considered when looking at research purporting to show relationships between stress and illness. We always have to ask, "What kind of stress, how intense and prolonged, on what kinds of illness?"

It is fundamental when thinking of stress to realize that, except for biophysical stressors, no life event has any inherent stressor value in itself. Only when an event is perceived by a human being, evaluated and appraised as dangerous, or a threat to self-esteem or loss of personal resources, does the stressor elicit distress. While this personal factor has proven a tenacious impediment to a systematic classification and measurement of universal stressors, it also is the key to how to cope with stress, for appraisals and evaluations of life events can, in principle, be changed. If what was once a stressor can be converted into a challenge, eliciting energy and commitment, then stress has been replaced with a new, presumably more healthy response.

Significant Recent Life Events

About thirty years ago Professor Thomas Holmes and R. H. Rahe, two medical stress researchers at the University of Washington, devised what has become a classic schedule of 42 potentially stressful life events.[1] These range from cataclysmic events such as the death of a partner or being fired at work, to more minor but still problematic situations such as moving, changing jobs and run-ins with the police. Most of the

42 events have a harmful quality about them, although there are a few that are normally considered positive, such as marriage, holidays and unusual financial success. These were included in the original schedule because strong positive events require adaptation (recall Selye's definition of stress), and anecdotal tales tell of people collapsing upon winning a lottery.[2] Each of the 42 items is assigned an adaptation value, with death of partner anchoring the high end of the scale at 100, and the minor events less than 20 (i.e., they require less than one-fifth as much adaptation on average as death of partner). Point values for each item were scaled based on the relative amount of change in one's life that must be made because of the event. Every aspect of life is disrupted when one loses one's intimate, but only one or a few aspects are disrupted by the minor events.

In Holmes and Rahe's original study with their *Schedule of Significant Recent Life Events,* a thousand United States Navy personnel reported the frequency of each of the 42 events experienced during a one year period. The number of reported events multiplied by the scaled adaptation value for each event was summed to get a total. It was found that those sailors who scored above 300 were about twice as likely on average to fall ill in the next six months than those who scored less than 150. Notice that in this study a test was given and scored, and then used to predict illness *before* it happened. This is an example of a *prospective* research design. In other research[3] the Schedule of Significant Recent Life Events was administered to hospital patients, and to healthy individuals matched to each patient for age, sex, marital status, social class and job salary. In that study test scores were found to be significantly higher for the patients than their matched healthy controls. This latter kind of research is an example of a *retrospective* design because the stress levels were ascertained after the illness had occurred. The retrospective studies suffer from the difficulty that since many people believe that stress is related to illness, once having fallen ill they tend to go back and find something that, after the fact, seems a significant life event. A healthy person, on the other hand, might not even consider that item a significant life event, since they didn't associate it with illness. Also it is known that healthier people tend to forget past events more frequently than ill people.[4]

The Schedule of Significant Recent Life Events, along with the scoring key, appears below in Project 5. In evaluating scores on this instrument, bear in mind that a high (>300) score does not necessarily mean that illness is imminent and inevitable. This scale is a *statistical* predictor. Furthermore, a high score implies nothing about the seriousness of any illness that does transpire, since colds, diabetes, indigestion and terminal cancer were all scored equally in developing the scale. A high score does suggest that one's life this past year has been rather full of events that for most people require adaptation. Such an individual might be recommended to consider some of the stress reduction techniques described in Chapters 6 and 7 in an attempt to balance out an unusually high number of recent potential stressors. Conversely, a low score will not guarantee health. These qualifications of the Schedule of Significant Recent Life Events scale are typical of the rather rough quality of group studies that correlate group average stress levels with average illness frequencies.

In another study, a consistent relationship between recent life changes and coronary accident was found when 279 survivors of myocardial infarction and the spouses of 226 victims of abrupt coronary death were interviewed.[5] Survivors and widowed spouses attested to a significant increase in life changes for themselves and the victims, respectively, in the six months before infarction as compared to the same interval a year earlier. In a second study, 18 men and women with myocardial infarction who ultimately died from the disease were compared with 18 matched subjects alive six years later. There was a significantly greater life events score in the diseased group.[6]

Although the life change schedule is attractive because of its simplicity and directness, it is actually a relatively weak predictor of disease. This is hardly surprising since the scale values are based on an *average* respondent. In fact, everyone responds distinctively to their "life events" in terms of the meaning of these situations to them personally. None of the 42 items on the schedule is inherently stressful, and the actual stress values for any particular individual will be unique to that person. The power of the schedule increases considerably if personality characteristics, such as "propensity to react" or "hardiness," are incorporated into the interview.[7] Thus if the propensity to react is low, or stress hardiness is high, an individual can experience many concomitant life changes without suffering pathophysiological consequences.

Because the schedule of life events scale tends to assume that its events are equally stressful for everybody (clearly false), other workers in stress research have evolved more personal scales designed to tap the minor idiosyncratic stresses, strains and pleasures of an individual's life referred to in colorful language as "daily hassles and uplifts."[8] The questionnaire given as Project 4 in the last chapter, designed to tap stress at work, is yet another example of a more personal stress inventory that some clinicians have found useful to administer to patients.

Occupational Stress

For many people work is stressful. An American study of university teachers found that the more the instructors felt pressured to achieve, the higher was their serum lactic acid level (an indicator of the activity of stress-induced muscular tension).[9] When work overload and pressure involve responsibility for people's lives, rather than responsibility merely for products, stress potential increases. Air traffic controllers have been the subject of considerable stress research since they are under very high pressure and have heavy responsibilities. Illness rates of air traffic controllers and airforce pilots was compared. Although both jobs are very challenging, the controllers have great responsibilities to other people, whereas the pilots' responsibilities were to themselves and their equipment. Hypertension was four times more common among the air traffic controllers, and diabetes and peptic ulcers were twice as common. All these diseases were apt to be diagnosed at a significantly younger age in the controllers. Moreover, in one of the few studies where quantitative differences were studied in the stressor itself, the controllers' incidence of disease was positively related to the degree of traffic at their airport. The busiest airports were more of a health risk than the quiet, backwater fields.[10]

Although great responsibility and heavy work loads seem to be health risks, so too is monotonous, routine, boring work. Occupational stress research has been advanced significantly by a group of Swedish investigators who have convincingly demonstrated that not only overwork, but also *underwork* is a powerful stressor. Moreover, their studies have shown that work environments giving rise to feelings of powerlessness and alienation are intrinsically stressful for the majority of workers.[11] In a classic study of sawmill workers planing, edging and grading in repetitive, dull work requiring quick decisions but little social contact and no control over the work process, it was found that these workers' urinanalyses showed elevated levels of metabolic by-products of stress; in particular, there were increased catecholamines, indicating sympathetic and adrenal medulla hyperactivity. Also, compared with other workers in the same mill who had more creative and interesting jobs, the repetitive workers had high rates of headaches, hypertension and gastrointestinal disorders, including ulcers.[12]

Can we draw any general conclusions from the stressful nature of the *overwork* experienced by air traffic controllers, in which job responsibilities are very high with frequent demanding decisions, and the equally stressful *underwork* environment of the Swedish sawmill workers, in which demands of a different sort are high, yet control over the work process is very low? The best generalization we have at present is that extreme values of work demand (high *or* low) are associated with high stress values, as measured by cortisol elevations and by susceptibility to illness; and this propensity can be accentuated by low control over working conditions. Conversely, a job with a moderate to high work demand is likely to be growth-promoting, associated with a sense of accomplishment, and relatively stress-free whenever the worker has high control over the work environment.[13]

Clinical Observations and Case Histories

The preceding sections illustrate how behavioral scientists and medical epidemiologists attempt to measure psychosocial stress and relate physical illness to it. It should be emphasized that the associations found between disease and such variables as significant life events, number of daily hassles or job demands are purely correlational. Thus, however suggestive, the results of such studies cannot definitively establish causal links between stress and disease for the simple reason that some other unnoticed variable also associated with the experimental variable could be the basis for the correlation. For example, although the air traffic controller studies seem to point to job pressure as a disease pathogen, the possibility cannot be ruled out that some other unmeasured variable (such as increased air pollution at busy airports) is the actual causal variable in the observed health risk.

Can the general practitioner himself, often knowing the patient's life and family situation well, carry out a program of stress research based on detailed analyses of single cases? Certainly the clinician is often able to pick out suggestive stress factors that correlate with the patient's presenting illness. Desmond O'Neill has presented a number of stress-related cases from his own family practice that illustrate the general approach. These range over a very wide class of ailments, from abdominal pain through premenstrual syndrome, migraine, to upper respiratory disease. Traditionally the narrative case history is considered by social scientists to provide only anecdotal or suggestive evidence, which in itself cannot prove cause-effect relationship. However, case histories are not to be lightly dismissed, especially when collected by experienced practitioners who are concerned with objective reporting. In fact, most of our hypotheses about stress and disease come from such "anecdotal" observations. And even though O'Neill is approaching his patients from the standpoint of allopathic medicine, his consistent psychosomatic viewpoint has much in common with our psychobiosocial framework. The practitioner of natural medicine can learn much from such old-fashioned family doctors. A few of O'Neill's cases are briefly described below in order to communicate the sensitivity and flavor of the individual case history approach.[14]

Nasal Symptoms. The syndrome of sneezing, running of the nose, nasal blockage and headache takes in some people the role of a stress disorder. When symptoms appear in the pollen season the disorder is often termed "hay-fever," but this name is misleading, since it implies that exposure to the antigen, pollen, is the sole causative factor.

> A woman of 30 had suffered from attacks of "hay-fever" during the season May to August each year from the age of 14. Her home was in the north of England, and at interview she admitted to feeling most unhappy and frustrated in London. She was kept under observation for some months, and it was observed that she had "hay-fever" symptoms only while in London, and not while staying with her relatives in the north.[15]

Skin Disorders. Itching is a common and important symptom in skin disorder. Indeed, it is the core of the illness in many patients. Few sufferers from eczema would trouble to come to the clinic if the skin did not itch. In other skin complaints it is the cosmetic aspect that troubles the patient.

> A woman of 50 noticed outbreaks of acne necrotica after a fight between her own pet dog and one of his enemies; after falling downstairs; after nursing a sister who was ill; and after a period of depression and poor sleep due to domestic difficulties. She said: "If I get agitated, the spots come out and start itching."[16]

> A man of 36, a taxi-driver, said of his psoriasis: "I feel self-conscious about it. This is the root of the matter. I feel miserable and tensed-up." Although the patches were not large, he felt sure that people noticed them. In public places, he thought himself conspicuous, felt very uneasy, and itched. The psoriasis was worse if he were depressed, and better if he were contented. It was not easy to be sure which was cause and which

effect. On the whole, the mood change seemed to come first. Sound sleep and freedom from worry made the lesions paler. A fall in trade and anxiety about money made it more red, and the lesions spread. So also his awareness of the eruption and the guilt-feelings aroused by it influenced the disorder for the worse.[17]

Hypertension. The following case record shows how a situation charged with resentment can affect a rise of pressure at medical examination.

> A 29-year-old advertising supervisor in a large concern was referred because his diastolic pressure was found to be 105 mmHg when he presented himself for the job. When seen one month later his pressure was 138/80 and his cardiovascular system was normal. It transpired that his previous employer, a choleric individual, had kept him hard at work by promises of high reward but always evaded giving him the security of a contract. This deception had aroused the patient's wrath so that eventually he decided to quit. The interrogation for the new post was long but very friendly. In a final session immediately before the medical examination which disclosed the high diastolic reading, he suddenly had a disconcerting question fired at him—what was wrong with his job that he should be considering one with a lower salary? At this point in his narrative, as he re-experienced his resentment towards his former employer, his blood pressure was found to have risen to 170/104.[18]

Animal Models of Disease

Animal models of human disease represent another, quite different way to investigate relations between stress and disease pathology. Although such experimentation is fraught with problems of generality, the best of such studies can help us to understand better the psychogenesis of human disease. We noted that humans show great individual differences in physiological response to environmental stress events that are consistent, and may even be inherited. A series of exemplary animal studies looked at the relationship between inherited and environmental factors in the genesis of hypertension in the rat.[19] Two genetically different strains of rats were bred from individual rats who were either (*a*) very susceptible or (*b*) very resistant to the hypertension that can be induced by a high salt diet, administration of adrenal cortical hormones, or by renal artery occlusion. Hungry rats from both genetic strains *a* and *b* were then trained to press a bar for small pellets of food, all animals earning their daily food ration from bar pressing. After the bar-pressing behavior was well learned, the food reinforcement schedule for bar presses was reduced and made unpredictable, a food pellet being available for a bar press only once a minute on average. At the same time, however, brief aversive electric foot-shock was also scheduled unpredictably for bar presses, the shocks arriving on average one out of every eight bar presses. Thus the experimental animals were in a conflict situation: they had to work to obtain their daily food supply, but this work incurred self-induced foot shocks. The metaphorical similarities of this regimen to many human work environments is quite obvious.

The experiment was continued for 13 weeks with the results shown in Fig. 5.1. During the first week of the experiment when shock was absent, both the hypertensive-susceptible strain (*a*) and the hypertensive-resistant strain (*b*) (called normotensive in Fig. 5.1) showed comparable (low) blood pressure levels. But beginning in week two when conflict was introduced, blood pressure rose sharply for the susceptible strain, reaching a high plateau by the fifth week, where it stayed for the remaining eight weeks of the experiment. Three months after the end of the experiment, blood pressure levels in the stressed sensitive group had returned to normal.

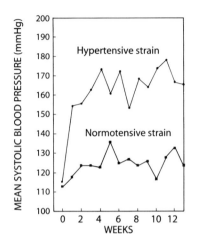

Fig. 5.1 Raised Blood Pressure in Rats over 13 Weeks of Conflict Training[20]

This animal model highlights the interaction of two of the key variables believed to be associated with essential hypertension: (1) inherited differences in responding to stress, and (2) an environment containing stressful events (the electric shocks combined with the demand to work to produce daily food).

Although no animal study can ever provide more than suggestive evidence for the pathogenesis of human disease, this very clear experiment done with good controls[21] reinforces our intuitions about the causal role of conflict-stress in hypertension.

Mechanisms Linking Stress to Disease

Stress-Induced Behaviors. Given that prolonged or intense stress (distress) can predispose to physical disease, what are the pathways over which this interaction takes place? One mediating pathway is via the behaviors that people use to mitigate stress, which actually themselves create health risks. Using alcohol to dull the senses, thereby reducing perceived stress and lowering felt distress, can lead to alcohol addiction with consequent liver damage and increased susceptibility to many other illnesses. Stress can induce anxiety and depression, both of which reduce activity and the motivation to keep physically fit, again raising the chance of falling ill. It is well known that some individuals cope with stress by overeating, thereby becoming obese with its health risks and increased incidence of disease. Others, however, eat poorly, neglecting nutrition, and again put themselves at risk. In general people under stress tend to engage in poor health practices. They may smoke more, eat poorly, drink more alcohol, and sleep less, all of which can influence immune response.[22] Health-promoting behaviors to cope with stress are discussed more thoroughly later. But for now the crucial point to note is that a patient's illness symptoms may well be related to poor habits of coping with the stresses and strains that are indigenous to modern human life.

Direct Physiological Links. Essential hypertension in humans is defined as persistent elevated diastolic arterial blood pressure greater than 100 mmHg of an unknown origin, and is a serious risk factor for coronary heart disease and stroke. Early psychoanalytic studies characterized the hypertensive patient as filled with unexpressed (repressed) hostility and anger. These people did not dare to express their feelings because it was believed that in childhood they experienced losing their parents' love when they expressed anger. As adults, their repressed angry emotions rarely rise to the surface, but they do result in low grade chronic tension and sympathetic nervous system activity, one consequence of which is elevated blood pressure. However, the underlying conflict between wanting to express anger and the anxiety about doing so is not completely hidden. It leaks out in exaggerated levels of annoyance to minor life events such as difficulties in finding parking spaces, waiting in supermarket queues, coin telephone failure, delays in traffic and at airports. The proclivity to make such stress responses has been combined in a *Daily Hassle Scale.*[23]

Hypertensive patients do tend to be more emotional, excitable, guilt-ridden, timid, insecure and sexually inhibited than normotensive patients. They appear over-deferential to others, anxious and tense, and actually the more they exhibit these qualities, the greater their peripheral resistance and blood pressure levels. When emotionally stimulated, their diastolic and systolic blood pressure increase more than normal individuals. Those hypertensive patients who express an interest in members of the opposite sex have exaggeratedly high heart rates and diastolic blood pressure levels. Also it appears that the typical hypertensive individual has relatively few intimate and confiding interpersonal relationships. Apparently the hypertensive individual feels less comfortable in social situations than the normotensive. One reason may be that the hypertensive's struggle to suppress hostility and angry aggression is picked up by others, who then tend to withdraw or deny intimacy to the individual. If so, this would act as a positive feedback loop leading to additional frustration, which would be expected to amplify the person's already exaggerated level of tension.[24]

The studies of essential hypertension confirm that the typical hypertensive person lives with a strong current of underlying stress which may well be an etiologic factor in their condition. The animal model of hypertension discussed in the section above is additional circumstantial evidence that conflict can bring out a latent susceptibility to high blood pressure. So how could chronic stress actually produce essential hypertension? Cannon's wing of the stress response (see Chapter 4) involves activation of the adrenal medulla with increased adrenalin secretion. This leads directly to increase in stroke volume of the heart and increased capillary resistance, both raising blood pressure. But Selye's pituitary-adrenal-cortex axis also contributes because mineralocorticoids (aldosterone) act on the kidney to retain salt and water, also increasing blood pressure. Moreover, if the stress response is prolonged or repeatedly evoked, leading to the resistance phase of the General Adaptation Syndrome, fats are mobilized to the blood stream partly to provide energy for the organism, but also to serve as a precursor for cholesterol plaques, which are created to repair microscopic tears in peripheral blood vessels subjected to the elevated pressures caused by the high pressure. But these plaques narrow the vessels, thereby providing one possible mechanism for a permanent change in the blood pressure set point that is characteristic of the gradual development of human essential hypertension, which develops insidiously over many years. While the account just given is speculative—there is controversy as to the precise roles of neurogenic, renal and vascular feedback mechanisms—it is offered here to show that in principle there is nothing mysterious or esoteric about the ways that psychogenic factors can influence the etiology of physical disease.

Modifying the Immune System. Consider this case history. Norman Cousins, former editor of *The Saturday Review*, fell ill with a serious autoimmune collagen disease, ankylosing spondylitis. Working in partnership with his doctor (whose main job was to clear the medical bureaucracy), Cousins evolved his own treatment protocol, based on the assumption that his illness was the result of stress, and that therefore energizing, positive emotions ought to assist his recovery. Cousins ordered films of Charlie Chaplin and Laurel and Hardy to be played at his bedside in the hospital and measured blood sedimentation rates before and after viewing these funny films, which, despite his serious illness, made him roar with laughter. Blood sedimentation rates systematically and permanently declined after each film session, and Cousins went on to fully recover and write a book about his experience.[25] Cousins' experiments on himself constitute a fascinating example of single-case scientific studies in which the research scientist is simultaneously the subject of his own experiment, a novel design that ought to commend itself to us in natural medicine. The only follow-up study so far to be reported of these intriguing results showed that laughter can indeed increase salivary immunoglobulin A, implying that B lymphocyte activity can be enhanced by positive emotions.[26]

In Chapter 4 we reviewed evidence supporting the notion that psychosocial stress is in fact able to bring about immune suppression. As noted there, medical students taking examinations not only show consistent changes in immune function, they also reported concurrent increase in acute upper respiratory infections at exam periods.

Providing care over a period of years for a relative with senile dementia or Alzheimer's disease has been characterized as profoundly stressful.[27] Care of a family member undergoing progressive senility entails coping with severe behavioral problems that include wandering, incontinence and the loss of ability to communicate or recognize familiar family members. Such caregivers have the misfortune of observing a loved one progressively deteriorate over a period of years. As might be expected, the stress of watching a partner change from a caring, loving individual into an empty shell of a human being is profound.

In addition to the strain of providing care, caregiving affects many other facets of caregivers' lives. One study found that on average, Alzheimer's caregivers spent over eight hours per day in caregiving activities, thus leaving little time for the caregiver's independent activities. As the dementia progresses more care is required, and it may come as no surprise to find that Alzheimer's caregivers suffer higher rates of depression than matched non-caregivers, and that immune functions are affected. A study by the Glaser/Kiecolt-Glaser team in Ohio found that Alzheimer's caregivers showed decrements on three functional immunological measures compared with matched control subjects. Additionally, compared with matched non-caregivers, individuals caring for Alzheimer's relatives had longer lasting upper respiratory infections, which occasioned significantly more visits to their physicians, implying that they were more severe.[28]

Forty first-year medical students were monitored for colds, influenza and general upper respiratory illness during an entire academic year. Students reported more activity-limiting acute infectious illness during exam periods than out of exam periods. Other retrospective studies show that people visit health clinics more, and have more severe upper respiratory disease, during periods when their Significant Life Event Scores (see Project 5) increase. At least one study showed that increased stress is reported three to four days preceding upper respiratory infection, nicely matching the 24-72 hour incubation time of many common cold viruses.[29]

There are a number of studies implicating stress as a risk factor in the development and control of herpes virus infections. Cellular immunity is believed to be a critical factor in both the onset of infection and subsequent clinical symptomatology. Compromised cellular immunity, as in patients with AIDS or those undergoing chemotherapy, is associated with reactivation of latent herpes virus. That this is due to impaired immunity is suggested by characteristic elevations in antibody titers, indicating an attempt by humoral immune components to offset the reduced powers of the cellular immune system.[30]

Epstein-Barr virus (EBV), a member of the herpes family, is the etiologic agent for common infectious mononucleosis. Like other pathogens, EBV need not result in actual clinical disease. Nevertheless, by their mid-20s nearly 90 percent of adults will show IgG antibodies to the virus, indicating a past controlled immune response to exposure to the virus.[31] In a prospective study of psychosocial risk factors in the development of infectious mononucleosis, the medical records of a class of 1400 cadets from the U. S. Military Academy were monitored for four years.[32] Presence or absence of the antibodies to the Epstein-Barr virus was used to distinguish, respectively, those cadets already possessing acquired immunity to mononucleosis, and those still potentially susceptible to the disease. New infections were identified by the appearance of Epstein-Barr antibodies. It was found that cadets under high stress due to a combination of high motivation along with poor academic performance were more likely to acquire the virus, more likely to develop clinical mononucleosis when they did, and then to spend more time in the hospital than cadets not experiencing that stressor combination.[33]

We conclude this brief review of studies implicating psychosocial stressors in both immune system *and* health changes by noting that there is virtually no information on human bacterial infections and stress. At present we can take it as a working hypothesis that psychosocial stressors can, acting through immune mechanisms, influence health. Stress, of course, cannot be a cause of infectious disease. What it can do, however, is to compromise the competence of the immune system by its ability to marshal energy resources elsewhere in the body, thereby disrupting many basic immune mechanisms. As psychoneuroimmunological research continues to clarify those mechanisms we may hope to be able to follow with some precision the biological pathways through which the stress response acts to influence the likelihood, severity and course of not only infectious disease, but any other disease influenced by changes in immune function.

Sociocultural Stress, Health and Illness[34]

Sometimes it is possible to see the effects of psychological stress on an entire society or subculture undergoing rapid social change. Harold G. Wolff made notes of conditions in central India where society was undergoing rapid changes after Independence. A growing number of Indians had become relatively affluent, well-nourished, educated, hygienically conscious and Westernized. Living conditions for these upwardly-mobile Indians in developing suburbs were far superior to Indians living in impoverished villages and overcrowded, unhygienic city ghettos. Nevertheless, it was amongst those wealthier Indians that such diseases as diarrhea, ulcerative colitis and asthma were prevalent. Apparently, in adapting to new circumstances and Western values, many individuals had lost the security of the old social system, but had not found a sense of community in the new social order. There was tension and anxiety, and many individuals exhibited offensive and defensive protective patterns of behavior, indicating a high level of stress that predisposed them to a higher incidence of psychosomatic disease.

Navajo Indians taken from their homes and put onto reservations only a few miles away suffered an appalling increase in mortality from tuberculosis after they had been moved. Although the new physical environment appeared highly similar to that from which they had come, and food, hygiene, clothing and shelter were actually better, the social disorganization which resulted from the move over-burdened the adaptive capabilities of many of these people who fell seriously ill. Similar results have been found in South America when peasant farmers moved from the countryside to shack ghettos in crowded cities.

On the other hand, a very insular community can sometimes protect its members from stresses. Roseto, Pennsylvania was established in 1882 by Italian immigrants. Snubbed by their Anglo-Saxon neighbors, the Rosetans clung closely together for support, and over the years maintained a tight-knit, homogeneous and relatively closed community. The Rosetans kept to many of their old ways, and tended to shut themselves off from the on-going changes in the wider American culture around them. Because of their mutual supportiveness and tight family structure, crime and poverty became almost unknown in their small subculture. Over the years many Rosetans prospered and grew wealthy, yet no class divisions were created. Everyone in Roseto dressed similarly and socialized freely, and surplus wealth was invested back into the community. In 1962 behavioral scientists made a study of this insular community and found that despite high intake of animal fat and widespread obesity, these people suffered an incidence of death from myocardial infarction and coronary artery disease less than half that of the surrounding county. Conversely, Rosetans who had moved away to nearby urban centers had the usual high illness rates of these diseases. Evidently, in the social homogeneity and close-knit social support system of Roseto, where one's place in life and relationship to others are well-defined and accepted, psychosocial stress is substantially reduced with a prevailing beneficial effect on health.

Research Designs in Stress-Disease Relationships

This chapter has presented scientific studies purporting to identify and clarify the role of stress in human disease. The evidence has been drawn from a number of different medical and behavioral research designs whose advantages and weaknesses are summarized below in Table 5.2.

Advantages	Disadvantages	Examples
Animal Models:		
Independent variables can be measured and manipulated. Extraneous factors can be controlled.	Problems of generalizing to human psychosocial stress.	Animal model of hypertension as a function of inherited predisposition and conflict.
Retrospective:		
Natural setting, subjects undisturbed by arbitrary experimental conditions.	Yields only correlations which cannot establish cause-effect; some tendency for research hypothesis to influence measurement of variables; need large groups. Stress may have been produced by the illness rather than vice versa.	Examining the personality factors of persons who have already developed hypertension.
Prospective:		
Same as above.	Need large groups; correlations only.	Significant Life Events Score predicts illnesses of sailors up to six months after taking test.
Group Experimental:		
Independent manipulations of antecedent and consequent variables permit causal inferences. Double blind matched control groups possible.	Experimental laboratory stressors may not be comparable to real-life stress; statistical results will not apply to every case.	(No human group experimental studies discussed in this chapter.)

Advantages	Disadvantages	Examples
Anecdotal, Speculative:		
Natural setting, practitioner can collect data in normal course of treatment.	Bias of investigator-practitioner confounded with research hypothesis being tested. Replication difficult. Spurious correlations possible.	Cases presented by Desmond O'Neill looking at life stress in patients with a variety of complaints.
Single-Case Experimental:		
One subject studied in depth; flexible treatment plan permits investigation of any potentially effective variable(s).	Exact replication of idiosyncratic treatment sequence difficult. Failures not often reported. Role of stress in disease inferred.	Norman Cousin's treatment of his own case of ankylosing spondylitis with laughter (plus high doses of intravenous vitamin C).

Table 5.2 Types of Medical and Behavioral Research Designs

Research in complementary medicine itself is still in its infancy, partly due to poor funding, and partly due to the paucity of qualified research workers. Practitioners tend to regard research as a low priority, even though, as noted above, they are often in the best position to undertake it. Doubtless, as the complementary and holistic viewpoints begin to penetrate establishment medicine, this situation will change. There is much valuable information for the holistic practitioner in mainstream medical journals, reference volumes and textbooks, as well as in the literatures of health psychology and behavioral medicine. To be able to evaluate that literature and the scientific studies of stress and other psychosocial factors in health and disease, practitioners of natural medicine, like their more orthodox colleagues, will need to acquire a modicum of skills in interpreting the common medical research designs which appear in Table 5.2.[35]

Project 5

Schedule of Recent Life Events[36]

PART A

Instructions: Think back on each possible life event listed below, and decide if it happened to you in the past year. If it did, check the box next to it.

☐ 1. A lot more or a lot less trouble with the boss.
☐ 2. A major change in sleeping habits.
☐ 3. A major change in eating habits (a lot more or a lot less, or very different meal hours or surroundings).

☐   4. A revision of personal habits (dress, manners, associations, etc.)

☐   5. A major change in your usual type and/or amount of recreation.

☐   6. A major change in your social activities (clubs, dancing, films, social visits, etc.)

☐   7. A major change in church activities.

☐   8. A major change in number of family get-togethers.

☐   9. A major change in financial state (a lot worse off or a lot better off).

☐ 10. In-law troubles.

☐ 11. A major change in the number of arguments with spouse (a lot more or a lot less than usual regarding child-rearing, personal habits, etc.)

☐ 12. Sexual difficulties.

PART B

Instructions: In the small box indicate the number of times that each applicable event happened to you within the past two years.

☐ 13. Major personal injury or illness.

☐ 14. Death of a close family member (other than spouse).

☐ 15. Death of spouse.

☐ 16. Death of a close friend.

☐ 17. Gaining a new family member (via birth, adoption, oldster moving in, etc.)

☐ 18. Major change in the health or behavior of a family member.

☐ 19. Change in residence.

☐ 20. Detention in jail or other institution.

☐ 21. Minor violation of the law.

☐ 22. Major business readjustment (merger, reorganization, bankruptcy, etc.)

☐ 23. Marriage.

☐ 24. Divorce.

☐ 25. Marital separation.

☐ 26. Outstanding personal achievement.

☐ 27. Son or daughter leaving home (marriage, off to college or university, etc.)

☐ 28. Retirement from work.

☐ 29. Major change in working hours or conditions.

☐ 30. Major change in responsibilities at work (promotion, demotion, transfer).

☐ 31. Dismissed from work.

☐ 32. Major change in living conditions (building new house, remodeling, deterioration of home or neighborhood).

☐ 33. Marital partner beginning or ceasing work outside the home.

☐ 34. Taking on steep mortgage.

☐ 35. Taking on small mortgage.

☐ 36. Foreclosure on mortgage or a loan.

   ☐ 37. Vacation.
   ☐ 38. Changing school.
   ☐ 39. Changing line of work.
   ☐ 40. Beginning or ceasing formal schooling.
   ☐ 41. Marital reconciliation.
   ☐ 42. Pregnancy.

The "mean values" for each life event on the previous page are listed below. For items in Part A just write down the mean values for any of the events that happened to you. For Part B items, multiply the mean value by the number of times the event happened, and add up the sum. Then sum totals for Parts A and B.

Life Event	Mean Value	Your Score	Life Event	Mean Value	Your Score	Life Event	Mean Value	Your Score
1	23	_____	13	53	_____	28	45	_____
2	16	_____	14	63	_____	29	20	_____
3	15	_____	15	100	_____	30	29	_____
4	24	_____	16	37	_____	31	47	_____
5	19	_____	17	39	_____	32	25	_____
6	18	_____	18	44	_____	33	26	_____
7	19	_____	19	20	_____	34	31	_____
8	15	_____	20	63	_____	35	17	_____
9	38	_____	21	11	_____	36	30	_____
10	29	_____	22	39	_____	37	13	_____
11	35	_____	23	50	_____	38	20	_____
12	39	_____	24	73	_____	39	36	_____
			25	65	_____	40	26	_____
			26	28	_____	41	45	_____
			27	29	_____	42	40	_____

Total _____

The more change you have, the more likely you are to get sick. Of those people with a score of over 300 for the past year, almost 80 percent will get sick in the near future; with a score of 150 to 299, about 50 percent will get sick in the near future; and with a score of less than 150, only about 30 percent will get sick in the near future. So, the higher your score, the harder you should work to stay well.

Preventive Measures: The following suggestions can help you use the Schedule of Recent Life Events for the maintenance of your health and the prevention of illness.

1. Become familiar with the life events and the amount of change they require.
2. Put the schedule where your family can see it easily several times a day.
3. With practice you can recognize when a life event happens.
4. Think about the meaning of the event for you and try to identify feelings about it.
5. Think about the different ways you might best adjust to the event.
6. Take your time in arriving at decisions.
7. If possible, anticipate life changes and plan for them well in advance.
8. Pace yourself. It can be done even if you are in a hurry.
9. Look at the accomplishment of a task as a part of daily living and avoid looking at such an achievement as a "stopping point" or a time for letting down.

Annotated Bibliography

Everly, George S. Jr. *A Clinical Guide to the Treatment of the Human Stress Response.* New York: Plenum Press, 1989. An excellent sourcebook for an in-depth presentation of the topics treated in this and the next two chapters. Uniquely oriented towards holistic clinical practice. Highly recommended to any practitioner interested in incorporating psychological medicine into their clinical practice.

Harvey, Peter. *Health Psychology.* London: Longmans, 1988. A slim paperback primer with a short and readable section on psychoimmunology.

Norton, James C. *Introduction to Medical Psychology.* New York: Collier Macmillan, 1982. Most of the issues treated in this chapter are developed in greater detail here from the perspective of behavioral medicine.

O'Neill, Desmond. *A Psychosomatic Approach to Medicine.* London: Billing & Sons, 1955. (Also republished as *Doctor and Patient.* Philadelphia: Lippincott, 1955.) Excellent case history approach written from the point of view of the general practitioner. The cases show convincingly how stress can play a role in virtually any sort of disease.

Pelletier, Kenneth. *Mind as Healer, Mind as Slayer.* New York: Dell, 1977. Somewhat dated now, this classic still provides a valuable nontechnical account of stress and disease from the holistic perspective.

6

Behavioral Medicine

Grant me the courage to change what can be changed, the serenity to accept what cannot be changed, and the wisdom to tell the difference.

—ST. FRANCIS OF ASSISI

*B*EHAVIOR THERAPY AND behavior modification are professions that apply the principles and methods from the experimental analysis of behavior to psychopathology, education and rehabilitation. The further clinical extension of these professions to the evaluation, prevention and treatment of disease created behavioral medicine. Although the roots of behavioral medicine lie in the psychology of learning and conditioning, the new interdisciplinary field is rapidly expanding to include elements from social, physiological and cognitive psychology, as well as epidemiology. The great power and promise of behavioral medicine is to provide the practitioner with a practical methodology for assisting patients to make and maintain the behavioral and attitudinal changes that are essential in the creation of a healthy lifestyle.

This chapter and the next examine a variety of treatment techniques and therapeutic viewpoints which derive from sources ranging from the laboratories of experimental psychology to Eastern spiritual disciplines. What they all have in common in one way or another is the attempt either to ameliorate disease or to promote health through inducing behavioral change. Thus they may legitimately be regarded as falling within the scope of behavioral medicine.

Biofeedback

Biofeedback grew out of the experimental psychology laboratory in investigations directed toward extending operant (reinforcement) conditioning to physiological systems. These systems, which include variables such as heart rate, blood pressure, brain waves, muscle potentials and skin temperature, have historically been classified as "involuntary," and long been viewed as intrinsically beyond the direct control of the subject. However, computers made possible new experiments in which external auditory or visual information about the moment-to-moment state of these biological variables could be provided as *feedback* to human subjects. This *biofeedback* consisted of computer-generated tones, lights, digital displays and images on screens which conveyed continuously updated information to a seated or reclining patient about one or more of their own biological systems. Under those conditions of self-monitoring, it was found that subjects could in fact exert significant control over their own physiology. A typical biofeedback set-up is shown in Fig. 6.1.

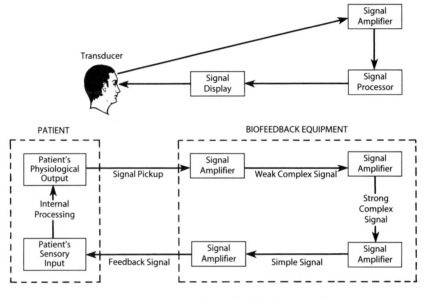

Fig. 6.1 Elements of a Biofeedback System[1]

The term biofeedback derives from "bio"—meaning that the information is biological, and "feedback"—meaning that the information is fed back directly to the subject's visual or auditory senses. In Fig. 6.1 a transducer taped to the forehead of the subject picks up the electrical activity of the frontalis muscle that is filtered and processed by a special-purpose computing system, which then displays it as a screen pattern to the subject. Instructions direct the subject to lower the value displayed to as low as possible. Analogous devices are used to detect and display heart rate, EEG alpha waves, palmar skin resistance, somatomotor activities, finger temperature and blood pressure. In all cases the visual or auditory information that is fed back to the subject is precisely coupled in time with the on-going state of the biological system.

For blood pressure feedback a pressure cuff is wrapped around the upper arm, and a crystal microphone is placed over the brachial artery. The cuff is automatically inflated to just the pressure where a Korotkoff sound is picked up from the microphone, which is then amplified and fed back to earphones worn by the patient. The subject then hears tones whenever blood pressure is just above the cuff pressure level. Instructions are given advising the subject to attempt to reduce the frequency of tones heard. Each time the electronic circuitry detects a Korotkoff sound, it automatically reduces the cuff pressure slightly. And when it hasn't detected a sound for a second or two, then it automatically increases cuff pressure just slightly. This continuous automated process keeps the cuff pressure oscillating just around the point where approximately half the heartbeats are heard and half are too low in pressure to be detected. To the degree that the subject is able to lower this point of oscillation he has succeeded in lowering his own systolic blood pressure.

In exactly this way biofeedback has been employed as a treatment option for essential hypertension and tension headaches. But it has also been used for a number of other disorders (see Table 6.1 below). Portable equipment has been developed for home and office, and some of the hardware permits independent recording and feedback from several different physiological systems. To date, the clinical results of biofeedback can be summarized as follows:

- Under optimal conditions moderate changes in the desired direction can be achieved by patients.
- In some (but not all) instances the acquired changes persist outside the training situation and remain durable over long-term follow-up.
- The same kinds of changes can often be achieved with other techniques, such as relaxation, visualization, diaphragmatic deep breathing and hypnosis (not to mention drugs) that do not require expensive and elaborate instrumentation.

Disorder	Biofeedback System
Asthma	Respiratory resistance
Hypertension	Forearm & frontalis EMG Dermal skin resistance Diastolic blood pressure Systolic blood pressure
Cardiac arrhythmias	Heart rate
Epileptic seizures	Expired air CO_2 levels EEG normalization
Migraine	Finger temperature Temporal artery vasomotor dilation EEG alpha waves
Tension headache	EEG alpha waves Frontalis muscle EMG
Raynaud's disease	Finger temperature

Table 6.1 Representative Disorders for which
Positive Results have been Reported with Biofeedback[2]

Biofeedback sessions require considerable motivation on the part of the patient, and considerable training on the part of the practitioner. Lastly, there is the question of how the subject actually achieves control over the physiological system. The best current evidence we have is that the subject is "controlling" his physiology by relaxing and visualizing, i.e., by actually "letting go." Thus, it appears possible that, in many cases, biofeedback may just be a very elaborate way to induce the same changes that traditional relaxation and meditative techniques produce. Paradoxically, one controls one's physiology by letting go of the habitually and unconsciously held controls.

Therapeutic Imagery

The use of the imagination to heal may be the oldest technique known for it underlies shamanistic practices in all ancient cultures. There is archaeological evidence from cave paintings suggesting that these practices, which are remarkably similar in Asia, Africa, the Americas and Europe, date back at least 20,000 years.[3] The origins of our own Western medicine are also closely connected with imagery. In the famous temples of Asclepius, which have been called the first holistic treatment centers,[4] diagnosis and treatment were based on induced dream imagery.

The images come and go with the times and with cultures, but there remains a common core: the belief of both practitioner and patient in the efficacy of a complex ritual involving suggestion and imagination in the context of authority and mystery. Later (in Chapter 13) we shall explore more deeply the ways that beliefs may harm or cure, and the power of the practitioner/patient relationship to heal. For now we look at a few clinical applications of imagery.

Philosophers and scientists alike have struggled to define the image.[5] The difficulty is that an image, like pain, is a private event. Whatever we do to the instructions "imagine a house," we alone know. Unfortunately it is not easy for us to say what we know, since language requires that at least two observers be able to point to the same thing or quality and assign it a word. For all the epistemological difficulties, the procedures for inducing imagery make remarkably effective cognitive-behavioral therapeutic tools. We may not know how or why they work, nor to what extent they are confounded with placebo effects, but their effectiveness has attracted practitioners from a wide spectrum of disciplines. Thus behavioral therapists have clients imagine a graded series of progressively more frightening scenes while in a state of relaxation. This procedure, known as *systematic desensitization,* is highly effective in alleviating many anxiety-based disorders. Wellness counselors direct patients to imagine themselves healthy and relaxed in delightful settings involving meadows, mountains, brooks, seashores and dunes. In the well-known imagery work of the Simontons, cancer patients imagined natural killer (NK) cells attacking cancer cells and macrophages engulfing metastases. Patients who worked persistently with this imagery had a mean survival time double the actuarial expectation.[6]

The various imagery procedures relevant to medicine can be categorized according to their purpose: diagnostic, treatment and treatment rehearsal. In all three the imagery may be more or less *guided*. Imagery as rehearsal plays an important role in behavioral counseling (see below) and stress inoculation training (see Chapter 7) because it provides a way for a patient to covertly rehearse various prescribed lifestyle changes or stress-coping techniques at home prior to implementing them in daily life situations. For instance, the covert rehearsal of (say) imagining chewing a stick of gum instead of smoking a cigarette in a given imagined stressor situation has a significant effect on reducing smoking behavior in the actual situation. Rehearsal imagery is also useful in ante-natal training, preparing the mother-to-be to anticipate the contractions of labor and to practice in imagination applying breathing techniques prior to the actual birthing.

Imagery techniques are used diagnostically to gain valuable information that is unavailable through routine history-taking. Thus the patient may first be relaxed and then invited to use free imagery to find a symbol or image that corresponds to a symptom, or to the illness as a whole. Once a symbol is found, the patient can be instructed to "give it a voice, ask it what it wants, what would be the implications if it got what it wanted?"[7] In this way the wider context or meaning of the symptom is often revealed.

Yet another powerful way of using imagery to obtain more diagnostic information about a condition is the invocation in imagination of an "inner advisor." In a relaxed state the patient is invited to close the eyes, and to bring a wise being/presence into the imagination. This presence could be a wise person, an historical figure or even a plant or animal. Once the patient is able to visualize this inner advisor, pertinent questions about the illness can be asked. The surprisingly informative and creative answers that often come are said to tap the unconscious, which is another way of saying that they are unreachable through the usual techniques of questioning, either by others or by self. The two case histories by Dr. Martin Rossman in Chapter 14 illustrate the inner advisor technique in detail.

In all imagery techniques the more vivid, detailed and durable the imagery, the more effective the procedure. For that reason, training in both imagery vividness and controllability is desirable.[8] In imagery training the patient looks briefly at an object. Then, with eyes closed, he is asked to describe the object in detail. With repeated practice the ability to describe details improves. The training can be extended to situations at large where sensations of touch, sound, smell and emotion must all be recalled. Imagery controllability can be improved by the use of covert positive reinforcement, that is to say, by immediately following the directed imagining of particular scenes or behaviors with a signal to image a second highly pleasurable scene.

Guided imagery as a treatment intervention was popularized in the late 1970s by the Simontons. Cancer patients formulated a series of images that included the destruction of their cancer cells. Typically this involves images of NK and cytotoxic T cells attaching themselves to cancer cells and then destroying them.[9] The original findings of a mean survival time almost double that of control subjects[10] are actually quite difficult to interpret because of the confounding of many other variables, including differential practitioner interest and attention as well as the expectation of positive results. The question that has intrigued researchers is whether the immune system can actually be influenced by such images. Although the evidence needs to be viewed cautiously, the most recent studies indicate that cancer patients who regularly (twice a day is typical) engage in such imagery protocols do show significant immuno-modulation: increased T cell responsiveness to mitogenic stimulation, raised titers of IgM and IgG antibody production, enhanced NK cell activity and elevated interleukin2 levels.[11] In another study healthy volunteers were able to change both the blood vessel adherence and site distribution of neutrophils by imagining such changes.[12] More-over, these remarkable results were only possible under the following conditions:

• Subjects must believe that they can influence their immune functioning.
• Detailed physiological knowledge of the cellular components and their role in im-mune defense function is necessary for effective neutrophil control.
• Subjects must be trained in relaxation/guided imagery.

Despite these provocative findings the clinician should view such results with caution. In the first place, no actual health outcomes have been measured in these im-munomodulation studies so we really do not know the clinical significance of these cellular changes. Moreover, nobody knows for sure whether in fact the immune system plays a major role in eliminating human cancer.[13] This uncertainty raises the unset-tling possibility that the imagery being used could be clinically effective (the Simontons' results) even though the immune system changes have nothing to do with it. At least one commentator has noted that the way images work in psychotherapy (when they do work) may primarily be due to the patients' and practitioners' "belief that certain images are causative."[14] That conclusion is probably applicable for their use in psycho-logical medicine as well. If so the efficacy of imagery procedures may well be occur-ring "for reasons unrelated to the image."[15]

Such considerations bring us full circle back to the magic of the shaman. Science is the religion of our times, hence our therapeutic images must be NK lymphocytes, antibodies, receptor binding sites and phagocytosing neutrophils. Our magic must be constructed from the latest research findings, and our shamans may wear white labo-ratory coats.

What, after all, lies at the core of imagery's effectiveness? Apparently all imagery protocols, past and present,

• Instill both hope and a sense of perceived control over the disease process;
• Displace the reverberating stress response of anxious worry with positive guided imagery;
• Entail the state of hypo-arousal called relaxation.

Hope, perceived control, stress reduction and relaxation in and of themselves consti-tute potent psychological medicine. In the final analysis the imagery procedures may simply be an exceptionally powerful way to harness them synergistically in the service of healing.

Self-Management

A guiding principle of holistic medicine and the biopsychosocial model of disease and health is that the management and prevention of medical disorders are more under the control of the individual than is usually credited. The way we eat, the degree to which we exercise and the attitudes which determine our stress reactions all relate directly to health. Although, to be sure, constitutional weaknesses and global ecological imbalances do constitute actions-at-a-distance that set limits on our personal control, we are coming to see that disease is frequently a result of a lack of health-enhancing behaviors. Indeed it is generally agreed among practitioners of natural medicine that a health-promoting lifestyle incorporates sound nutrition that is predominantly low in saturated fat, sugar, red meat and processed, devitalized foods, and is high in natural vitamins, minerals and fiber from organically grown produce, with protein mainly from vegetable sources. Regular aerobic exercise for the human body is also essential to counteract the sedentary occupations that predominate in the developed countries of the West. And because challenges, demands and their resulting tension are endemic to human life, the healthy person must acquire effective coping resources to deal adaptively with potential stressors, and so manage stress effectively. Thus, holistic medicine invites individuals to assume responsibility for maintaining their health through developing and sustaining healthy lifestyles.

Though the trend toward personal responsibility in health is relatively new—indeed the complementary medicine movement is itself a part of this emerging twentieth century outlook—the belief in the merit of self-knowledge is as old as the hills. The virtues of self-development were extolled by Plato, Shakespeare, Spinoza, Goethe and Buddha, just to mention a few historical figures at random. Indeed the close relationship between behavior and disease has also been mentioned over and again in history of medicine. But until recently, the methods for influencing our own conduct in the direction of long-term desirable health goals have been hit-or-miss, and notably unreliable. After preaching, lecturing, exhorting and pontificating on the virtues of exercise, whole foods and leading a balanced life, we are left with appealing to common sense or willpower to implement our fine philosophies. Evidence from the world around us suggests that these inner virtues are either of limited use or else are in scarce supply. The dire warnings of lung cancer on cigarette packages and advertisements, and the general knowledge that hypertension carries a high risk of coronary heart disease, has neither put the tobacco companies out of business nor brought about fundamental changes in our high-pressure, competitive and frenetic work habits. The practitioner of natural medicine cannot rely on chance that his client's willpower or good common sense will prevail. In natural medicine we have long looked for ways to assist patients to acquire and maintain the healthy lifestyles that we promote. Principles of self-management derived from behavioral medicine offer practical tools and an effective methodology for the creation of individualized programs designed to inculcate the lifestyle changes that we know foster health.

The clinician's job in a self-management (self-control) treatment plan is to guide the process and to insure that a good caring relationship (partnership) is developed with the patient. The practitioner serves as a faithful consultant who provides information and resources, teaches concepts and suggests techniques. The client, however, is the one who makes the final decision about the treatment plan, and carries out the active interventions in his own life. Moreover, although in the early stages of a program the professional may be very directive in training and providing active support for the client's behavior changes, the clinician must be prepared to gradually fade out her directive role if the client's changes are going to become autonomous and not dependent upon the practitioner for their long-term durability. A self-management, or self-control program in behavioral medicine begins with the client carrying out observations on his own behavior (self-monitoring) and passes through the series of five steps identified below. The entire process may encompass weeks or months during which new skills and attitudes are practiced and gradually learned.

Self-Monitoring. Self-awareness, insight and consciousness-raising are stressed in many psychological treatment models, from gestalt therapy through the self-help movement to psychoanalysis. In behavioral self-control, increased awareness takes the form of self-monitoring, or self-observation of explicit behaviors, noting the cues, stimuli or situations that occasion them. Golf counters, wrist timers, pocket notebooks and even beads are the tools of the trade for keeping track of heart rate, minutes of jogging, calories consumed, thoughts that arise when about to binge on chocolate, stress situations, times of lighting up a cigarette and so forth. It may not be obvious that self-monitoring is itself a skill that, like playing tennis or acquiring a foreign language, has to be learned. As the patient's consultant, the practitioner's job is to explain and demonstrate the technique(s) chosen, and on subsequent visits to go over the notebooks carefully, checking that they are being kept faithfully. External reinforcement—for instance, allocating privileges or rewards of one sort or another whenever criteria of success are met—may be added optionally as part of the patient/practitioner contract. A behavioral diary which records the time and place of critical antecedents and consequences is desirable. Self-monitoring was originally conceived as a way of gathering preliminary information and assessing the pre-treatment behavior to be changed, but it soon became apparent that patients just monitoring their own behavior is inherently salutary. Self-awareness has therapeutic powers in its own right, since some habits can be changed merely by attending closely to them and recording them.

Goal Specification. Deep-seated lifestyle changes, of course, require more than just close observation. The next step is for client and practitioner to establish concrete goals. Here the consultant has to insure that the goals are specified as behavioral objectives. A client will do what, when and where, and under what conditions. Note that the emphasis is on what *will* be done, not what won't be done. The practitioner's job is to help make the behavioral objectives explicit as well as realistic, bearing in mind what she knows about the client's patterns as revealed by the self-monitoring assessment in the previous phase. Clients wishing to lose weight may come in very enthusiastic and want to lose 40 pounds in two months. The practitioner must be the force which keeps the goals realistic, knowing that starvation diets are not substitutes for permanent lifestyle changes. The practitioner too will have to emphasize *behaviors*, since outcomes (losing 40 pounds) do not specify the means. A particular client may wish to stop smoking; the practitioner will have to work out together with the client precisely what behaviors are going to be acquired that will substitute for smoking. If a relaxation program is recommended, it will have to specify the amount of daily practice, and that must be a realistic and agreed upon figure, not one that is simply prescribed. Behavioral medicine challenges our traditional paternalistic role of "doctor knows best." And while that may be frustrating to a professional at first, in the long run the practitioner will reap the benefits of knowing herself to be a midwife assisting and empowering patients to make lasting and deep changes in their lives.

Situational Control. A key concept, which derives from the experimental lab, is to trace the stimulus or *situational antecedents* of behaviors. Behavior never occurs in a vacuum; it is invariably governed by the circumstances and situations in which it developed. Thus a cup of coffee is the situation that may control lighting up a cigarette, a frustrating situation at work can occasion a junk-food binge, and regularly setting aside a certain time of day for yoga or meditation can cause that time to become the stimulus for quiet contemplation and serenity. The practitioner will often suggest interventions designed to break existing situational controls that are associated with unhealthy habits. The patient will be supported in creating new situations that will come to control health-promoting behaviors. A very successful behavioral program carried out by Richard Stuart, in which patients lost an average of nearly 40 pounds and retained the weight loss on long-term follow-up, utilized a stimulus-control analysis based on a written record of daily eating and assessment of progress by monitoring weekly weight gained or lost.[16] Total caloric intake was reduced by limiting the number of situations in which eating was authorized (e.g., eating only at the table, focusing on the sensations of chewing of food, no books, newspapers or television to distract from the eating experience) and by enhancing stimulus control (e.g., food shopping had to be done *after* a meal rather than before, the fridge and larder could not be stocked with high-calorie snacks). Here desirable behaviors (slow, focused eating, attending to hunger cues from the stomach) were taught, and the cues for overeating (inattentive eating, shopping while hungry, eating at the fridge at night) were removed. In other treatments, insomnia has been treated by contracting with clients to use the bedroom for sleeping and sexual activities only, never for reading, arguing, watching television or working.

Incentive Modification. Individuals can present reinforcement to themselves in a variety of ways. Tangible rewards—prearranged forfeits deposited with the therapist that can be reclaimed, gift certificates, permission to take a weekend away—are sometimes effective, although seeing the desirable changes in health and feeling fit are effective inherent rewards. Often the therapist will encourage the client to include family and friends to insure social support of the new ways so that everyone in the patient's life will understand and reinforce the new stimulus controls and the new behaviors being practiced. The client, too, will be encouraged to seek added social incentives, such as finding a friend to share an aerobic exercise program.

Rehearsal. This is a crucial component of many programs in behavioral medicine. The rehearsal can be "covert" in the practitioner's office in the form of visualizations of the desired behaviors and the resulting good feelings when the patient imagines stepping on the scale and seeing a weight loss. In a stress management program a client may be asked to visualize encountering a potential stress situation developing at work or at home, then imagine applying a stress-reduction technique (relaxation, cognitive restructuring, positive affirmation) which is being learned, and finally to imagine a successful outcome. In behavioral medicine the practitioner assumes the role of a teacher or coach helping the client to acquire and practice skills that he will take out into the everyday world and use to foster healthy habits. These skills are necessary to counter the effects of future stress as well as the pulls (advertising, the media, social pressures) toward unhealthy behaviors that are still so prevalent in our society. Clearly, the treatments have to be eminently practical, easy to use and understand, capable of providing immediate results and able to produce changes which will endure beyond the immediate health problem which has brought the patient to the practitioner in the first place.

Behavioral Counseling[17]

Behavioral counseling offers the consultant in natural medicine a practical method for implementing the self-management principles given above. In behavioral counseling the clinician and patient, working together, problem-solve together how to replace an at-risk health behavior with a health-promoting one. In treating chronic disease, the practitioner of natural medicine is likely to suggest changes in four main areas that will probably involve lifestyle changes, hence the learning of new behavior patterns:

- Dietary changes
- Reduction or elimination of substance-abuse behaviors, such as drinking or smoking
- Development of an aerobic exercise program
- Acquisition of stress-reduction techniques.

By remedying health risk behavior patterns and learning new skills in any of these four areas, the patient may be able to influence health in a positive way.

Health behavior counseling is based on the empirically established behavior principles discussed in the section on behavior theory in Chapter 3, and elaborated in more detail below. Employing behavioral monitoring (see above), the clinician and patient together must first develop an understanding of the factors that tend to promote or suppress a particular health behavior in one of the four principal areas. Then the patient/practitioner team will develop a behavioral treatment plan or intervention strategy designed to favor new health-enhancing behavior patterns to replace old at-risk patterns. The collaborative effort involved in the intervention program is essential for maximizing the likelihood of a successful outcome. Once implemented, the program is then closely monitored by the practitioner. Difficulties encountered are brought up in subsequent consultations and the plan modified as required. In a successful program, which may take weeks or months, the practitioner is able to withdraw active support gradually, leaving the patient able to maintain the changes indefinitely.

These very direct steps, which are characteristic of behavioral counseling, set it apart from psychotherapeutic counseling approaches to be discussed later in Chapter 8. Health behavior counseling focuses explicitly on one or more particular target behaviors and does not go into an exploration of how the at-risk behavior began in the first place. The assumption is simply that the behavior is now being maintained because of factors currently existing in the patient's daily environment. Health behavior counseling seeks to identify these factors with the aim of developing an intervention to reduce or eliminate them. Concurrently, the treatment plan will target new health-enhancing behaviors to replace the old at-risk patterns.

In health-related behavioral counseling the practitioner must make a behavioral diagnosis which supplements the medical diagnosis. This behavioral diagnosis involves an analysis of the patient's various health risk behaviors, and the various environmental events and cognitive beliefs on which these behaviors depend. To develop this diagnosis the practitioner must collaborate closely with the patient in a true partnership. It is, after all, the patient who has the detailed information on his daily activities and interpersonal relations. Thus, in behavioral counseling the patient takes a very active role in helping to identify and solve the health problem. Not only does this active role optimize the chances of the patient's adherence to the program, it also reinforces one of the major goals of behavioral counseling, namely the patient's development of new self-management skills. If the practitioner does all the work of behavior analysis and diagnosis, as well as creating the treatment plan, the potential of behavior counseling for encouraging self-responsibility is considerably blunted.

Health-Related Behaviors: A Functional Analysis. Health-related behaviors are actions or activities made by an individual that affect health. Some health-related behaviors promote health, while others either directly undermine it or constitute risk factors that increase the probability of disease. Smoking, alcohol and drug abuse, a sedentary lifestyle and a diet rich in saturated fat, refined carbohydrates, red meat and sugar are common examples of health-risk behavior patterns. On the other hand, regular aerobic exercise, a diet high in natural fiber, unrefined carbohydrates and poly-unsaturated oils, and applying stress-reducing skills are health-enhancing behavior patterns.

Health-related behaviors function like other human actions such as walking, talking and playing the piano. They are acquired, maintained and controlled in the same way as any other behavior. Behavior is a term itself that is used to describe any recognizable unit of human activity that can be identified out of the continuous stream of activity that characterizes human life. Behavior units can be relatively long sequences of activities such as the actions involved in walking up a flight of stairs, reading this paragraph, cooking a meal or writing a letter. Or they may be very brief and discrete like the twitch of an eyelid, or the snapping on of a light switch. Moreover, behavior has an inherent hierarchical quality, such that long sequences can be arbitrarily broken down into smaller units when desired. Taking a homeopathic remedy can be a behavioral unit, but it is in turn composed of smaller units such as opening the bottle, extracting the pill so as not to touch it, popping it under the tongue and retaining it there until it has dissolved.

Even though typical health-promoting behaviors—optimum diet, regular aerobic exercise, stress management skills—involve very complex sequences of activities, they still are assumed, like all behavior, to be lawfully related to the environmental events that surround them. The principal events that determine such activities are the motivational needs (e.g., Fig. 3.2) on which they are based, the situational antecedents that make them possible and the consequences (benefits, gains, rewards) that maintain them. The exact connections, termed *contingencies,* between a particular health-related behavior and these events may be complex and obscure, and the patient in general may not be aware of many of these connections. It is in fact the clinician's job to help the patient identify these behavioral contingencies and to determine under what conditions they operate. In the case of health-risk behaviors, such an identification and determination forms the behavioral diagnosis.

Generally the practitioner can identify events or activities in the patient's everyday environment that have a direct influence on the health-related behavior of concern. For instance, the behavior of smoking a cigarette is frequently linked to the prior behavior of having a cup of coffee. It may also be linked to tension produced by the patient anticipating a stressful event at work. In both these examples a health-risk behavior is at least in part under the control of *antecedent* events that can be identified in the patient's environment. But behavior—including health-related behavior—is invariably under the strong influence of the events that typically follow it as well. These *consequences* may be either positive (pleasurable) or negative (aversive or unpleasant). Behavior that is followed by positive consequences or removes negative situations is reinforced and therefore tends to be learned and then sustained. Conversely, behavior that is followed by negative consequences or removes positive situations is punished, and therefore tends to be suppressed. Lighting up a cigarette is followed by the positive consequences of a pleasurable taste and a feeling of relaxation, and is also followed by a reduction of the negative tension. Smokers have learned this sequence on the basis of these sorts of positive and negative-reducing consequences having transpired in the past. Although it may involve considerable detective work to discover such details, a similar sort of analysis is assumed to underlie any sequence of human behavior, however complex or lengthy.

The concept of control by the antecedents and consequences that surround and interweave human action is, in principle, straightforward. However, the typical health-risk behavior is embedded in a complex context in which the controlling consequences and antecedents may be very subtle and difficult to tease out. Yet it is precisely this that the patient, knowledgeable about his own life, and the practitioner, skilled in behavioral analysis, working together as a team must achieve. Clearly, there must be considerable patient education here, for the practitioner has to teach the relevant psychological principles to the patient so that the partnership can evolve a program designed to alter either the antecedents or consequences of the current undesirable behavior to such an extent that alternative health-promoting behavior becomes more attractive.

One of the reasons why patients often find it difficult to change health-deterring habits, even when they wish to do so, even when they are well aware of the risks of such habits, is because of the relative power that *immediate* behavioral consequences have

	Immediate Consequences		Long-term Consequences	
	+	−	+	−
Current at-risk behavior	**many**	few	few	many
Desired health-promoting behavior	few	**many**	many	few

Table 6.2 Comparison of positive and aversive consequences for a patient who wishes to replace an at-risk behavior with a health-promoting behavior. The most powerful contingencies are shown in bold.[18]

over *delayed* or deferred consequences. Table 6.2 shows, for example, the difficulties in supplanting a current at-risk behavior with a desirable health-enhancing behavior. The typical current at-risk behavior, be it dietary, substance abuse, sedentary lifestyle, high pressure Type A behavior or whatever, has many positive immediate consequences and few negative immediate consequences. This is why such behaviors are maintained indefinitely in spite of patients' knowing that they are health risks. The many long-term negative aversive consequences simply lie so far in the future that they cannot disrupt it. Additionally, learning a new desired self-care behavior is difficult because, as Table 6.2 illustrates, any new behavior is likely to have few immediate positive consequences, and the initial effort of learning it is itself an immediate negative consequence. However, if a new self-care behavior *can* somehow be initiated and then supported—perhaps at first by the practitioner's encouragement, an immediate positive consequence—eventually its long-term positive consequences will materialize to maintain it. During this initial establishment period the professional's encouragement and support in getting the self-care behavior going is crucial to its long-term success.

Steps In Behavioral Counseling. The principles of behavioral counseling can be applied to any health-related habit or desired lifestyle change. Although there will be important differences in emphasis and in the particulars, depending on whether the behavior involves diet, exercising, learning to reduce stress or eliminating a substance-abuse habit, the sequence shown as a flow chart in Fig. 6.2 describes the general steps.

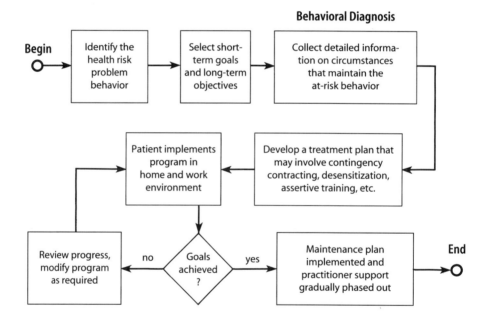

Fig. 6.2 Flow chart for implementing desired health-promoting behaviors. In every step the patient and practitioner are working together as partners in the behavioral analysis and decision making.

First, the patient/practitioner team identifies the health-risk problem behavior. They then discuss the desirable goals—short- and long-term—that a behavior program could realistically achieve over a given time span. Once these goals are agreed upon by both professional and patient, a period of self-monitoring begins. Usually at the next treatment session the team examines the results of the self-monitoring and develops their behavioral diagnosis. This diagnosis includes the behavioral analysis of the controlling contingencies. From the diagnosis an appropriate intervention treatment plan is derived which is designed to evoke and support new adaptive, healthy skills in place of old maladaptive, unhealthy ones. Although in some cases there may be behavioral practice (rehearsal) in the clinic, the bulk of the work is done by the patient implementing the plan into daily life. In later treatment sessions the practitioner reviews progress with the patient, identifies blocks or difficulties and, if necessary, suggests modifications to the treatment plan. At the point at which the treatment goals are close to being achieved, the partnership then develops a plan to maintain the goals as practitioner support is gradually withdrawn. In the typical case involving chronic illness, the consultant in natural medicine will be concurrently carrying out a program of treatment in any of a variety of medical modalities while engaged in this process of behavioral counseling.

Example: Creating a Physical Fitness Program. The process of behavioral counseling is best illustrated concretely. Since natural medicine views many chronic diseases as caused or exacerbated by a sedentary lifestyle, practitioners often suggest to patients that they take up some form of aerobic exercise.[19] Many patients agree in principle that they would like to do this, but in fact do not seem able to develop a regular program for fitting aerobics into their daily schedule. This is precisely the kind of problem that lends itself to the application of behavioral medicine in the form of behavioral counseling.

Following the flow chart in Fig. 6.2, the health-risk problem behavior is identified as a lack of physical (aerobic) activity that may have contributed to obesity or a variety of other somatic complaints. Physical fitness itself is associated with a reduced chance of cardiovascular disease. Regular exercise aids the treatment of sleep disorders and diabetes, and contributes to weight loss by suppressing appetite and expending calories, which in turn has a beneficial effect on blood pressure. An exercise program promotes feelings of well-being, and is a valuable stress reduction resource.

If the practitioner recommends a fitness program and the patient is in agreement, the patient-practitioner team must then select a realistic goal. Using a list such as that found in Table 6.3, the clinician and the patient will go over potential aerobic and nonaerobic activities and select some that the patient feels attracted to, and which could be realistically fitted into the patient's daily schedule. The patient may be referred to publications describing the benefits of aerobics. The clinician will inquire about weekends, vacations and trips to evolve a program that will be viable with changes in scheduling. Typically, the partnership might decide that a realistic long-term objective would entail engaging in an aerobic activity three to four times a week. This goal must, however, be approached gradually through a series of progressively more demanding short-term subgoals.

For instance, the patient may consider jogging 45 minutes three or four times a week to be his long-term objective, but the first short-term goal may simply be a 15-minute walk two or three times a week. Once this is achieved, he may, over the next few weeks, be able to increase the time and pace of his activity to 30 minutes of brisk

Aerobic	Nonaerobic
Walking	Baseball
Jogging	Bowling
Bicycling	Golf
Hiking up hill	Volleyball
Swimming	Football
Stationary cycling	Tennis
Skating	Sailing
Cross-country skiing	House or garden work
Jumping rope	Lifting weights
Aerobic dance	Surfing
Basketball	Shopping
Soccer	Horseback riding
Kayaking, rowing, canoeing	Water skiing
Ice hockey	Hunting or fishing
Calisthenics	Motorcycle trail riding

Table 6.3 Examples of Aerobic and Non-Aerobic Activities[20]

walking interspersed with a few minutes of jogging. In general, not more than a 10 percent increase per week in activity demand is recommended to allow the body time to accommodate to each subgoal.[21]

The progressive nature of the aerobics plan illustrates a general principle: virtually any lifestyle change must be implemented in small steps. The practitioner must insure that the steps are not too big, for if they are, patients may fail to reach the subgoals in a reasonable time period, become discouraged and discontinue the treatment plan. A patient may in fact come with a history of such failures from other, less systematic programs, and this history must be elicited by the clinician so that any pessimism and negative expectancy can be discussed. By explaining that the program will begin with a very modest activity demand, and that the expansion to the final objective will be very gradual and completely under the control of the patient, the practitioner may dispel such negative expectancies.

Having decided on the activity or activities, the patient is invited to imagine how to fit them into his current lifestyle. A rough agreement is made, a behavioral prescription written (see Fig. 6.3) and the patient instructed to collect data for the next treatment session. This data monitoring need be merely a week's recording of when the activity was engaged in, and for how long.

In the follow-up treatment session the patient/practitioner team will examine the activity log and work out whatever bugs have appeared. For instance, the patient may have programmed a morning walk before breakfast, but found in practice that there was insufficient time to do it. On inquiring, the practitioner may discover that breakfast involves reading the financial section of the morning paper. Obviously if new behaviors are going to be fitted into a patient's life, some other behaviors will have to be reduced or omitted. Perhaps three days a week the morning paper can be missed. Possibly the patient can go to bed 30 minutes earlier. Or perhaps the time for aerobics needs to be rescheduled.

As sessions progress, the team continues to monitor progress closely in the aerobic exercise program. Sometimes the original exercise activity becomes boring, so the practitioner may suggest more variety, inviting the patient to choose another activity

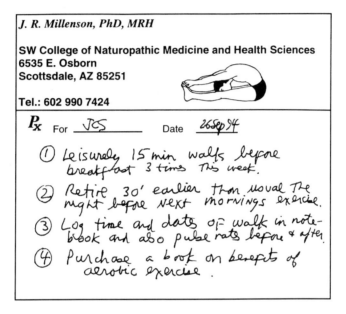

J. R. Millenson, PhD, MRH

SW College of Naturopathic Medicine and Health Sciences
6535 E. Osborn
Scottsdale, AZ 85251

Tel.: 602 990 7424

R_x For ___JCS___ Date ___26 Sep 94___

① Leisurely 15 min walks before breakfast 3 times this week.

② Retire 30' earlier than usual the night before next mornings exercise.

③ Log time and date of walk in notebook and also pulse rate before & after.

④ Purchase a book on benefits of aerobic exercise.

Fig. 6.3 Example of a Behavioral Prescription

or two from the list shown in Fig. 6.2. Clearly, some aerobic activities are suited to particular seasons, so the program may vary at different times of the year.

Unlike changes in diet, eliminating smoking or reducing alcohol or coffee consumption, an aerobics program usually can attract immediate positive consequences. Other behavior-change programs typically involve an initial period when there are immediate aversive consequences, e.g., nicotine or caffeine withdrawal, the bother, effort and time involved in learning new recipes and shopping for unfamiliar foods, and often some social disruption. During the initial period of most behavior change programs, the long-term positive consequences to come (weight loss, feeling fitter, having more energy) haven't yet emerged. In an aerobics program, however, right from the beginning there are potential positive consequences in the form of increased alertness, enhanced well-being and the sheer pleasure of movement. These natural consequences of exercise are immediate incentives that encourage patients to adhere to the fitness program. When failures do occur they are generally not because the patient has difficulties acquiring the new behavior, but because of problems in changing the lifestyle sufficiently to fit aerobics into it.

Common Problems. A variety of common problems must be anticipated. Some patients have difficulties getting started with their fitness program. The practitioner should insure that the activities chosen are indeed enjoyable, and not chosen simply because the patient thinks they are "good for him," or because he notices others doing them. A formal or informal self-contract, allowing himself a special treat upon completing a week's successful program, or conversely, having to pay a fine to a disliked organization if the week's program is not completed, may be of occasional value. Some patients need group support and should be encouraged to find a friend or a group to exercise with at least one exercise period per week.

Negative consequences of exercise—sore muscles, over-fatigue—should be addressed. The practitioner may prescribe appropriate low potency homeopathics and arnica or comfrey cream for muscle strain, aromatherapy massage or reflexology for relaxation, and advise the patient to cease the exercise before extreme tiredness develops.

Sometimes the patient will get the program underway, but then grow bored with it. Again the practitioner should review the chosen aerobic activities, perhaps suggesting more variety during the week. The pleasant aspects of exercising with a friend or family member should be stressed. Some patients like to jog in different venues, others enjoy a running track. In general patients should not be encouraged to continue an exercise that persists in being boring.

When a patient cannot find the time to carry out the treatment program, the clinician must be sure this complaint does not imply a loss of interest in the program. She should initiate a discussion to review the treatment goals and objectives, and the rationale for it, to be sure that the patient is still committed to it. Behavioral medicine requires full support of the patient throughout the treatment protocol.

If the practitioner is satisfied that the problem is one of time scheduling, then the team must review the patient's daily routine to see if the exercise period is placed at the optimum time, when the possibility of conflicts with other important commitments is minimized. Each time of the day—morning, lunch time, evening—will have advantages and disadvantages, and these will be different for each patient. So the practitioner must go over the pros and cons of the exercise time with the patient to reach an agreement on optimum scheduling. It helps to schedule a "back up" or secondary time in case the primary selected time is unavailable on a given day. Another flexible strategy is to have an alternative exercise that can be done at any time: jogging in place, jumping rope, brisk walking. Self-monitoring, of course, should continue regardless of the activity selected. The professional must always insure that the program is easy to engage in. Minor problems such as appropriate clothes and shoes should be anticipated and arranged for. The site of the activity should be identified: local park, swimming pool or health club.

Maintenance Program. Once the patient has succeeded in following the program for about six weeks the practitioner should develop a plan to insure that the program is continued indefinitely without her support. The practitioner may gradually space out treatment sessions, and withdraw any special contracting contingencies (e.g., patient permitting himself special rewards when the week's criteria have been successfully met) that had been introduced to get the program started. The clinician may ask the patient to anticipate potential future problems (family vacations, seasonal changes, job change) that might disrupt the program and invite the patient to propose workable solutions in advance. In this way, dependence on the practitioner is gradually eliminated.

Adherence to Treatment

Throughout the discussion of behavioral counseling the emphasis has been on the patient collaborating closely in an active role with the professional. One reason for this emphasis is to empower the patient to take personal responsibility for as many of the factors influencing health as practical. Another reason is that when the patient is a partner in the treatment plan, the likelihood of adherence to it dramatically improves.

Behavioral change programs involving lifestyle changes are complex interventions. They require changes to long-standing habits that have been established and sustained for many years. New health-promoting behaviors in diet, exercise and stress reduction invariably disrupt an individual's settled patterns. Moreover, many of these treatment programs involve changes in several lifestyle areas at once. The potential for nonadherence to treatment and patient drop-out is ever present in such complex and far-reaching changes.

Noncompliance with treatments is endemic in orthodox medicine. Various studies have shown that 20 to 50 percent of patients fail to appear for scheduled appointments, 20 to 80 percent make errors in taking medication, 25 to 60 percent stop taking medicines before the prescribed course has been completed, and 20 to 80 percent of patients drop out of lifestyle-change programs.[22] There are no comparable data available for complementary medicine, but my impression is that adherence to treatment recommendations is far from perfect. And the problem of noncompliance to physician's prescriptions and proscriptions is not of recent origin. Two thousand years ago Hippocrates mentioned it in his work *Decorum,* advising the physician to be alert to the faults of patients which make them lie or refuse to confess that they failed to take their prescribed remedies.

Two terms have been used to denote a patient's tendency to perform accurately a recommended treatment: compliance and adherence. *Compliance* connotes conformity and acquiescence to the authority of a health-care professional. *Adherence* suggests that the patient is choosing in a self-motivated way to carry out an agreed treatment. Whenever possible, holistic medicine is collaborative and emphasizes self-care and self-responsibility in health. Thus the term compliance has little place in the practice of natural medicine. On the other hand, the holistic practitioner must be concerned to optimize the conditions for adherence to whatever treatment plan is worked out between herself and the patient.

Both terms, compliance and adherence, seem to suggest that the ideal state is for the patient to follow the treatment. However, given the history of fads and fashions in medicine, and the once-approved use of poisons (mercury, arsenic and strychnine) and injurious treatments (blood-letting, emetics and purges), there is a strong case for the concept of intelligent noncompliance.[23] Patients are rightfully wary of new drugs whose side effects may be worse than the disease for which they are prescribed, or of remaining indefinitely on a course of medication whose long-term effects have yet to be evaluated. Interestingly, physicians themselves, when they are patients, have a far lower rate of compliance than the average patient. Do they know something others do not? To overemphasize patient compliance is to endorse a false concept of physician omniscience.

There are two principal variables affecting adherence to treatment. The first, to be discussed in detail in Chapter 13, is the degree to which the patient expresses satisfaction with his physician, that is to say, the degree of rapport established in the patient/practitioner relationship. The second principal variable in adherence is the way that the treatment is presented and then supported by the practitioner. The complex lifestyle-change programs previously discussed often contain important built-in contingency provisions to favor adherence. We've already discussed how ongoing problems with a program are solved collaboratively in behavioral counseling. But questions of treatment adherence in natural medicine extend beyond these programs to a variety of procedures that patients are asked to perform: many practitioners recommend a battery of nutritional supplements to be taken at precise times in relation to meals; medical herbalists prescribe tinctures, teas, decoctions, capsules and fomentations; naturopaths recommend sitz baths with special salts and minerals added, compresses, soaks, coffee enemas and castor oil poultices; aromatherapists prescribe self-massage and essential oil baths; homeopathic remedies must be taken at specific times in a special way and sometimes in conjunction with changes in symptoms; flower essence remedies should be taken three or four times a day, often with affirmations to be recited. These various natural medicines, remedies and treatments require considerable effort, time and expense, some are a nuisance (castor oil packs, coffee enemas) and others are noxious (unpleasant tasting herbs). Evidently, natural treatments are as likely as orthodox treatments to be subject to various degrees of adherence.

Practitioners of natural medicine generally endeavor to educate patients to the need for recommended treatments, medicines and prescriptions. However, research shows that patients forget much of what they are told, and the more they are told in any one visit, the more they forget. Furthermore, writing down the information does not improve their ability to remember it. On the other hand, the more medical knowledge the patient possesses, the more he will recall.[24] Nonadherence to treatment can occur because of external factors such as the expense of the medicines or treatments, as well as from difficulties incorporating the treatment plan into the daily rhythm. But nonadherence can also occur because the patient is not fully convinced of the efficacy of the treatment, or has a different belief or philosophy about his illness than the practitioner.

In general, adherence to treatment is something that the practitioner of natural medicine cannot take for granted. If the practitioner addresses the issue in the initial interview, indicating that nonadherence may occur for various reasons, and if she creates a nonjudgmental climate about it, patients are more likely to be honest and report nonadherence when it occurs. In that climate of openness, treatment nonadherence can be problem-solved like any other behavioral symptom, namely by reviewing the treatment rationale, providing information about the condition including diagnosis and prognosis, and endeavoring to modify the situational antecedents and consequences so as to shift the balance in favor of adherence.

Self-monitoring alone is often enough to tip the scales to satisfactory adherence. If the patient logs the time of each dose of herbal medicine or each homeopathic pill, and the log is reviewed at the next treatment session, adherence will be enhanced. In a study of vitamin C's effects on colds, in which one tablet four times a day was prescribed over a three-week period, nearly 80 percent of the 71 subjects failed to adhere satisfactorily to the treatment.[25] Yet when these same subjects were then instructed simply to record the time of taking their vitamins (self-monitoring) and also forfeited a small monetary deposit for failing to comply, marked improvements in adherence were achieved.

The patient who consistently declines to adhere to a treatment plan to which he has agreed, and continues to affirm his agreement to, can be extremely frustrating. The practitioner may then wish to revert to a simple caretaker function, indicating to the patient that when he is ready to keep his commitment to the plan, she too will be ready to participate actively. Until then she keeps the door open for the patient to return to his role as a full, active participant. Such a stance is in keeping with holistic medicine's emphasis on the patient's responsibility as an equal partner in the treatment. The patient should certainly never be coerced into a treatment, but the practitioner should expect the patient to do the work the team has agreed will likely re-create the balance and harmony that favor health. Failing to set this expectation would belie a holistic medicine that addresses not just the symptoms of disease, but its causes, which are often rooted in psychosocial dimensions.

Project 6

Devising a Self-Management Program

Utilizing the five phases of self-control strategy (self-monitoring, goal specification, stimulus control, incentive modification, and rehearsal) as described in the text, design a self-management program for a lifestyle-related health problem of your own (or that of a patient).

Annotated Bibliography

Antonovsky, Aaron. *Health, Stress, and Coping.* London: Jossey-Bass, 1979. In contrast to most of the medical literature—natural as well as allopathic—Antonovsky takes the long-neglected position of "What causes health?" (salutogenesis) rather than "What causes illness?" (pathogenesis). His distinction between tension and stress, and his conceptualization of generalized stress-resistance resources, are fundamental.

Doleys, Daniel M., Ron L. Meredith, and Anthony R. Ciminero, eds. *Behavioral Medicine: Assessment and Treatment Strategies.* London: Plenum Press, 1982. An excellent reference source for the practitioner requiring information on the many topics which behavioral medicine is now encompassing. The chapter on pain is recommended, but there are also useful chapters on obesity and anorexia, biofeedback, substance abuse and addiction.

Pomerleau, Ovid F., and John P. Brady, eds. *Behavioral Medicine: Theory and Practice.* Baltimore: Williams and Wilkins, 1979. The first and the classic text in the field. The chapters on self-management, smoking, obesity and biofeedback are notable for their clarification of key conceptual issues.

Russell, Michael L. *Behavioral Counseling in Medicine.* New York: Oxford University Press, 1986. A very practical text for the practitioner interested in assisting patients to reduce their health-risk behaviors and develop health-promoting behaviors. Techniques of interviewing, behavioral analysis of problem behaviors, formulation of treatment protocols and objectives, and ongoing monitoring of behavior change are described for enhancing adherence to, and success of programs for, dietary reform, aerobic exercise and stress reduction.

7

Managing Stress and Pain

After rising from a night's sleep, assisted by over-the-counter sleeping pills because of difficulty sleeping as a result of increased caffeine consumption while watching the World Cup on television, Jones sat down to a breakfast of bacon, eggs and coffee. Running late, he ran for his car, lit a cigarette and drove to work along with thousands of others (it took him 40 minutes to travel about 15 miles, even though most of the route was on the expressway). While driving to work, he experienced chest pains and a slight lightheadedness. He drove to his underground parking space (polluted with carbon monoxide), then took the escalator to the main elevator of his large office building into which he had to squeeze along with 15 others, five of whom were smoking, despite the No Smoking sign. He finally arrived in his office, lit a third cigarette, picked up a cup of coffee and began to work. During the late morning his boss called him into the front office to complain about an assignment still unfinished. After sitting at his desk most of the morning, he went out for lunch. Lunch consisted of a ham and cheese sandwich on white bread, chips and a piece of pie. Jones returned to work and sat at his desk the remainder of the day aside from a late afternoon coffee break, and a dispute with one of his colleagues over responsibility for a certain job not yet accomplished. Following the dispute he experienced heartburn, which he ignored. After work he took the elevator and escalator down to his car, drove home in rush-hour traffic and entered a house full of screaming kids. He ate a large dinner and sat down in front of the television with a cup of coffee and a piece of chocolate cake. His day was over at 12:30 A.M., and he again experienced difficulty falling asleep.[1]

*T*HE ABOVE DESCRIPTION OF "A typical day in the life of the 'Healthy Western Person'" is by no means as much a caricature as it ought to be. With such lifestyles we may indeed echo Antonovsky's (1979) question: "How do any of us remain healthy?" In the three previous chapters we looked at the psychophysiology of stress, how stress can create illness and the principle of creating stress-resistant resources. We now turn to very practical ways of creating those resources to manage tension and keep it from leading inevitably to stress. Finally, because chronic pain is one of the chief complaints that the practitioner of natural medicine sees, and because many of the same techniques that help with stress are useful for chronic pain, some contributions of behavioral medicine to the theory and management of pain are assessed.

Model of Stress Management

The nature of the stress response and its intimate relationship to disease challenges psychology to evolve a stress-management technology that clinicians can draw from. The stress-retarding resources of any such psychotechnology must come from one of the three fundamental strategies people use to cope with stressful circumstances:

- Stressors can sometimes be avoided, either directly or by modifying the external situation in which they lie. The stress of a polluted city might be eliminated by a move to the countryside. A point is reached in a stressful relationship or job where the individual decides to end it. On another level we can work to change a political system that ignores the environment and creates global sources of stress. Such coping strategies are *problem-focused*.
- When the stressor itself cannot be eliminated or reduced, it is still possible to *adopt counter-measures* to minimize or mitigate our responses to it. Relaxation training, meditation, yoga, biofeedback, eating more healthily, getting more exercise, going to bed early, having a massage are all important stress-reducing resources. None of these will affect the external situation, but they will all be valuable for minimizing its effects. This coping strategy is *emotion-focused*.
- Finally, one can work on *changing oneself* either by learning new skills to bring to bear on the situation to control it better, or by changing one's attitude toward the stress-producing situation. This coping strategy is *self-focused*. Thus, a challenging job situation may at first be stressful. As the individual learns ways to cope with the demands of the new work, stress is reduced and may eventually be completely eliminated. Feeling obliged to stick with a job that is detested, suffering through a difficult period with a partner, or bowing to financial adversity, it is still possible to change the way one responds to such problems. People can learn to accept what they can't change, can learn to channel their creative energy into new places and to teach themselves to *release* many of their expectations that the world must be a certain way in order to be happy in it.[2]

Life is inevitably full of challenges, demands and threats. The initial response to these ubiquitous events is *tension*—the body's initial alarm response to a demand, Selye's first phase of the General Adaptation Syndrome. This initial stage of tension is not in itself a health risk. Indeed we thrive on challenges and a paucity of them is probably itself a stressor. It is only when severe tension is prolonged, due to the individual's failure to cope with or manage it, that we begin to speak of stress. Strictly speaking, the field of stress management ought properly to be called *tension management,* because coping ideally means keeping tension from progressing to stress.

What can we say in general about whether potential stressors will lead to actual stress? Certainly psychosocial stressors depend for their potency on our interpretation and appraisal of them. But this *transactional* view of stress as depending on both the situation and the person is too general to give much practical help in managing stress. The practitioner wants general purpose *stress-resistant resources* (Antonovsky, 1979) for patients to use to steer their way through the rocky passages of life.

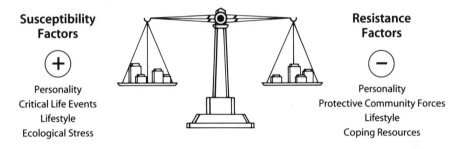

Fig. 7.1 Model of Health Risk[3]

The availability of such resources will counterbalance stressors. The balance in Fig. 7.1 shows symbolically some of the cogent forces that act in a person's life situation to determine the degree of health risk at any given time. On the left pan of the balance are any dysfunctional personality traits that the individual brings to the challenge, any critical life events (see Project 5) currently or recently operating in the patient's life, health risks in lifestyle and whatever ecological stressors might be concomitantly operating.

Pitted against these health risk factors are the health-promoting and stress-resisting factors shown in the right pan: adaptive personality traits that help transform demands into positive challenges, healthy lifestyle elements, the support that comes from being a valued and integrated member of a social community of friends and relations, and any specific coping resources such as knowledge, skills and information that the individual can bring to bear on the current challenge.

When the resistance factors exceed the susceptibility factors, the scale tips to the right and the disease risk is lowest (Fig. 7.2). Conversely, when the susceptibility factors exceed the resistance factors, the scale tips down on the left, and the risk of disease is increased (Fig. 7.3).

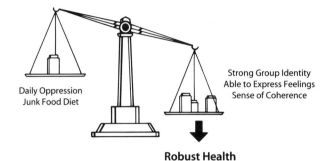

Fig. 7.2 Resistance Factors Exceed Susceptibility Factors

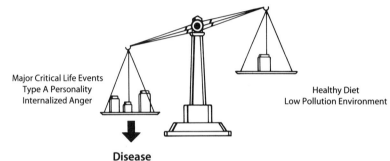

Fig. 7.3 Susceptibility Factors Exceed Resistance Factors

The practitioner wants to be able to assist the patient to develop stress-resistant resources, for according to the balance model, that will help the patient to minimize health risk factors. One of the most important of these resources is in fact the caring, trusting relationship that the professional will strive to create with the patient. The practitioner should become a resource to whom clients can come at the time of increased stress to seek out practical assistance and support for self-management. The informed practitioner therefore needs to possess either the knowledge and skills in stress management to work directly with clients, or know enough about the options to refer patients to qualified specialists in behavioral medicine.

Progressive Relaxation

One of the most generally useful and easily implemented stress management techniques is that of progressive relaxation.[4] The principle behind relaxation to counter stress is easily understood. The physiological response to a stressor includes, among the various measures described by Selye and Cannon, a state of muscular tension in the skeletal muscle system. This is a perfectly adaptive mechanism, preparing us for fight or flight. But when the stressors are psychosocial and the tension remains unrelieved, we may rightly speak of a tension having progressed to stress. The relaxation response is physiologically opposed to tension. A muscle cannot simultaneously be relaxed and tense. Hence the acquisition of the skill of being able to relax selective muscle groups at will amounts to a stress reduction skill.

This is the theoretical rationale, and the evidence for the practical value of relaxation is extremely supportive of the theory behind it. In general, relaxation programs have been shown to be as good or better than biofeedback, meditation, hypnosis and some forms of psychotherapy for a variety of stress-related complaints; used in conjunction with biofeedback and cognitive-behavior self-management programs, it enhances their stress-coping effects. Progressive relaxation therapy of the abbreviated version to be described below has been successfully used alone, with both children and adults, or in conjunction with other techniques, to deal with general tension, insomnia, hypertension, asthma, migraine, tics and other disorders. Of course relaxation is not a panacea since not all clients will maintain the motivation required for sustained practice, which is required if the technique is to have lasting and broadly general stress-retardant effects, i.e., to become a general stress-resistant resource. Nevertheless whenever a patient's physical problem seems to be stress related, progressive relaxation is one of the first techniques the clinician will think to try since it requires no instrumentation, the instructions are simple and easy to follow, it is a benign and pleasant procedure and there are few if any contraindications. The guidelines below are illustrative. Each therapist will present the material in their own natural style.

The patient should first be given a brief theoretical rationale of relaxation, as just described. The complexity and interrelationships of the skeletal muscle system as a whole—there are over a thousand different muscles, each able to be in any degree of tension at any given time—is explained. Part of the technique consists in making the patient aware of tension being held in various muscle groups. The general way that awareness is brought to a group, and the way tension versus relaxation is taught, is to identify some dozen or more muscle groups beginning with the dominant hand and forearm and working gradually along the body, selecting one group after another, first tensing the muscles in that group as forcefully as possible, holding the exaggerated tension for 8-10 seconds, and then releasing it completely for a longer period of about 30 seconds. (Some salient groups and the method of tensing are shown in Table 7.1.)

Muscle Group	Method of Tensing
Hand and forearm	Make tight fist.
Upper arm	Press elbow down against chair.
Forehead	Raise eyebrows as high as possible.
Upper cheeks and nose	Squeeze eyes tightly shut and wrinkle nose.
Chest, shoulders	Take deep breath, hold it, pull shoulder blades together.
Abdomen	Hold stomach out, and then simultaneously try to pull it in.

Table 7.1 Sample Muscle Groups and Ways of Achieving Exaggerated Tension

It helps to suggest to the patient that in the release the muscle be allowed to relax back to a state of zero tension, and then to pass through zero to the negative side: even more relaxed than relaxed, as it were. Generally the practitioner will go through the dozen or so muscle groups one at a time, repeating the tensing and relaxing instructions about three times for each group. Allowing 10 seconds for tensing, 30 seconds for relaxing, 3 repetitions and 15 muscle groups results in a 45-minute session, which is quite sufficient. Patients are generally encouraged to practice the progressive relaxation sequence twice daily for 15-20 minutes. Some patients will find it hard to relax a certain group completely. They should be reassured that tension habits of a lifetime may take more than a single session to be unlearned, but that they will see value, even in partial relaxation, very soon.

After a few sessions, as the patient learns how to bring about a fully relaxed state in any of the selected muscle groups, she can be encouraged to combine groups in different parts of the body, and to experiment with relaxing muscle groups whenever demands are encountered in daily life. The patient should be able to relax without the preceding tension instructions as she comes to learn the subtle body signals of a relaxed state. Rehearsal can be done by requesting the patient to visualize potentially stressful situations. Eventually, muscle groups can be combined into four broad classes: (1) arms and hands, (2) face and neck, (3) chest, shoulders, back and abdomen, and (4) legs and feet. Gradually, the tension stage of the training can be eliminated altogether and the patient can relax on a "count" (e.g., "1, 2, 3, 4, 5, totally relaxed"). About ten sessions should suffice to reach a satisfactory level of proficiency.[5] To provide extra incentive for practice at home, some practitioners prepare individualized relaxation cassettes for their patients.

Meditation and Yoga

Records of meditative practice date back thousands of years. Although there are many forms of meditation, the most widely known in the West are Transcendental Meditation (TM) and various forms of the method taught by Gautama the Buddha about 2500 years ago in North India. In the Eastern tradition the meditator works towards an altered state of consciousness, actually a state beyond consciousness, known variously as satori, jnana or enlightenment. While there are such sincere and dedicated seekers in the West, a rather more limited goal of many who have been introduced to the practice of meditation is the introduction of tranquility and balance into an otherwise hectic and busy lifestyle; in a word, meditation as stress reduction.

In meditation practice one selects an "object" on which to focus the attention. In TM the object of meditation is a verbal sound, called a *mantra*. In one form of TM the sound is selected from one of 16 sounds (most of them resonant sounds with no meaning to the Westerner, such as nama, ram, omm . . .), and while maintaining a comfortable yet erect, alert sitting position, the sound is repeated rhythmically over and over for 20 minutes. In another form of TM the sound is the English word "one," and it is repeated silently on each in-breath and again on each out-breath. In the two well-known Buddhist meditations (Zen from Japan and Vipassaña from Southeast Asia), the meditator usually sits on a cushion in the cross-legged position (the difficult lotus, or the easy Burmese style), or on a low bench, or even in a straight-backed chair. In both Zen and Vipassana practices the initial object of meditation is the rise and fall of the abdomen in breathing; later, when the meditator is consistently able to hold attention to the breath, the field of attention is widened to encompass whatever stimuli are salient, whether street noises, visual events, nearby voices, aches and pains, thoughts and feelings. The meditation practice consists in attempting to remain dispassionately aware of whatever is happening and not to be deflected or submerged in reveries about these stimuli. At all times one attempts to keep the body completely still and to remain detached from all the thoughts, sensations or emotions that arise and pass away. One reason this is called a practice is because it takes practice. The beginner spends most of the meditation time constantly dragging the attention firmly but gently back to the object of meditation. For most of us, the internal dialogue goes on continuously, largely out of our control. Gradually and with practice, however, thoughts begin to subside and this emergence of voluntary control over thinking may be one of the most important effects of meditation as a stress-control technique.

All the varieties of meditative practice induce a state which may be characterized as "relaxed alertness." From the point of view of behavior theory, meditation is a form of self-induced extinction (auto-desensitization). One allows whatever images, sensations and thoughts that arise to come and go as they will, doing nothing about them, neither judging them nor condemning them, neither allowing oneself to be drawn to them nor consciously pushing them away. This is, in effect, an extinction process in which no reinforcement is ever given for these mental acts; instead, everything is consistently paired with a state of relaxation. Of course, to reach such a state requires considerable practice and perseverance for most. Many meditation disciplines recommend a once- or twice-daily 20 minute or longer practice, although there is evidence that even sitting quietly this way once a week is beneficial as a stress reducer.

The two practices described are suitable for Westerners because they minimize the cultic and cultural trappings that many forms of Eastern religion carry with them. However, the calm and peaceful surroundings of a retreat setting are also conducive to success in holding one's attention steady, and for inducing tranquility in the meditator. The burning of incense and the chanting of repetitive, unfamiliar sounds may come to serve as stimulus controls that cue the meditative situation and thus, through conditioning, become linked to the state of relaxed alert awareness that characterizes meditation. Once such conditioning takes place, these trappings of the meditative situation can themselves induce the meditative state.

Research has confirmed that during TM meditation the body enters a state of profound rest, accurately described as a hypometabolic state. Oxygen consumption is lowered in 20 minutes of meditation to a degree reached normally only after six hours of sleep. Heart and respiration rates slow, skin temperature increases (characteristic of parasympathetic relaxation) and a decline in blood lactate concentration occurs, indicating deep skeletal muscle rest. The EEG suggests that the meditative state has unique qualities combining both sleep and wakefulness. There is also evidence that meditation involves a shift in hemispheric dominance, which in most cases means an emergence of right-brain intuition and holistic thought. A number of stress-related illnesses have been affected positively by meditative practice: improvement in breathing patterns of patients with bronchial asthma, decreased blood pressure in hypertensive patients, reduced premature ventricular contractions in patients with ischemic heart disease, reduced serum cholesterol levels in hypercholesterolemic patients, and amelioration of stuttering.[6] These beneficial effects on disease may be the result of any one or a combination of the known effects of meditation practice. Thus the resting state of meditation conserves energy that may later be used for healing. The nonjudgmental attitude practiced can generalize to daily life so that the meditator is less disturbed by formerly stressful situations. If the ability to focus and hold one's attention learned in meditation generalizes to life off the cushion then the meditator's ability to remember the tools of self-management programs at the moment when they are needed should be enhanced. Interestingly enough, the sheer self-discipline of learning to sit immobile with fixed attention for 20 to 60 minutes seems to strengthen will power. The resultant increased ability to keep one's personal resolve is helpful to the individual in every other area of life, e.g., in strengthening determination to give up smoking, to eat more healthily and to make the time for aerobic exercise.

Thus, meditation is a very general behavioral medicine that the practitioner of natural therapeutics may suggest to patients who desire to make health-enhancing changes in their lifestyle. The basic instructions are simple and can be given and assimilated in a single session; but they do need to be given preferably by a reputable meditation teacher, or at the very least by someone who has practiced meditation sufficiently to have obtained at least a hint of the potential benefits.[7] Because the work is the patient's, the technique is likely to appeal to those with an independent, inquiring mind who are receptive to taking responsibility for their own health. A certain healthy skepticism is useful, but of course it must be combined with an open mind.[8] Many students of meditation find it helpful to join regular weekly sitting groups for group support, and also for the inspiration of a teacher who has practiced extensively for some years. Highly religious patients should be assured that a non-cultic practice will not interfere with any of their personal beliefs, and indeed the forms of meditation most popular in the West are compatible with all forms of organized religions.

Meditation can bring up strong emotions, and, although rare, even frightening hallucinatory experiences, so it is useful to have an experienced meditator to consult to get through any difficulties. The general advice given for all phenomena is to "just watch" and not get involved. However it is probably wise for those patients who are bringing up powerful negative feelings to refrain from sitting longer than 15 or 20 minutes until they are fully grounded in the practice. The goals of meditation of course go well beyond stress reduction, but it is the free choice of the student to decide toward what level to strive. Many medical practitioners may feel satisfied if the technique proves salutary in relieving stress-related symptomatology, and in helping to amplify and strengthen any other prescribed stress-resistant resources.

Meditation, however, is not a cure-all and has contraindications too. Many people use meditative techniques to relax, but if what the person really needs is extroverted social involvement, meditation may merely compound a problem. For such individuals the indiscriminate use of meditation may further reduce the opportunities to interact with others and so increase loneliness and isolation.

Hatha yoga, which combines a series of precise postures known as *asanas* with relaxation and focused breathing, can be considered a special class of meditation. The resulting suppleness and body awareness has the ability to relieve a number of musculoskeletal complaints. In addition, many yoga postures succeed in massaging and exercising individual organ systems in such a way as to comprise a complete system of physical medicine. Yogic therapy has been found to be a useful adjunct in the treatment of bronchial asthma, insomnia, headaches, stuttering and the management of tension. Unlike simple relaxation techniques and meditation, however, the postures of hatha yoga do need close supervision at least in the beginning, and there are cautions and contraindications for hypertensive patients and others with cardiovascular disorders.[9] Yoga is best done at least an hour and a half after a light meal. Practice can be typically 15-20 minutes daily. Occasional group sessions with a trained teacher are useful to correct problems and to provide extra incentive. One of the simplest and yet most beneficial poses is the "corpse" posture, in which the fully relaxed body is stretched out, lying prone on the back, breathing slowly, deeply and regularly. As in other meditation techniques the attention is focused and held on an object—often the breath, or the muscle stretch in holding a pose—for a period ranging from a few seconds to some minutes. The technique is gentle and progressive in that the student, breathing into the posture, begins at whatever is the comfort limit in a stretch. Over time the student will be able to approximate more and more the classical form of the asana, although this may take sustained practice for many years. The benefits extend well beyond body training, for hatha yoga, like all yogas, is designed to lead to unity consciousness.

T'ai chi ch'uan is a classical Chinese form of moving meditation. The roots of t'ai chi lie in the philosophy and medicine of Taoism, associated with the legendary figure of Lao Tzu, who is reputed to have been born in 604 B.C. To the ancient Taoists, wisdom and health lay in following nature and doing nothing to oppose her. Thus t'ai chi—the series of exercises which arose from this tradition—emphasizes soft, natural movements, smooth, effortless breaths, and a stance firmly grounded on the earth, with explicit attention paid to unifying the sequence of movements. Ta'i chi aims to focus thought on this series of movements, simultaneously maintaining continuity from one movement to the next, so as to create the sense of a continuous movement. This moving meditation is designed to teach a state of relaxed wholeness, encompassing emptiness and fullness through change and movement. As in other meditations, a variety of health benefits are achieved over time, the practice is easily learned and can be carried out anywhere, and is well-suited to any age in life.[10]

Stress Inoculation Training

This colorful phrase—stress inoculation training—comes from cognitive behavior therapy, and combines elements of Socratic teaching, cognitive restructuring of beliefs and attitudes, behavioral rehearsal, self-monitoring and problem solving. The training is meant to "inoculate" individuals against stressful situations by creating "psychological antibodies," i.e., general purpose cognitive and behavioral skills that can be used to resist potential psychosocial stressors. The training is a kind of "learned resourcefulness" in how to cope successfully with manageable levels of stress so as to build a defense system usable in the future against even more stressful situations.

Devised for ameliorating pathological effects of stress—chronic headache, irritable bowel syndrome, peptic ulcers, hypertension and other functional complaints—stress inoculation training is in fact a kind of counseling. The training consists of three major phases. In the initial phase the practitioner and the client work together to create a collaborative partnership out of which they *conceptualize* the stressful problem. The practitioner endeavors to pinpoint the sources of stress in the patient's environment, and may introduce the patient to some of the principles described in this and the previous chapters. The ideas of stress resistance resources, and the ways that potential psychosocial stressors become stressful depending on one's evaluation and appraisal of situations, help to demonstrate to patients that they have more control over stress than generally imagined.

In the second phase, called *skills acquisition and rehearsal,* the practitioner works with the patient in teaching and rehearsing a variety of coping skills. The particular skills to be taught vary widely depending on the presenting problem jointly identified in conceptualization phase one. Stressed parents might be trained in parent effectiveness communication skills. An individual stressed at work might be taught simple assertiveness skills. A person in a relationship crisis that appears to be a significant health risk factor might be taught conflict resolution skills. Many patients will be taught relaxation. But in addition to these behavioral skills, the practitioner will be teaching new positive self-esteem beliefs.

Each person's psychosocial stress tends to occur in patterns which, although they vary in details from situation to situation, frequently have a common theme. The practitioner looks to see what "self-fulfilling prophecies" the client has which are actually dysfunctional ways of viewing the world:

- I'm not good at meeting new people.
- You need a lot of money to be happy.
- Nobody cares for you unless you can prove your worth.
- I'm not attractive so I can't create an intimate relationship.

Once an individual begins to believe such negative judgments, these beliefs actually act to create consequences that are consistent with and reinforce them. With such beliefs one can easily create the very situation and conditions that are most dreaded.

A key way to detect such self-fulfilling prophecies as the first step to countering them is for the practitioner to ask patients to report on their "self dialogues," i.e., what they say to themselves when actually under stress. When the internal dialogue is stress-engendering or stress-magnifying as, for example,

- I'm not as good as others.
- Everything I do turns out badly.
- What's the use?
- Life has no meaning.
- There's nothing I can do to control it/them.
- It's all my fault again.

then the practitioner points out the factual errors in these global judgments and invites the client to replace them as they arise with positive and accurate judgments:

- I'm actually quite good at . . .
- Yesterday I cooked an excellent meal which turned out very well.
- There are a number of things I can do which have an impact.
- Life has the meaning that I choose to give it.
- I may not be able to control it/them, but I can control what I think about it/them and consequently what I feel about it/them.

In this work the practitioner is not merely giving lectures on the virtues of positive self-esteem or how to view the world more realistically, but is working in a detailed way with the client to *rehearse and practice* these new self-beliefs.

The final phase of stress inoculation is the *application* beyond the actual presenting problem. In phase two the development and rehearsal of skills took place mostly in the office or clinic. Now in phase three, through homework assignments, the skills acquired are carried out into the client's real-life environment. Among other things, the patient is trained to detect a potential psychosocial stressor before it becomes full-blown, to monitor the positive effects of the various coping skills and to maintain the positive belief system acquired in phase two without the support of the practitioner.

Stress inoculation training is quite appropriate for a practitioner to carry out to complement whatever natural medicines and treatments are prescribed for the presenting problem. The training can be as short as a single session for a client about to encounter a known stressor (e.g., before hospitalization and surgery), or as long as 20 to 40 sessions for patients with deep-seated and multi-causal clinical problems, such as chronic back pain. Follow-up sessions are useful to ensure retention and continual usage of the skills so that they become a routine part of the individual's lifestyle. The training is quite compatible with all the other stress-reducing techniques discussed earlier.

Pain

A substantial number of patients attending a natural medicine practice will present with chronic pain. Almost by definition these are cases that allopathic medicine

Case History of Impact of Chronic Pain on Lifestyle

Ruby was a 42-year old woman who experienced three years of severe pain following a whiplash sustained in a car accident. Her pain was severe enough to disrupt all aspects of her life. Ruby reported that her pain did not allow her to get a good night's sleep. Consequently, she was fatigued most of the time. She neglected her husband, children, friends, and home.

Her husband, Jack, was fed up with her complaints. The expense of Ruby's medication and medical treatments drained the family's finances and curtailed vacations and other pleasures. Ruby had no interest in any previously enjoyed activities, including sex. She wanted to be left alone.

Ruby's teenage children, Jennifer and Roy, were equally troubled by her behavior. They felt she had become a different person since the accident and were demoralized by her unpredictable behavior. She would belittle them for no apparent reason, and they felt they could not please her. Confused and angry, the children began staying away

from home as much as possible.

Ruby then became angry because they stayed away and accused them of lack of caring. She was depressed and guilty about her behavior.

Jack, who was a salesman, also spent more and more time away from home, often volunteering for extended selling trips. His inaccessibility led to more anger on Ruby's part. The continual conflicts served to drive Jack further away.

Jack and Ruby's former friends no longer visited them because Ruby constantly talked about her pain and suffering and complained that no one understood her condition. Friends stopped inviting the couple out because Ruby's pain was unpredictable, and she often had to back out of plans at the last moment.

Ruby's life had "collapsed" (to use her word). She spent her time lying down, in bed, or seeking new medical treatments. The boundaries of her existence were restricted to home and physicians' offices or hospitals.[11]

has been unable to help. Often these patients have suffered for months or years, been on hypnosedatives or minor tranquilizers, may have had anesthetic blocks or neurosurgery to sever nerve pathways, and whose lives have been profoundly disrupted by their constant unwanted companion. Chronic pain is usually defined as pain that has persisted for at least six months. In many cases it is no longer clearly related to an underlying pathology, though it may have begun from an injury or once had a detectable organic component. Thus in chronic pain there is often either a negative medical workup, or a static pathology (see box).

Despite the apparent absence of pathology in such chronic pain cases, often the trained hands of a practitioner in complementary medicine can detect imbalances and blocked energies.[12] In many cases natural medicines alone are sufficient to bring about significant alleviation or even elimination of a patient's pain. Acupuncture and osteopathy are notable for their usefulness in pain alleviation. Herbalists have an armamentarium of nervines and botanical tranquilizers which are often helpful. Many homeopathic remedies have unique pains as their keynotes. And yet, at the end of the day there still remains a residue of patients whose suffering is unmitigated. For them, behavioral and psychological methods may usefully augment natural therapeutics.

Our cultural predisposition is to regard pain as a wholly negative experience, something to be avoided and eliminated as soon as possible. This attitude accounts for the huge trade in over-the-counter pain "relief" drugs. In fact, pain is nature's signal to an organism that there is something wrong somewhere. What is wrong may or may not be tissue damage. Pain is our warning signal, analogous to the red light that comes on when our automobile's oil pressure is dangerously low. Would we be content to fix the problem in our car by putting a piece of tape over the oil light or by cutting its wire to the oil reservoir? That in fact is the equivalent of taking aspirin or surgically severing nerves for a pain whose origins and maintaining conditions we have been unable to trace.

In dealing with pain the practitioner will, as usual in holistic treatment, attempt to discover the underlying initiating and maintaining causes of a patient's chronic pain—be it tension or migraine headaches, rheumatic joint pain, sciatica, lower back pain, temporal-mandibular pain, trigeminal pain, neuralgia or whatever. And it is generally when the clinician can find no satisfactory pathological explanation from extensive laboratory tests that he is likely to turn to the psychology of pain for further help.

The Gate Theory of Pain. The psychology of pain begins with a refutation of the very simple and commonly held belief in which the experience or sensation of pain is as-sumed to arise from a one-to-one correlation with stimulation of certain peripheral nerve fibers specialized for pain. Although it is indeed true that there are such specialized pain fibers, and although it is also true that excessive stimulation of other sensory nerve fibers can result in pain, the experience of pain is far more complex, and far more multi-determined, than any such simplistic view can explain.

We know there is no one-to-one correlation with tissue damage because a simple cut can give a more painful sensation than a deep-seated invasive cancer. Then too, we've all experienced in the heat of an active moment how we may have injured ourselves and not noticed it until much later. A recent newspaper report told of a child who was caught in a gang war and was machine gunned in the belly, who came home and said, just before collapsing, "Mommy, I don't feel so good." (Happily, she recovered fully after emergency surgery.) During World War II, wounded soldiers were studied and it was found that they required far less morphine and reported much less pain than did civilians who incurred injuries of comparable severity. In general the wounded soldiers were relieved and elated because their wound meant their safe return home was guaranteed. The corresponding injury to a civilian meant a disruption and cessation of normal life, with anxiety and fear over the financial, social and personal consequences of long recuperation and possible disability.

There appears to be great individual variation from person to person in the experience of pain with similar pathology due to factors we can only guess at. In general terms, emotional distress from social, interpersonal and spiritual sources summates or potentizes pain of physical origin to produce the experience of *total pain,* or what we might simply call suffering.

Thus pain is a complex multi-determined experience with *sensory, affective* (feeling) and *evaluative* components. The so-called *gate theory* of pain is a model that endeavors to encompass these complexities and interactions.[13] The gate theory recognizes that incoming stimuli from certain nerve fibers have the potential to produce pain experience *if* the impulses from these fibers are allowed to pass a "gating mechanism" located in the spinal dorsal horn that allows them to continue on up to higher levels of the cerebral cortex. However, the gate can be open, closed or partially open depending on various factors which are listed in Table 7.2.

	Factors that open the pain gate	Factors that tend to close the pain gate
Physical factors	Locus & extent of injury	Sedation medication
	Readiness of nervous system to send pain signal	Counter-stimulation (e.g., massage, acupuncture)
	Muscle tension	Muscle relaxation
		Brain endorphins
Emotional factors	Anxiety & worry	Calmness, serenity
	Depression	Positive emotions (joy, optimism)
Cognitive factors	Focusing on the pain	Distraction
	Lack of engaging life activities	Involvement in life activities
	Catastrophizing about the pain	Adaptive attitudes

Table 7.2 Factors Influencing the Experienced Intensity of Pain[14]

The gate theory helps to explain why negative emotions such as anxiety, worry and depression can augment pain; and correspondingly, it provides a conceptual structure that suggests procedures such as relaxation, counter-stimulation and cognitive reconceptualization that are likely to push the gate closed, thereby actually reducing the experienced pain intensity.

The term *brain endorphins* appears in Table 7.2. These are opiate-like neurochemicals recently discovered in the brain that have powerful mood-altering properties, one of which is an analgesic, pain-modulating effect. Endorphins—short for *endogeneous morphine*—are the body's naturally produced tranquilizers. Although first discovered in the brain, they are in fact found in considerable concentration in the immune and endocrine systems as well as other tissues. Moreover, since virtually every cell in the body has receptors for picking up endorphins and responding to them, the view is developing that they are the messengers of an intricate intercellular communication network responsible for generating and transmitting emotional and motivational states throughout the body.[15] We are just beginning to learn about the endorphins, but we do know that their concentration levels are elevated during relaxation, meditation and after aerobic exercise, as well as other techniques that reduce stress.

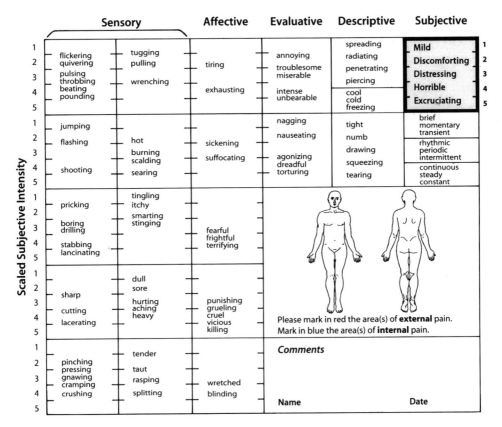

Fig. 7.4 The McGill Pain Questionnaire. Highlight no more than one word per box that describes your pain. (Note: Any box except that in the top right corner can be left empty.)[16]

Measuring Pain. Clinicians require a way of measuring the various dimensions of pain in order to evaluate the effects of whatever interventions they are making. Fig. 7.4 is a questionnaire devised by one of the co-creators of the gate theory of pain, Professor Ronald Melzack of Canada. The questionnaire contains a table of some 87 adjectives set in small-scaled boxes in four main categories of experience. The three basic categories of pain described above—sensory, affective and evaluative—occupy the first four columns of the table reading from left to right. Notice that the adjectives located within the small boxes are aligned at the exact level of their scaled value from 1 to 5.

Where did these scaled values from 1 to 5 come from? Look up at the top right shaded box. This contains the scale from 1 to 5 (mild to excruciating) that a large group of pain patients and their doctors used to assign numbers to each of the words in the three categories. The words have been entered at the average rated value. Thus, e.g., if a patient fills out the McGill Pain Questionnaire by circling pulsing (2.4), shooting (3.9) and lacerating (4.0) from sensory column 1, smarting (2.0) from sensory column 2, frightful (3.5) from affective column 3, and miserable (2.7) from evaluative column 4, these six scores are summed and then divided by 6 to get an average of 3.08 for the patient's rated pain. Of course, the patient also checks in the top right shaded box, and that value gives a second personal pain index. (Note that there are two columns, the *descriptive* and the lower three-tiered *subjective,* that are unscaled simply because they contain essentially neutral adjectives.)

Out of this questionnaire one gets three measures: (1) the personal pain index, which is the level of pain on a scale between 0 and 5 marked in the shaded top right box; (2) the total number of words checked in the three categories (six in our example); and (3) the average scaled value of the checked words (3.08 in our example). In research to date it has been found that these variables do respond in a favorable direction to certain behavioral techniques: hypnosis, relaxation, biofeedback, reinforcement of wellness behaviors and cognitive-behavioral therapy.[17] It is important of course to do long-term (up to a year or longer) follow-ups to monitor the durability of the selected treatment(s).

Pain Behavior. In many cases of chronic pain that has persisted over years, the patient will have adopted habits in which the pain has become integral to the person's lifestyle. Something of this sort seems to have happened with Ruby, described above in the case history (see box). Family members come to treat the patient with kid gloves, and the disability becomes a way of being for the patient. Nevertheless, if the patient presents for treatment it may be assumed that this lifestyle is not really working. What we usually find when we look into the patient's family and life situation is that the patient's behaviors originally induced by pain (protecting a sore muscle, grimacing, wincing, expressions of pain, complaints, restricted movements) have eventually become ways of relating to the world and are now reinforced by the attention of others (even if it is negative attention, as it was in Ruby's family).

Thus, many pain clinics work on *extinguishing* these pain behaviors and *reinforcing* wellness behaviors: talking about other subjects, increased activity and exercise, returning to work, taking up hobbies, helping others. Generally the clinic systematically withdraws the patient's pain medication over a 2-month period, since addiction to pain killers is considered part of the pain syndrome. It is important to keep in mind when encouraging such wellness behaviors that the patient's experience of suffering is not invalidated. In fact, nobody but the experiencer really knows how much pain they feel. That is the nature of a purely private sensation of which pain is an exemplary example. It is useful to reassure the patient that while it may not be possible to find the precise cause for the pain, nonetheless a combined program that encourages wellness behaviors and works with the factors that close the pain gate will afford help in coping with the suffering. Perhaps to put pain in a more philosophical context, we might take courage from the words of a famous man who suffered for years from jaw cancer and many operations. When asked about how he could work with the pain, Sigmund Freud responded: "There is a tiny island of pain surrounded by a sea of tranquility."

Hypnosis. There is considerable mystique about hypnosis due both to the sensational stage effects produced from time to time, and also because so far science has failed to fit the phenomenon into a coherent theory that relates it to the main body of psychology. No doubt hypnosis is one of those scientific anomalies that one day, when we fully understand it, will help to revolutionize our way of thinking about consciousness. For now, however, perhaps the most useful way to view hypnosis is to say that although the hypnotic trance is best viewed as an altered state of consciousness manifesting deep calm, highly focused attention and heightened suggestibility, nevertheless it may only be qualitatively different from similar states which are approached in a less sensational way by other relaxation and visualization techniques.

In any event, ever since 1829 when the French surgeon Dr. Cloquet performed a successful mastectomy without the use of drug anesthetics on a 64-year-old hypnotized woman, there has never been doubt that under optimal conditions the hypnotic state can block pain. During the surgery, as incisions were made from the armpit to the inner side of the breast, and as a malignant tumor was cut out, the patient's heart rate and respiration remained stable and she conversed normally with the surgeon, showing no signs of experiencing pain.

Why then isn't hypnosis in general use for all pain? Unfortunately, only a small proportion of the population is able to enter a deep enough trance to allow such feats as Dr. Cloquet's. Nevertheless, as one of the tools in the practitioner's armamentarium it can be effective, especially when combined with other therapeutic procedures.

The eminent American hypnotherapist Theodore X. Barber has described the use of hypnosis in the treatment of tension headaches. In the exploratory interview the therapist gathers information about the typical antecedents of headaches. After explaining to the patient that self-hypnosis, or self-induced relaxation, can be effective in modifying the patient's typical tension responses to stressors, the therapist induces trance or deep relaxation state. Here are typical suggestions for deep relaxation, modified slightly from Barber:

> Get into a comfortable, relaxed position. Just let yourself feel totally calm, relaxed, and completely at ease. Now close your eyes, and take a deep breath and hold it momentarily . . . Now let it out, and as you do, feel all the tensions of the day expiring with it . . . And now as you breathe calmly and peacefully, you begin to let go of all tensions, all worries and concerns, any frustrations are left behind . . . You're becoming even more calm. Imagine yourself [floating on a soft cushion of cloud / lying on a warm, sunny beach / lying on a warm, soft grassy meadow / floating down a lazy river

> in a canoe] . . . and as you do you're becoming even more comfortable, even more
> relaxed, tranquil, serene . . . Breathing slowing and gently, your thoughts begin to slow
> down . . . Time is slowing down, lots of time, so much time . . . Your mind and body
> slowing down, totally relaxed . . . Arms relaxing . . . legs relaxing, face relaxing . . . Body
> and mind relaxing . . . warm and comfortable . . . Totally at peace now, becoming
> more and more relaxed, becoming drowsy . . . Limbs heavy . . . Peaceful, quiet, calm,
> drifting and floating still deeper . . . and deeper . . . utterly relaxed now.[18]

In the state of calm that results the therapist can now go over the conditions that
have been worked out in advance with the client that typically precede the onset of
tension headache: rejection by a significant person, a quarrel with one of the children,
a difficult interaction with a colleague at work, a traffic jam, time pressure of work
and so forth. The therapist will suggest that the client visualize a potentially stressful
scene while in the deeply relaxed state, and then point out how calm, relaxed and
tension-free the client feels in that situation, not the slightest hint of a headache. The
therapist may suggest that the next time such a potential stressor situation occurs the
client will relax in this same way and avoid the tension that leads to the headache.
The session may include a number of such visualizations and suggestions for future
encounters, after which the therapist gently brings the client back to the normal
"waking" state of consciousness:

> Now I'm going to count down from 10 to 1 and as I count you'll find yourself slowly
> coming back to this room, to your normal active state: ten, nine—starting to stir—
> eight, seven . . . leaving the [beach/cloud/meadow/river] . . . six . . . gradually coming
> back (therapist may raise his voice slightly, speaks more insistently) five, four, three . . .
> feeling your body in the chair . . . two . . . legs solidly, firmly on the floor . . . one! FULLY
> HERE, as you open your eyes, stretch your body, and look around the room, feeling
> alert, active, refreshed.

Typically the therapist will make a 7- to 10-minute relaxation cassette tape (also called
a self-hypnosis tape) for the client to use at home to practice the relaxation/trance.[19]

Wellness and Preventative Medicine

In providing stress-resistant resources the practitioner of complementary medicine is practicing preventative medicine. In our culture this is relatively rare, for we
are accustomed to asking, "Why am I sick?" and only seldom asking, "Why am I
healthy?" Health and illness are two ends of a spectrum, but which end we focus on is
critical. Our Western "health-care" establishments are in reality disease-care institutions, and as such they are concerned far more with the mechanics of disease than
with the conditions that foster health. As I write this chapter I am working in the
stacks of a distinguished Western university health sciences library. Glancing around,
I see books on infectious illness, the history of venereal disease, morbid anatomy,
psychopathology, mental illness, brain tumors, the management of juvenile diabetes,
textbooks of internal medicine. Contrary to what the name on the library door might
suggest, there are few books or resources on health science.

Focusing on health, or *wellness,* means asking new questions. Some of the known health-risk factors are poverty and great social disruption, yet in every disenfranchised, impoverished group a significant proportion of individuals remain healthy no matter how difficult life seems. Why? What kept some concentration camp survivors healthy and balanced? The poor and oppressed all over the world are at greater health risk, yet many individuals come through harsh and brutal conditions healthy and hale. Why? Indeed, when you consider the stressors with which each and every one of us is constantly bombarded, it is not a trivial question to ask how any of us stays healthy.

In Chapter 9 we will discuss the kind of personality that, because of its ability to cope well with demands and challenges, has been called the *stress-hardy personality.* For now, however, we can take note of what, from both intuition and research, appears to be one of the most powerful general stress-resistant resources of such a personality. This resource is appropriately called a *sense of coherence*: the conviction that however rocky the road, one still "retains a dynamic feeling of confidence that one's internal and external environments are predictable and that there is a high probability that things will work out as well as can reasonably be expected."[20] It is probably not an exaggeration to say that the relative success of any stress management technique depends on the degree to which it succeeds in instilling a new and more holistic way of viewing problems of living.

> For every human being life has undesirable aspects. Aging and death are inevitable for me and you and every person we care about. Also either we or people we love will experience birth defects, paralysis . . . severe pain, bodily disfigurement, and many other undesirable happenings. Every human being will also experience other unwanted events, such as loss of a job or loss of financial security, rejection by parents, lovers, children, or friends; unsavory encounters with others . . . who are not the way 'we want them to be,' and encounters with many undesirable external events (ranging from inclement weather to traffic jams to wars or a world in turmoil). The first and most essential facet of wisdom and ability to live happily is fully to accept at a very deep level that life inevitably has problems and virtually every day we will encounter events and behaviors from others that we do not like at all and wish would never occur. This philosophical attitude, which is found in those who have attained wisdom and the ability to live at a high level, is quite different from the implicit philosophy adopted by the great majority of individuals.[21]

Project 7

Creating a Personal Stress Inoculation Program

In coping with their own potential stressors, practitioners have the opportunity to set an example for patients in how to manage stress successfully.

Each of us must evolve our own particular program that we set into effect when we encounter significant challenges in our life. Our personal program will reflect our own strengths and weaknesses.

The first step is to begin to monitor our own stress responses. We have to see what situations we find most taxing, and then pinpoint how our body reacts to those situations. What are we telling ourselves (our "inner dialogue") when these situations occur, and how does that dialogue actually magnify rather than diminish the stress? What are our particular stress patterns?

Then we have to look carefully to see what role we ourselves might be playing in bringing about the situations that lead to stress. Often there is a conflict of motives involved, e.g., "This work is tedious and boring and unfulfilling, but I don't want the hassle of looking for a new job or being out of work for an unknown period."

But even if there are no conflicts, challenges and demands are endemic to living. How do we counterbalance stress? The text describes some techniques and resources. Which one(s) appeal to you personally? Project 7 invites the reader to create a personal list of both general and specific stress-resistant or stress-retardant resources, and describe how and when these have been used. It is suggested that the reader choose a particular technique from the lesson (meditation, yoga, relaxation, autogenic training, self-control, self-hypnosis, visualizations . . .) which has some intuitive appeal, obtain more information about it, practice it, and record how successful it proves in coping with stress in your own life.

Start by going over the three basic ways to cope with a demand:

(1) What can I do to change the situation?
(2) What can I do to minimize and counterbalance my own stress responses?
(3) What can I do to change myself: either through acquiring new skills to cope with the challenge, or by changing how I think about it?

▆▆ Annotated Bibliography

Antonovsky, Aaron. *Health, Stress, and Coping.* London: Jossey-Bass, 1979. **Daniel A. Girdano**, and **George S. Everly**. *Controlling Stress and Tension: A Holistic Approach.* Englewood Cliffs, NJ: Prentice-Hall, 1979. A very practical book with exercises, illustrations and techniques described in sufficient detail for the interested student practitioner.

Hoffmann, David. *Successful Stress Control the Natural Way.* Wellingborough, Northamptonshire: Thorsons, 1986. A holistic approach to stress management with emphasis on botanic medicine. Most of the "alternative" techniques that have proven of value in mitigating stress are described.

Kabat-Zinn, Jon. *Full Catastrophe Living.* New York: Bantam-Doubleday-Dell, 1990. A practical sourcebook documenting the power of the meditation practice of "mindfulness" as a stress-reduction resource, and its value in medicine in general.

Meichenbaum, Donald. *Stress Inoculation Training.* Oxford: Pergamon Press, 1985. Provides the essentials of a cognitive-behavioral training program designed for teaching individuals behavioral and conceptual coping skills. The intent is not only to help individuals to resolve specific immediate problems, but to provide them with a set of general coping skills to deal with future challenges.

Pelletier, Kenneth R. *Mind as Healer, Mind as Slayer.* New York: Dell, 1977. The chapters on biofeedback, meditation, relaxation and autogenic training are all relevant to stress management, and delve into these topics in sufficient depth to give the practitioner a feel for how to use them.

West, Michael A., ed., *The Psychology of Meditation.* Oxford: Clarendon, 1987.

Woolfolk, Robert L., and **Paul M. Lehrer,** eds., *Principles and Practice of Stress Management,* 2nd ed. New York: Guilford, 1993. Useful chapters on relaxation, yogic therapy, biofeedback, autogenic training and hypnosis.

8

Psychological Counseling

If a man does not keep pace with his companions,
perhaps it is because he hears a different drummer.
Let him step to the music which he hears, however
measured or far away.

— HENRY DAVID THOREAU (1841)

*E*VERY PRACTITIONER OF natural medicine treats a significant proportion of patients whose symptomatology seems to be associated with significant emotional dysfunction. The patient comes complaining of backache, headaches, chronic indigestion, arthritis, rheumatism, asthma, hypertension or chronic fatigue, yet either at the initial visit or sometime later it becomes clear that all is not well on the emotional plane. The patient may be concerned with apparently intractable problems on the job, persistent difficulties at home with partner and children, lack of a meaningful creative life, a disappointing love affair or perhaps no love life at all, a recent or not so recent death of a loved one to which adjustment is proving difficult, a mid-life crisis still unresolved.

Even when such feelings are not antecedents to the physical illness, they are commonly secondary byproducts of it. A sudden stroke or heart attack that leaves a formerly vigorous and active person partly crippled affects all aspects of life, and depression is a natural response to the loss of physical and intellectual powers. But no less debilitating are surgical operations that change physical appearance, or ones whose long-term prognosis leaves the person in the limbo of uncertainty for many years. Infirmities such as arthritis and diabetes progressively limit abilities, and are associated with ever-increasing pain and immobility. These and other long, chronic illnesses that constrain the patient's ability to do many forms of productive work, or which reduce strength sufficiently to eliminate the possibility of once enjoyable activities, often generate psychological as well as physical burdens.

The pervasiveness of the interaction between the physical and the emotional

131

means that the professional cannot avoid questioning the role of emotional factors and psychosocial etiology in many patient problems. Aside from the homeopath—who will examine these factors as a matter of course in taking the case, and in part base the selection of the remedy on them—every other natural practitioner will have to choose how to respond, if at all, to whatever emotional/psychological sides a case presents.[1] Prior chapters have illustrated how psychosocial factors can indeed be health factors, for diets, lifestyles and personalities can either be relatively healthy or relatively pathogenic. Chapters 5 through 7 emphasized that a prolonged stress response to challenges and significant life experiences acts through neural, endocrine and immunological pathways to constitute a definite health risk. If the practitioner of natural medicine elects to work explicitly with the emotional aspects of a patient's imbalance she will be taking on some of the functions of a counselor or psychotherapist. This is what the ancient Greeks called "medicine by words," or simply, psychological medicine.

In this chapter we'll first discuss how to begin, then speak briefly about the differences between counseling and psychotherapy, and then complete our introduction by focusing on empathic listening, a skill that underlies virtually all counseling modalities. With this background in hand we next take a deeper look at five modern schools of psychotherapy. These five—Rogerian person-centered, gestalt therapy, reality therapy, multi-modal behavior therapy and existential therapy—comprise a representative sampling from a spectrum containing literally dozens of currently fashionable schools and psychotherapeutic systems. The intent of the presentation is to give the practitioner a sense of the very different possible ways of working with psychological medicine. In selecting these five from among the many systems available there is no implication that they are the "best" or necessarily the most fundamental. They are simply ones whose value I have personally experienced through teaching and in my own practice.

How to Begin

Merely listening empathically with caring interest and close attention to the patient, taking the time to understand fully the context and implications of his physical symptoms, is already a first and very important step in the counseling process. In considering the suffering patient as a whole person and not just a diseased or dysfunctional bit of physiology, the professional is already practicing elementary psychological medicine. Indeed, the need to be heard and understood is an important reason why the patient has come in the first place. For as religion loses its vitality and its connection with the living truth, doctors have come to occupy more and more the traditional roles once held exclusively by priests and the clergy. Unfortunately, the technical-scientific training of the orthodox physician offers little preparation for this task, and the assembly-line health system of institutionalized medicine allows little or no time for it. Thus, consciously or unconsciously, many patients come to alternative and complementary practitioners hoping that they can find a sympathetic ear. Patients frequently expect alternative medicine to help them gain insight into what is wrong with their lives, for they already sense that the presenting physical complaint may only be the acceptable tip of an otherwise frightening and incomprehensible iceberg of difficulties. Since part of the job of the holistic practitioner is to help the patient find "the healer within," there will often be times when it is impossible to separate the practice of complementary medicine from something very like psychotherapy.

But even if the propensity for counseling is there, what is the practitioner's training for it? Fortunately, it is not necessary for the practitioner of natural medicine to devote years of formal study acquiring a higher degree in clinical psychology or psychiatry to be of use to her patients. As oncologist Carl Simonton has noted, we can be of great value merely by learning to listen, to assure our patient that his "negative" feelings of anger, anxiety or depression are very natural ones, appropriate to the situation in which he finds himself, and not something to be hidden or suppressed out of shame.

> [B]asic counseling skills are not difficult to acquire. Teaching people basic assertiveness, for example, is an important skill that is easily taught. How to deal with resentment is fairly easy to learn; or how to deal with guilt. There are pretty standard techniques for these situations. And most important, just to be able to talk to somebody about one's problems is of tremendous help. It leads one out of the sense of helplessness that is so devastating.[2]

To the degree we can manage to be open, accepting and genuine human beings ourselves, and not hide behind professional roles, we can model the kinds of attributes that psychotherapeutic research has found create positive changes in clients' self-esteem, increase their ability to handle potential stressors, induce greater flexibility in the face of unpredictable life events, and lead clients to greater acceptance of themselves. It is the very acceptance and integration of our own life experience, the congruence between our own feelings and behavior, and our own self-esteem—in short, our own being—rather than any set of techniques, that proves the most valuable asset in assisting patients with their problems of living.

Practitioners vary in the extent to which they are likely to feel drawn to work directly with the patient on the emotional issues around the illness. Furthermore, counseling has to be a consensual agreement. Some patients are eager to explore difficult personal areas of their lives, and are quite open to the idea that there could be an interaction between their physical symptoms and emotional issues; indeed, they may be the first to suggest it. But others will resist to the bitter end the notion that there is or could be any relation between the two. Unfortunately, in common parlance the very word *psychosomatic* connotes both "imaginary" and "moral weakness." Pushing an unwilling or unprepared patient to accept a relation between the mind and body that he does not feel or dares not consider will be fruitless and probably counterproductive. Still, some alternative practitioners regard psychological medicine (i.e., medicine with words) as important as their own therapeutic modality, routinely supplementing treatment with counseling. Others will not find that the patient's emotional issues specifically require their focus, but rather see them as resolving concurrently with the physical symptomatology, requiring no special attention or techniques. Occasionally a case presents where the emotional side is so clearly pathological, or the patient so obviously out of contact with reality, that the professional will feel obliged to refer the patient to a qualified holistic psychotherapist or psychiatrist.

Ultimately it is the professional's own healthy personality and healthy lifestyle, her own self-esteem and self-acceptance that are the most important "techniques" in counseling. That having been said, there are a number of useful qualities and concepts that have evolved which do characterize the successful counseling relationship, and which can be effectively taught. These therapeutic attributes derive from a variety of different "schools" of psychotherapy, most of which have developed over the past 25 years. Not so very long ago there was in the West only one school of treatment: psychoanalysis, occasionally combined with hypnosis.[3] Now, as the twentieth century draws to a close, there are literally hundreds of different schools and theories of psychotherapy, many of them quite chauvinistically trumpeting their own unique panaceas. What we will do here is to consider some basic attitudes towards problems of living and imbalance derived from a representative handful of the currently influential schools. Such a comparative approach illustrates the common threads from which all therapies are woven. Moreover, it provides an eclectic sampling of useful counseling qualities, techniques and attitudes from which each practitioner can create her own unique set of therapeutic tools, choosing those which seem the most valuable and personally congenial.

Counseling and Psychotherapy

In practicing psychological medicine, is the practitioner of natural medicine doing counseling or psychotherapy? Appearances to the contrary, there really is no fundamental difference between what counselors do versus what psychotherapists do. The term counselor is of course much broader, since the field is represented by a variety of professions ranging from school counselors, social workers, career counselors, the clergy, psychologists and psychiatrists, to lawyers engaged in divorce and dispute mediation. Despite this great range of professions, the differences among individual counselors is greater than the differences among the particular professional umbrella under which the practitioner works. This suggests that counseling is a highly individual endeavor. Counseling has the connotation of being short-term and not as "deep" as psychotherapy, but that distinction is actually unsupported by what the workers actually do.

In fact, the difference between the two enterprises—counseling and psychotherapy—turns out upon close investigation to be a quantitative difference in how counselors and psychotherapists distribute their time in sessions with clients. The appropriate comparisons are made in Table 8.1 below. Both counselors and psychotherapists engage in the same set of activities. But whereas counselors spend more time advising, informing and explaining, psychotherapists spend a greater proportion of their time listening, supporting and reflecting back what they have heard. We

Activity	Psychotherapists	Counselors
Listening	60	20
Questioning	10	15
Supporting	10	5
Evaluating	5	5
Explaining	5	15
Interpreting	3	1
Informing	3	20
Advising	3	10
Prescribing/ordering	1	9

Table 8.1 Relative Percentage of Time Spent by Counselors and by Psychotherapists[4]

might characterize the difference, then, as saying that on average, counselors are more directive and inclined to give advice and explanations, whereas psychotherapists are more nondirective, listen more and give considerably less advice and explanation. Despite the averages, however, there are many nondirective counselors, and quite a few directive psychotherapists. Individual counselors and therapists develop their own style, which may deviate considerably from the averages shown in Table 8.1.

Active Listening

Table 8.1 indicates that psychotherapists spend much of their time listening. A considerable amount of that listening is purely passive listening. They are in good eye contact, giving close attention to what the patient is saying and doing, occasionally nodding, ah-ha-ing and um-hum-ing. Passive listening is not to be underestimated because often all a troubled person needs is a sympathetic ear. Just knowing that another person is interested enough to be willing to listen can allow feelings to be ventilated, after which the person can very often bring their own intelligent solution to the problem with no help from the counselor or anyone else. Passive listening is supplemented by various neutral, invitational "door openers" such as:

- "What's on your mind today?"
- "Would you like to talk about it?"
- "I'd be interested to hear how you feel about it."
- "Tell me more."
- "Sometimes it helps to get it off your chest."

Valuable as passive listening and door openers are for opening up communication lines, there is another kind of special listening that therapists do which is far more active; it is a skill that counselors generally have to work at to acquire. This special kind of listening is known as *active* or *empathic listening,* the importance of which for helping relationships was first emphasized by the distinguished humanistic psychologist Carl R. Rogers.

In active listening the counselor is listening not just *to* the words, but listening *through* the words for the feeling tone or emotion that lies behind them. Once having picked up that feeling tone, the counselor will feed it back to the speaker. How does this work? First of all, since it's impossible to get inside another's skin, note that no one, not even the most sensitive and skilled friend, lover or counselor, ever knows exactly what another person is experiencing. However, by listening closely to what is heard and how it is said, as well as by attending closely to gestures and other nonverbal signals that can be picked up from the patient, one is able to make plausible inferences about another's feelings. Consider for a moment the patient as a sender in a communication system with you as the receiver. He has an experience or a feeling that he wishes to share with you, so he has first to select the appropriate words, which constitutes a *code* that will represent these inner feelings. On hearing those words, you—the receiver—have to decode them to guess or infer the sender's experience.

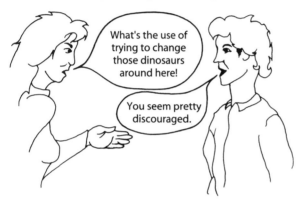

Fig. 8.1 Active Listening:
Picking Up the Feelings Behind the Words

In the example of Fig. 8.1, a patient has been speaking about her job and explaining how difficult it's been for her recently trying to deal with a new and very critical supervisor. It was your door opener, "So how are you feeling in yourself?" that initiated the conversation, and so far you have been passively listening with a few "uh huhs." Abruptly she says to you, in a very disgruntled tone of voice, "What's the use of trying to change those dinosaurs around there!"

When the listener feeds back what he has decoded, the sender gets tangible evidence of listening (see Fig. 8.1). The sender may confirm it ("I am discouraged, it's true") or correct it ("Well, actually I'm more angry than discouraged"), but in either case the listener's response is likely to facilitate further disclosure and open up even deeper feelings.

If active listening were just a skill to ensure that speakers and listeners communicated effectively it would be a valuable tool for minimizing misunderstandings. But it is far more than that. What active listening does is to foster two of the most important ingredients for any growth-fostering or health-enhancing human relationship. These ingredients are *empathy*—the ability to put oneself in the shoes of another and to understand their personal world—and *acceptance.* Knowing we are understood and accepted allows us to open up and to explore even deeper feelings, and when we do that our rational intellectual resources for problem solving become more accessible.

Why as counselors do we have to *learn* to listen actively? Why doesn't it come naturally? One reason has to do with a general lack of emotional literacy in our culture. Whereas we routinely describe our environment with a variety of colorful adjectives, making the finest distinctions and indicating subtle shades of meaning, we seldom employ many words to describe our feelings. How many times do we ask a patient "How are you feeling today?" and get answers such as "Okay," "Not too bad," "Not so good." We speak as though there were a poverty of feeling words. Thus, to practice active listening it helps to try to describe feelings in two, or better, three descriptive emotion words. (To assist with that process, see Fig. 8.2 which illustrates a variety of emotions, and Appendix A to this chapter, which lists a range of emotional words.)

Aside from a general lack of emotional literacy, our typical, culturally learned reaction to a person expressing a problem in emotional code is usually very far from empathic and accepting. We are much more likely to respond automatically with one of a dozen typical responses, which generally communicate our desire to influence or *change* the other person in the way that we think appropriate. These responses usually come from our own need to get the other person to change their way of thinking, feeling or behaving to conform to what we believe is appropriate. Sometimes we give such responses simply because we are uncomfortable with their feelings. Because these typical automatic responses (1) inhibit the person from getting in touch with deeper feelings, (2) retard their natural problem solving ability, and (3) often engender resentment and anger directed back at the listener for trying to control them, these responses are appropriately called roadblocks to communication, of which twelve have been identified.[5] They are also roadblocks to creating the kind of patient/practitioner relationship that will both create a healing climate and optimize the patient's adherence to whatever treatment plan evolves. So it is vital to recognize and avoid them wherever possible.

Let's examine the *communication roadblocks* to our patient's disgruntled expression that was coded as a speech about dinosaurs, although it clearly has nothing to do with biology.

1. **Ordering, directing**
   "Take some initiative on your own and stop worrying about others around you."

2. **Warning**
   "If you don't develop a more positive attitude there, you're going to get fired, that's obvious."

3. **Moralizing**
   "Listen, you're lucky you've still got a job in these hard times."

4. **Advising**
   "Why don't you just go in and sit down with your supervisor and tell her exactly

Feelings Likely When Wants Are Being Satisfied:

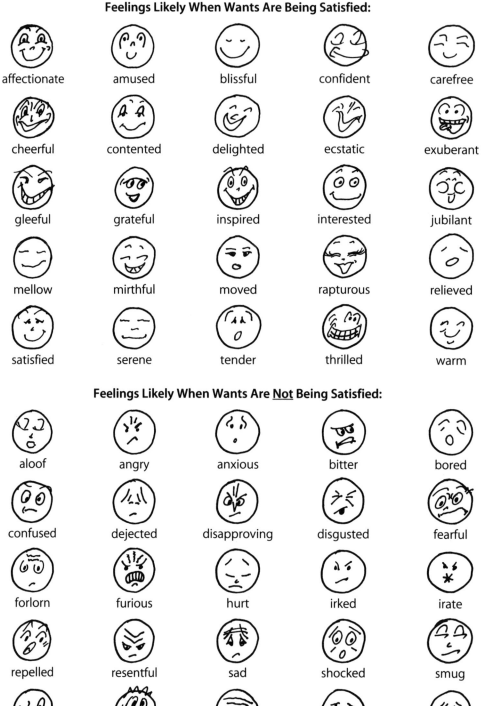

Feelings Likely When Wants Are <u>Not</u> Being Satisfied:

Fig. 8.2 How Do You Feel?

what you feel. After all, she's a human being too, and I'm sure she'll understand and help you to work it out rationally."

5. **Logic**
   "Well, if you're right, in time she will certainly come round to seeing it your way."

6. **Judging, criticizing**
   "Frankly, anyone who complains as much as you do has got to expect trouble."

7. **Praising, agreeing with**
   "I agree entirely. That's what I like about you, you are so perceptive. She certainly is a rotten supervisor, and you are to be congratulated for having the courage to call her on her insensitivity."

8. **Name calling**
   "Aha! Yet another 'whistle-blower' about to stir up the office and make life difficult for everybody, including yourself."

9. **Analyzing**
   "No doubt your supervisor reminds you of your mother, and so brings up these infantile responses of inadequacy in you that you are still working out."

10. **Reassuring**
    "Well, hard as it seems today, by tomorrow you'll have completely forgotten the whole episode. Time heals all wounds, you know."

11. **Questioning, probing**
    "Is this the first time you've had difficulties like this? What other things there are bothering you?"

12. **Distracting, tangenting**
    "Think about the challenge you're being offered there. That reminds me of the time when I . . ."

It is instructive to carefully read each of the twelve responses above and let ourselves experience how we might feel if someone had responded this way to a statement we made, similar to the patient in Fig. 8.1. More than likely we will feel defensive, want to close down or to lash out at the person who made them. (This is even true of statements 7 and 10, agreement and reassurance.) Yet all these are very common ways that we all respond to friends, colleagues, acquaintances and casual strangers. Not only that, the roadblocks include the responses most typical of physicians' communications to their patients, advice and reassurance.[6] Indeed, so long as the speaker does not have strong and unresolved emotions behind their words, these twelve responses are *not* necessarily roadblocks. It's when affect or *emotional charge* lies behind the speaker's words that these responses become roadblocks, communicating nonacceptance. Of course, there are times when reassurance about a diagnosis or prognosis is just what is appropriate. And certainly there are other times when patients definitely expect advice from their practitioner whom they have consulted as an expert in natural medicine. It is when a practitioner intentionally moves from a problem-solving, solution-oriented mode into "counseling mode" that she must be extremely cautious about sending a message of nonacceptance. For each of the roadblocks conveys the listener's intent to *change*, rather than to *accept*, the speaker. Such a climate of non-acceptance is not conducive to personal growth, development and emotional health because when people feel judged, analyzed or put down, they become defensive, closed and resistant to change. This is not a mood conducive to healing, and if the patient generates stress responses to his practitioner's nonacceptance of his feelings, physical problems can definitely be exacerbated.

There is a very profound paradox here and it lies at the basis of what is appropriately referred to as *counseling mode,* as opposed to the fix-it mode from which the health practitioner often (and rightly so) works. Committed to assisting our patient's healing process to restore wholeness, we *do* want to initiate changes that will help him to move towards psychological and physical health. Clearly, the various natural therapeutics and medicines were developed in order to help bring about physical and emotional changes in the direction of health. Yet as counselors, working in the emotional plane, if we employ these twelve roadblocks as bulldozers, we are very unlikely to create a helping relationship. Conversely, to the extent that we can learn to listen actively, to practice empathy and acceptance of where the patient is at the moment, we create the very climate for the desired changes. There is no special magic here. It is simply that in this climate of empathic listening and acceptance we are removing the hindrances impeding the patient's own inner healer, *vis naturae medicatrix,* from operating.

Person-Centered Psychotherapy

Beginning in the early 1940s the American psychologist Carl Rogers began to develop what first became known as *non-directive counseling* as a reaction to the then-dominant directive and interpretative psychoanalytic therapies. Challenging the conventional wisdom that "the doctor knows best," Rogers' approach to counseling emphasized the creation of a therapeutic climate of openness, genuineness, acceptance, unconditional regard and empathy. Employing little technical props beyond reflection, paraphrase and (especially) active listening, the therapist totally eschewed all of the commonly accepted practices of advice, suggestion, persuasion, teaching, diagnosis and interpretation. As we have seen above, in actively listening the counselor attempts to put herself in the patient's shoes, to see and imagine the world as the patient experiences it, from his perspective. In that sincere attempt of the therapist to empathize, a climate of safety, trust and acceptance is created between therapist and patient, which is a necessary condition for positive therapeutic change and personal growth.

The basic premise behind Rogers' non-directive approach to counseling is that troubled patients (clients[7]) possess within themselves everything they need to resolve problems, fulfill needs and grow more whole. The therapist's job is merely one of releasing the barriers to self-actualization. And because the therapist cannot judge for the client what is best for him or what needs to happen in therapy, the non-directive approach is best characterized as *person-centered therapy*. It is the client, not the therapist, who determines both the course and duration of the therapy.

In medical practice we have a patient who has presented with a physical illness, yet for one reason or another we have decided that, along with our other natural therapeutics, counseling is an appropriate intervention that we wish to offer. From the person-centered point of view something has gone wrong with the natural process of self-actualization, and if we can help the client get back on the track of being true to himself, this will be a valuable aid to health. Why do some individuals become "stuck" in their growth and live unfulfilled lives, full of anxiety, tension, lack of meaning, punctuated with overwhelming depressions and burdened with chronic stress to which they feel helpless victims? The question is vital to health psychology because this constellation of stress and helplessness is a severe health risk. Person-centered theory suggests that the core of the problem of the distressed individual begins in early childhood as the infant attempts to please its parents. In healthy development that tendency gradually gives way to a balance with one's own needs for authenticity and relative independence from others. But if that normal development is arrested for some reason, one may continue into adult life compulsively endeavoring to please others, trying to be the self that others want, not the true self. Though it may be years ago, the shadowy figures of our early authority figures lie deep within us, sometimes still pulling us to be what we are not.

The role of the person-centered therapist is radically different from the way we are accustomed to thinking of a counselor. In fact, the person-centered therapist's role is precisely to have no role! Techniques are less important in person-centered counseling than a *way of being* with clients that is facilitative in getting the client in touch with their own deep experience and organismic knowledge, that is to say, in touch with who they really are.

What is that facilitative way of being? Carl Rogers has distinguished three qualities that promote growth: (1) the therapist's ability to be genuine, authentic, *congruent*; (2) the therapist's caring, *unconditional regard,* prizing, respect and acceptance of her client; and (3) the degree that the therapist can succeed in "getting into the client's world," in *empathizing* with her client. Of the three attributes, Rogers regards genuineness as paramount. The person-centered therapist does not hide behind a professional role; her own behavior must be as congruent as possible with her own feelings. Above all this will mean an active interest on the part of the therapist to know the client, to be there to hear and to watch the client unfold and grow. But it can also occasionally mean the therapist showing her own insecurity or uneasiness, annoyance or frustration about the therapy, even if these feelings temporarily clash with unconditional regard. Of course, the therapist who finds herself persistently judging a client would be wise to refer that client to a colleague. Moreover, being real doesn't mean that the therapist burdens the client with her own personal problems. Nor does it mean that the therapist will blurt out impulsively any feeling that arises.

> This stress on realness, deeply contrary to earlier ideas of the therapeutic relationship, sometimes involves statements such as, 'I'm not listening to you very well this morning because there are some problems on my mind and I can't concentrate.' 'I'm afraid of you at this moment—afraid of what you might do to me.' 'I feel uncomfortable with what you just said.' In each instance I would be expressing a feeling within myself, not a fact, or supposed fact or judgment about my client. To say, 'I feel bored at the moment. I wish I didn't feel this way but I do,' does not pass judgment on my client as a boring individual. It merely adds the basic data of my own feelings to the relationship. As I share this boredom and sense of remoteness from him, my feelings change. I certainly am not feeling bored as I try to communicate myself in this way. I am, in fact, likely to be quite sensitively eager to hear my client's response. As contact with him returns, my empathic understanding begins again to be experienced. To be real is to reduce barriers in the relationship. My client is now likely to find himself speaking more congruently because I have dared to be real with him. It now becomes a genuine person-to-person relationship between two imperfect human beings.[8]

In a therapeutic climate of genuineness, sincere interest, acceptance and empathy the client's trust and safety are enhanced, and he is given a model for his own genuineness, self-honesty, acceptance of all parts and sides of himself. Because another person, the therapist, accepts and respects him, is genuine with him, so the client's own self-esteem is enhanced in successful therapy. In addition, as the client begins to allow himself to experience all aspects of himself, he begins to become more autonomous in judging himself, less dependent on what others think about him. He can embrace his own polarities as he hears that love and hate can coexist, weakness does not preclude strength. He begins to change his own concept of who he is, and as he does so he becomes more open to the world, more flexible in dealing with it, more present-centered, more in touch with feelings from moment to moment, better able to manage stress, to accept both failure and success, to trust his own being, to appreciate his own uniqueness. In short, the client's emotional/psychological health improves markedly, thereby optimizing the likelihood that physical health will also improve.

The real work of the person-centered therapist is in active listening, entering into the world of the client fearlessly and enthusiastically. Yet understanding the client's world is more than just capturing the content of the client's words. It includes picking up the feelings from the client's tone of voice and bodily gestures, feeding back responses which reflect what the client is feeling at the moment, as well as feelings lying just beyond the hazy edge of awareness. We could call this "leading" the client slightly, tentatively, cautiously—for active listening will always involve an element of guesswork—into deeper and deeper levels of the patient's own awareness, to insights and discoveries lying just beyond the last edge of awareness. The therapist's reflections will not always be accurate, yet where there is sincerity, where the client experiences the therapist as earnestly trying to come into his world and experience, the inaccuracies are seamlessly corrected by the client and turned to facilitate deeper experience. Active listening is a real skill that beginners often parody with simple re-phrasing. The difference between a dry rephrase and a true empathic response is the client's corresponding dry response: "Yes, that's what I just said," versus a warm "Yes! *That's* what I really meant. And moreover . . ."

The following example from a therapeutic group illustrates the dramatic differ-ence between clinical probing and an empathic listening response, and demonstrates the liberating effect of being fully and deeply understood when that empathic response is finally found. Doug, a 38-year-old professional man, has just told the group about losing his business, wife, family and credibility in his community, and then, after sev-eral years of painful struggle, slowly rebuilding his business and working his way back to solvency.

Therapeutic Group Dialogue[9]

Dialogue:

Comments and **Roadblocks**:

Group Member1: You mentioned the divorce and being separated from your children and the sadness that brings you. It seems like you have some hang-ups you aren't telling us about.

Note the implicit **judgment** in "hang-ups."

Doug: Well, that just happened to be a very painful experience in my life and I was just trying to relate that that's what happened. To me it was very sad and it will always be sad, but I feel like I was able to go through that experience and am a better man for it.

Member2: Do you feel that it was a lack of strength that caused this breakup?

Another **judgment** and Doug begins squirming and frowning.

Member3: I feel like you are carrying a burden from that event that's holding you back. Like you have not made your peace with this—a scar that you keep rubbing. It seems like you have a lot of hurt under the surface.

Now Member3 begins **analyzing.** The result is that Doug crosses his legs, folds his arms and looks detached and uninterested.

Doug: You are probably right in a way. I am a very volatile person. (*In a low voice*) I still feel very guilty about my children, coming from a puritanical background.

Member2: I wonder how much you let yourself feel your hurt . . . just let yourself feel it fully?

The group is fishing and **probing,** trying to get him to express his "obvious" pain or feelings. Doug is not, at this point, close to his felt meanings. Instead he's becoming more and more defensive and further from exposing his deepest feelings to the group.

Member1: Did your wife leave you? Did she walk away from you?

Member2: What feelings do you have about that?

> The group resumes **questioning** and **probing**. **Asking** for feelings is not the same as actively listening for them.

Doug: (*without affect*) Well, we had some hard times.

Member3: Why did she leave you?

> More **questioning.**

Doug: I lost all my money and she didn't feel like she could stay in the community and face the creditors, so she split . . . I chose to stay and pay back all the money we owed—to rebuild. She had her feelings about a certain lifestyle. Social acceptance was very important to her—more important than me.

> Yet in spite of their roadblocking, Doug lets it be known that he does want to be understood. So he tries to explain.

Member2: You still seem to have a lot of pain. It seems essential to your being. You haven't let it out.

> But Member2 comes back with an **opinion, analysis** and a **judgment**.

Member1: How long ago did this happen?

> And here's Member1 with more distracting, irrelevant **questioning.**

Doug: Four years ago.

Member1: Wow! A long time to carry it [the pain] around.

> This is Member1's **projection** of what it'd feel like for him. He is not, however, in Doug's world.

Member3: Have you had any other relationships?

> More tangential **questioning.**

Doug: Yes.

Member3: How are they going?

Doug: Fine (*very defensively*). I think the group is right about my anger and pain. But I feel good. I've dealt with my ex-wife and I've dealt with the anger. I don't feel I am so bad off as you are suggesting.

> The group's **probing, questioning** and **projecting** their feelings onto Doug have led to little empathy and no therapeutic movement.

Therapist: It must have taken tremendous courage and strength to fight your way back and build your life after being so devastated.

> At this point the therapist, who had remained silent throughout the above dialogue, steps in with empathic active listening and some sensitive, "leading" guesswork.

Doug: Well, you know it was damn painful (*his eyes growing moist*), the emotional and physical pain. My whole world collapsed . . . rejected by the community . . . after she left me. Just the sheer damn *effort* of a couple of years fighting back . . . (*sobbing now and relating the story again* . . .) It's just been the last year that I've been able to laugh and feel secure financially. (*With anger* . . .) And I supported my children all through that period and still do!

> Simply understanding Doug's feelings brought the release that the group could not shake out of him, no matter how well-meaning their intentions.

This dialogue is worth detailed study by the practitioner who is considering counseling patients. We all are accustomed to probing and questioning, imagining how we would feel in the situation our patient may describe to us, but going into counseling mode requires that we step back and try to see the patient's world as he sees it. The excerpt shows how not to do it; and then finally how, with dramatic effect, it can be so simply, but skillfully, done. The vignette also shows the fundamental difference between projecting your opinion on a patient ("You haven't let it out," says Member2) and a sensitive, "leading" guess ("It must have taken tremendous courage," says the Therapist) that assists the patient to contact a deeper layer of feelings.

Gestalt Therapy

Gestalt therapy was the creation of Berlin-born Fritz Perls (1893-1970), a medical doctor originally trained in psychoanalysis. Like many of the innovators of the modern therapeutic schools, Perls became dissatisfied with the emphasis on the patient's past childhood and what he saw as psychoanalysis' limited goal of helping people adjust to a sick society. Perls began to focus on the present, the here and now, and gradually developed a unique perspective on the therapeutic process which involved creative "exercises" and "experiments" carried out with the client. These techniques were designed to help clients get in touch with unacknowledged and unintegrated sides of themselves. Through dialogues, clients contact opposing and alienated sides of their personality: e.g., the authoritarian, shouldistic "top-dog" versus the wimpy, poor-me, victim-consciousness "underdog"; they learn to embrace opposite polarities within themselves such as love and hate, weakness and strength, anger and sadness, grief and joy. In emphasizing that the patient must bring to awareness and embrace all aspects of his here and now experience, Perls introduced the notion that the healthy person was a complete "gestalt," that is to say, an integrated whole being. Conversely, dysfunction and pathology were merely the results of fragmentation and alienation of parts of self. Thus the role of therapy is to bring the parts back into awareness. Integration follows naturally once we are aware of our total being.

Gestalt therapists insist that their therapy is not merely these awareness techniques and exercises. Rather, gestalt therapy is about fostering a present-centered, process-oriented (as opposed to content-oriented) *way of being*. Nonetheless, gestalt therapy is definitely identified by its unique techniques, which psychotherapists and counselors from various therapeutic orientations have adopted freely. Below are described some of the most characteristic of the gestalt exercises in consciousness-raising.

- In the *empty chair dialogue* the patient carries on a dialogue between polarities of his personality, e.g., top-dog self speaking to the imagined underdog self sitting opposite in an empty chair. The patient moves back and forth from chair to chair, always assuming the appropriate personality for the particular chair in dialogue with himself. The therapist's job is to keep the patient in the present, and to keep reminding him to stay with his experience rather than talking *about* it.

- The client is asked to append every statement he makes with "and I take responsibility for it." For instance, "I feel wounded and hurt and I take responsibility for it." "I'm fed up and I take responsibility for it." The idea of taking responsibility for our own feelings, actions, thoughts and their consequences in the world is basic to gestalt therapy, for it counters the victim consciousness and sense of helplessness that underlies self-defeating behavior.

- Clients may be asked to *play out their projections,* as when they play their parents, their partners or their colleagues. In so doing they act from an internalized picture in themselves (called an *introject*) which they project out onto others.

- Or, they may be asked to *act out the very opposite of how they feel,* as a way of experiencing what it feels like to be on the other side. Often deep emotional release (*catharsis*) can be experienced by verbalizing the opposite of a present feeling, for indeed, however suppressed, the potential for that opposite is in us too.

- Sometimes the therapist may invite the client to *exaggerate or emphasize something they feel or think or say.* Suppose that the patient is dialoguing to her top-dog in the empty chair opposite and says, "I want you to leave me alone." The therapist may ask her to say it again, louder, with more feeling and with body expression. "Leave me alone," repeats the client. The therapist shouts, "Leave me alone!" And the client screams out, "Leave me the hell alone!" Again, the object is to become aware of what it feels like to really take a stand, to be fully present in the moment, and to take personal responsibility for a feeling.

- Gestalt therapists work persistently to bring the patient into a present-centered, here-and-now mode. Thus, the tendency for the patient to speak "about" things, to talk about "one does this, and one does that," to talk about how he felt yesterday or last week or someplace outside the office, is always countered by the therapist inviting the patient to speak from the point of view of "I feel," to replace a discussion of how they felt yesterday with their partner to how they feel right now, here with the therapist, in this room, in this very moment. If they need to talk about other people, the other people are "brought into the present" and placed in the empty chair and their projections allowed to speak for themselves.

- Dream work is particularly effective acted out in present-centered dialogue. The patient retells a dream not as a narrative of something that happened during a night past, but by acting out the characters or even the objects in her dream, letting them speak to each other right here and now in the present. The idea is that anything we have created reflects a fragment or piece of us, and bringing the pieces together in the therapy session is a way of becoming whole, of completing our own personal gestalt.

The perspective behind gestalt therapy is humanistic, for it sees the suffering or symptomatic individual as blocked in his growth. The function of therapy is simply to show him that he does not need anything (including the therapy!) he doesn't already have. The philosophy of gestalt therapy is very close to Eastern mysticism in its view that only the present is real, and that the sole necessary therapeutic tool is awareness of what is. The past is only real insofar as we bring it into the present, which all of the exercises are designed to do. So, too, the future is only a rehearsal in our imagination, and preoccupation with rehearsal prevents us from experiencing the freshness of the moment, the healing quality of what is in and around us right here and now. Talking *about* an oppressive, abusive, dismal childhood is considered one of the ways that patients stay stuck in victim-consciousness, and why gestalt therapy focuses on process and on the body, which does not lie. Postures carry a message, and the therapist may ask the patient's folded arms, crossed legs or furrowed brow to speak for themselves.

Most of the goals of person-centered therapy apply to gestalt work as well—increased self-acceptance, flexibility and awareness, plus a more autonomous personality less dependent on external support. Like person-centered therapists, the gestalt therapist is above all congruent and real. But gestalt empathy takes the form of the therapist's intuitions about what the patient's nonverbal cues are trying to say. Gestalt therapy has been criticized as being narcissistic, encouraging people to do their own thing at the expense of others, but that tendency is an exaggeration of an early phase of therapy which is a corrective to the more usual tendency of people to please others at their own expense, with devastating consequences for their self-esteem and their health as well. As we get more in touch with the complexity of all our parts, as we are able to embrace our contradictions, oppositions and polarities, to be more fully human in all the complexities, so too do we actually come to see ourselves as part of the planetary gestalt with our own unique cooperative, highly social role to play. Our social self is just another part of ourselves, and one that we cannot embrace fully until we experience and accept its polar opposite, our individuality.

Reality Therapy

In the early 1960s the American psychiatrist William Glasser began to develop a new model of psychotherapy.[10] Working first with delinquent adolescents, and later with alcoholics and drug addicts, Glasser's attention was drawn to the persistent fact that virtually without exception, his suffering, unhappy, dissatisfied, socially failing clients seemed to feel themselves the powerless victims of circumstances beyond their control. Certainly many of them did come from broken homes, many had suffered child abuse, and others were deeply enmeshed in dysfunctional family situations from which they could see no escape. Nevertheless, Glasser became convinced that the way back to emotional and physical health for his patients lay in their recognizing that however devastating their past, it was over and done with. Glasser adopted the existential position that every person is constantly choosing moment by moment to take the most effective control of their lives that they know how, although that on-going choosing process is obscured and compromised by patients' beliefs that they are the hapless victims of circumstances.

Working from this position Glasser began to see that people remained entrenched in self-defeating and self-hindering behavior patterns, stuck with feelings of anxiety, depression, guilt and resentment—all feelings that invariably they said were unwanted, but felt to be out of their control—because these were actually the best ways that patients knew of getting their basic needs met. By depressing, anxietying,[11] self-blaming and developing a variety of psychosomatic complaints, such a person manages to gain some attention, sympathy and connection to others. But at the same time such connections invariably reinforce a stance of powerlessness, stamp it in and prevent the individual from having healthy relationships, healthy commerce with the world. Thus the basic needs to feel free, to have a sense of mastery in the world, and to be valued for our strength are compromised because we believe ourselves to be controlled by the past and by external events.

Glasser realized that to break this vicious cycle of victim-consciousness, a therapy was required that taught patients how to get their basic needs met effectively in the world as it is. This focus on *the world as it is* and the patient with his unique abilities and limitations *as the person he is* comprises the essence of a therapy which could be called ultrarealistic, or as Glasser eventually called it, *reality therapy*. This approach is very utilitarian. It concerns itself essentially with assessing the patient's basic needs and wants, and helping them to see that they alone are responsible for operating in the world so as to get these needs met. Reality therapy emphasizes above all personal responsibility, by which is meant that each of us has the ability to choose what we do and to use our choices to operate upon the world so as to get our needs met in a way that doesn't prevent others from getting their needs met. Contrariwise, we do not have the ability to control anyone else's behavior. So we must give up our struggle to make others be what we want them to be. The best we can do with anyone else in a free world is to act in a way that might predispose them to take us into account in choosing behavior that gets their needs met.[12]

The process of this therapy can be described in a straightforward way, but acquiring the skill, delicacy and persistence to conduct reality therapy with patients usually requires a two-year professional training course. There are seven basic steps carried out in a course of therapy lasting weeks or months, and although the steps proceed roughly one after the other, any given session may have elements from any of the seven.

1. The therapy begins with the therapist making friends with the client. This is done by *listening,* actively and passively, and also by the therapist exploring the client's likes, what he enjoys, and what feels truly fulfilling to him. Insofar as the past is discussed, it is in this initial stage, and then only in order for the therapist to find out what actually worked positively in the person's life. All attempts by the client to talk about how bad life is and was are deftly parried by the reality therapist who consistently focuses on what *did* work in the patients life, what skills he *has* got, when he *was* happy. Feelings are discussed in reality therapy, but never processed nor encouraged as they are in gestalt or person-centered therapy. Rather, negative feelings are considered as signs that basic needs remain unfulfilled and that something needs to be done to get them fulfilled. Once needs are met, the feeling signals will disappear naturally. Focusing on the emotional signals themselves is like focusing on the red oil signal light on our car dash panel. What we need to focus on is not the light (the feelings), but on the oil (needs) deficit. In summary, this first stage of therapy is just the establishment of a warm, trusting, empathic relationship that we recognize as the *sine qua non* of all psychotherapy, whatever the particular theoretical bent.

2. Next the therapist gets down to the business of exploring the patient's wants, needs, desires and how he perceives the world. Needs are considered to be the general hierarchy of motives that we considered in Chapter 3, common to all human beings and existing at various levels. Wants and desires are the particular objects and relationships that each of us seeks in fulfilling these needs. Safety, security, love and identity are universal needs; each of us will find different and to some extent unique ways to meet these, hence everyone's list of wants, desires and values will be different.

3. Then therapist and patient look at just how the client is currently living his life, what he is actually doing to get these basic needs fulfilled. Here the therapist's job is to convince the patient that his dysfunctional behaviors, negative feelings and psychosomatic symptoms are all personal choices and not things happening *to* him out of his control. This *reframing* of the patient's ways of being is actually an instance of what is called more generally in psychotherapy an *interpretation*. Leading a client to an interpretation in such a way that he himself imbibes it, sees its basic truth and acknowledges its implications takes great persuasive skill, persistence and patience accompanied with empathy, unconditional regard and a sense of humor.

4. Now comes a crucial, distinctive stage of reality therapy: the therapist must get the client to evaluate the effectiveness of his ways of getting his needs met. If therapy is to proceed further, the client must personally acknowledge of his own volition that these ways are in fact not very effective. This personal judgment needs to be a crucial bit of insight towards which the therapist must skillfully lead the patient, and then wait patiently for him to choose to embrace it deeply and fully.

5. Once the client makes the clear judgment that what he is doing is not working for him, the stage is set for the therapist to suggest that the patient make a plan to im-

plement new behaviors that are likely to be more effective. There can be no coercion by the therapist to implement a plan that she might use in her life, because the therapist's values and desires will not be the same as the patient's. The therapist's role is that of a skilled resource person, able to see the reality of the patient in this world as it is, ready to give information and advice. Nevertheless, it is the client who must choose what he wishes to do.

6. Once a plan is formulated, the therapist will now insist upon an agreement that bit-by-bit will be carried out by the patient. A patient who has been frightened to go out with the opposite sex may make a specific commitment to initiate contact with a particular person at such and such a time on such and such a day. A patient drinking twelve cups of coffee a day with milk and three sugars commits to reducing this to five cups a day starting tomorrow morning. The agreements made are quite specific. There may be behavioral practice (rehearsal) in the therapist's office, and there will generally be homework assignments (e. g., "speak to five strangers about the weather or something else inconsequential before the next session," or "replace two daily cups of coffee with herbal teas," or "walk two miles on Monday, Wednesday and Friday of the coming week"). Once the agreements stage is operative, at each session the therapist checks to see how they are going, and, if necessary, suggests modifications and amendments to the cooperative treatment plan. Reality therapy is very explicit that excuses for failure to carry out agreements are neither accepted nor even discussed. The therapist must impeccably model personal-choice responsibility and the view that she believes that her patient can operate upon the world successfully. Accepting excuses, even the most innocuous, would merely collude with the patient's old belief that he is a victim of circumstances and delay his personal empowerment.

7. Not only will the therapist accept no excuses for why an agreement wasn't carried out, she also remains steadfast in her commitment to the client. She will never punish nor negatively judge the client for his failures. To do so would reinforce the client's "failure identity," which, according to reality therapy, is ultimately the cause of all psychological, emotional and psychosomatic problems. She will simply cheerfully insist upon a new realistic commitment for the next session, emphasizing her belief that this patient, like every person alive, can successfully operate upon the world to get their basic needs met.

Perhaps of all the therapeutic schools, reality therapy has been the most explicit about the connection between psychosomatics and counseling. Glasser regards the emotions that arise when our basic needs go unmet as creative ways that our nervous system has evolved over millennia to generate physiological and sensory effects in us to try to help us get our needs met. So when we become angry when frustrated, anxious when we are about to lose love or can't get it, guilty when we hurt others, or depressed when we lose people, material possessions and opportunities, these feelings (and the physiology that goes with them) increase the likelihood of new adaptive behaviors that will better meet our needs in the newly changed situation. Anger focuses and energizes strong commitment and persistence to a goal we believe in strongly, fear prevents us from venturing into danger, shame insures that the next time we will be more cooperative, depression dampens ongoing action and encourages us to pause and think about new ways of solving a problem we are stuck with. But just as we discussed in our chapters on stress, if these emotions are prolonged, or if they do not in fact eventually lead to effective behaviors that fulfill our basic needs, then physical illness can develop. This is simply because of the body's wired-in structure that connects emotion with tissues, organs and the immune system. Once we do get symptoms, if we then get sympathy, attention and human connection for complaining about them, illness behavior may be reinforced and maintained. In this way psychosomatic disease becomes a perverted way that our needs for attention, human involvement and connection with others will be partly met, albeit at the expense of our needs for freedom, personal power and happiness.

Eclectic Multimodal Therapy

The psychotherapeutic schools and techniques described in the previous three sections represent a small sampling from literally dozens of different systems. No practicing clinician can hope to be conversant, much less possess expertise, in every technique and every viewpoint. Nevertheless there is much to be said for the gadfly who can pick and choose from whatever source provides useful ideas and techniques. For not only does human disquietude come in many forms, so too different personalities respond selectively to different treatment styles. Some patients respond well to active listening and the gentle, passive, unconditional regard of the person-centered approach. Others are brought out by gestalt awareness exercises, whereas some clients definitely need the responsibility and boundary-setting of a more confrontational counseling such as reality therapy.

Actually, the majority of practicing counselors and psychotherapists identify themselves as "eclectic," meaning that most do indeed draw upon diverse sources of therapeutic techniques. Perhaps the most clearly defined and consistently integrated eclectic approach is that developed by South African-born psychotherapist Arnold A. Lazarus. One of the original pioneers of behavioral therapy,[13] Lazarus was troubled by the experimental data from long-term follow-up studies after successful therapy that indicated that the benefits of behavior therapy on its own were often short-lived. Only when the entire spectrum of the patient's behaviors, feelings, sensations, beliefs and thought processes were evaluated and explicitly involved in the treatment protocol were the benefits of therapy durable. Drawing on the traditional psychological view of an individual's personality being made up of behavior, affect, sensation, imagery, cognition, interpersonal relationships and biological functions, Lazarus broadened behavior therapy to include all seven of these basic modalities. The resulting *multimodal therapy* consists of a comprehensive assessment and eclectic-based treatment of any or all of these seven modalities that are dysfunctional, deficient or maladaptive. The first letters of each of the modalities form the acronym BASIC IB. Calling the biological modality "D" for "drugs," but remembering that it includes nutrition, hygiene and exercise as well as medicines, medications and physical interventions that affect personality, we get the more compelling acronym BASIC I.D.

The seven modalities that help define a unique person do not form a static portrait, but interact sequentially. Consider a patient who presents with headaches without underlying organic pathology. The initial interview is conducted in such a way as to elicit characteristic ways that the patient responds in the seven BASIC I.D. modalities. Say it transpires that when the patient has a headache (sensation) he becomes quiet and withdrawn (behavior), starts feeling anxious (affect), pictures the pain as an "internal hammer with hot spikes driven into the skull" (imagery) and starts imagining himself dying of a brain tumor at the age his father died (more imagery), while convincing himself (cognition) that the doctors have probably missed something seriously wrong. Here the modality sequence is SBAIC and the treatment protocol will address that sequence, since it is important to break the dysfunctional chain of events which constitutes a positive feedback loop that turns a small, acute pain into a major, chronic one.

Assessing the BASIC I.D. profile essentially constitutes a psychotherapeutic diagnosis, but a far more detailed, personal and useful one than the dehumanizing categories (e.g., neurotic, character disorder, hysteric, paranoid schizophrenic) of the well-known *Diagnostic and Statistical Manual of Mental Disorders* (DSM-IIIR), which have been created through analogy with physical disease categories. As discussed in Chapter 2, the biomedical model behind such diagnoses fails to recognize not only the multicausal nature of illness, but misses all the subtle but pervasive interactions between body and mind. Conversely, although the BASIC I.D. diagnosis will not yield a single, simple diagnostic name tag, when constructed skillfully and thoroughly it creates a complex and faithful picture of the major modalities making up the whole person.

The BASIC I.D. is assessed during the initial counseling interview from questions (Lazarus, 1981) such as the following:

B   1. What behaviors are getting in the way of your happiness? What would you like to start doing? What would you like to stop doing? What would you like to do more of (increase)? What would you like to do less of (decrease)? What do you regard as some of your main strengths or assets?

A   2. What makes you laugh? What makes you cry? What makes you sad, mad, glad, scared? How do you *behave* when you feel a certain way (e.g., sad, mad, glad or scared)? Are you troubled by anxiety, anger, depression, guilt or any other "negative emotion"?

S   3. What do you especially like to see, hear, taste, touch *and* smell? What do you dislike seeing, hearing, tasting, touching and smelling? Do you suffer from frequent or persistent unpleasant sensations (such as aches, pains, dizziness or tremors)? What are some sensual and sexual turn-ons and turn-offs for you? What bearing do your sensations have on your *feelings* and *behaviors*?

I 4. What do you picture yourself doing in the immediate future? How would you describe your "self-image"? What is your "body-image"? What do you like and dislike about the way you perceive yourself to be? How do these images influence your behaviors, moods and sensations?

C 5. What are some of your most cherished beliefs and values? What are your main "shoulds," "oughts" and "musts"? What are your major intellectual interests and pursuits? How do your thoughts affect your emotions?

I. 6. Who are the most important people in your life? What do others expect from you? What do you expect from others? What are the significant people in your life doing to you? What are you doing to them?

D. 7. What concerns do you have about the state of your health? What are your habits pertaining to diet, exercise and physical fitness? Do you take any medications or drugs?

Table 8.2 below summarizes the results of a typical assessment with some indicated treatments for a man with alcohol dependency.

Modality	Problem or Deficiency	Proposed Treatment
Behavior	Avoids confronting most people Negative self-statements Drinks excessively when alone at home at night Screams at children	Assertiveness training Positive self-talk assignments Develop social outlets Learn active listening skills to use with children
Affect	Suppresses anger (except to children) Anxiety reactions Depression	Assertiveness training Gestalt exercises to express anger Self-hypnosis
Sensation	Butterflies in stomach Tension headaches	Abdominal breathing exercises Relaxation training/biofeedback
Imagery	Being locked in bedroom as child	Guided meditation with visualizations
Cognition	Self-talk about low self-worth Numerous regrets	Positive affirmations homework Reality therapy for basic needs
Interpersonal relationships	Ambivalent responses to wife and children Secretive and suspicious	Possible family therapy, support group such as AA Bibliotherapy (books to read on the power of self-disclosure)
Drugs/biology	Reliance on alcohol to alleviate depression, anxiety and tension Junk-food diet No aerobic exercise	Meditation, relaxation training, self-management program Nutritional counseling Contingency contracting for exercise plan

Table 8.2 BASIC I.D. Modality Profile of a Man with Alcohol Dependency

Once the BASIC I.D. assessment data are gathered and the profile assembled, the therapist and patient are in a position to work out a cooperative, detailed treatment plan to address the deficiencies, dysfunctions and excesses in the profile. (See the right column in Table 8.2 above.) Both the assessment and the proposed treatment are carried out with the active cooperation of the patient; indeed, the patient himself can be instructed to construct his own BASIC I.D. profile at home and bring it in to compare with the one that the therapist has constructed from the initial interview.[14]

If the case and proposed treatments listed in Table 8.2 are examined closely it will be observed that the eclectic therapist employs techniques drawn from all the psychotherapies discussed above, as well as those from the stress-management programs of Chapter 7. The eclectic multimodal therapist must be flexible enough to be able to use diverse techniques without necessarily subscribing to their theoretical underpinning. In formulating a treatment plan the practitioner will recognize the unique strengths, skills, weaknesses and limitations of each patient, and so select treatments that are individually tailored to the particular client's personality and needs. The structure provided by multimodal therapy gives the practitioner of natural medicine a basic holistic framework of operation without in any way constraining her choice of treatments or her philosophy of healing.

The Existential Approach

Existential psychotherapy is not a specific technical approach that presents a new set of rules for therapy. Rather, existentially oriented counselors and therapists continue to bring the therapy back to the deep questions about the essence of the human condition and the nature of anxiety, despair, grief, loneliness, meaning and isolation. The approach deals centrally with the fundamental questions of creativity and love. Out of the understanding of the meaning of these human experiences, existential psychotherapists have created a perspective on the process of therapy that goes beyond particular techniques and transcends therapeutic schools.

> The spirit of existential psychotherapy has never supported the formation of specific institutes because it deals with the presuppositions underlying therapy of any kind. Its concern was with concepts about human beings and not with specific techniques. This leads to the dilemma that existential therapy has been quite influential, but there are very few adequate training courses in this kind of therapy simply because it is not a specific training in technique.[15]

Existentially oriented therapists identify four ultimate concerns that recur over and over again in deep psychotherapy: death, freedom, isolation and meaninglessness. The patient's confrontation with and resolution of each of these fundamental human concerns constitutes the existential framework. "Death . . . haunts the individual as nothing else. It rumbles continuously under the membrane of life. The child at an early age is pervasively concerned with death, and one of the childs' major developmental tasks is to deal with the terror of obliteration."[16] To cope with this terror, we erect denial defenses against death awareness. Yet eventually we must come to terms with the reality of death, for psychopathology is to a large extent the result of failed death transcendence. Symptoms and maladaptive character have their origin in the individual terror of death. Because the individual is responsible for and the author of his own life design, freedom itself can be terrifying. If all authorities and all social structures are only real to the extent to which we invest them with power, then we are ultimately going to have to work out for ourselves the meaning of our own lives. Following an authority is to cling to something that itself, like ourselves, has feet of clay. Nobody can tell us what life means; in this freedom we are alone, and only we can construct our own meaning for life. But this pervasive aloneness also means that any attempt to link ourselves to another for our own meaning is ultimately doomed to fail, and we must come to terms with our own existential aloneness from which no relationship, however close, can rescue us. Here too the patient's attempts to deny this essential aloneness through compulsive sexuality, through endeavoring to fuse with a partner, or even the opposite, trying to prove that he can exist totally independently of others, all of these are devices with which we try to deny our essential aloneness. Ultimately we are going to have to find a resolution to the dilemmas of death, isolation, freedom and the paradox of finding meaning in a universe that has no inherent meaning beyond the one that we ourselves create in it. These are the questions the existential psychotherapist retains permanently in her consciousness when working with patients, no matter what therapeutic techniques and no matter what treatment goals have been agreed. And only to the extent that the practitioner herself has resolved these existential questions can she assist another with these great universal human dilemmas and paradoxes.

Although existential counseling implies no set of formal techniques, this is not to say that it is devoid of guidelines for working with clients. Quite the contrary, as European existential counselor Emmy van Deurzen-Smith has emphasized, the existential counselor works from a very distinctive framework of values and assumptions. As van Deurzen-Smith has pointed out, existential counseling, in its concern to assist clients to clarify their own values, assumptions and intentions, is akin to a philosophical investigation of an individual life, and the sessions are not unlike Socratic dialogue.[17] The basic assumption of this philosophical approach to counseling is that it is always possible to make sense of a life, to discover how a person is in the moment the author of his own experience, however distasteful and apparently unwanted that experience seems to be. When the counselor can assist the patient to see exactly the implications of what they are choosing and creating, the possibilities for meaning, and a sense of purpose, re-emerge.

The existential counselor is unlikely to be interested either in behavior change techniques or in providing empathic reflections of feelings. Rather her emphasis will be on a dispassionate examination of the way that the patient is living his life, what hidden assumptions and unperceived intentions lie at the base of it, and to show how in all of this the individual is exerting considerable personal power and employing numerous positive strengths and resources of which they are perhaps only dimly aware. Van Deurzen-Smith likens the existential counseling session to a tutorial on the art of living, where the counselor is an expert on unraveling difficulties, pointing out contradictions and hidden assumptions, and in perceiving clients' positive resources that are implicit in how they are already living. In this kind of investigation, a patient's physical complaints and negative emotions reflect difficulties in solving current problems of living, and are never the direct focus of treatment interventions. Rather, these symptoms and distressful emotions are considered signs that the client needs to re-examine his way(s) of living with the aim of assessing to what extent he is really living authentically, in keeping with his own deepest and truest values. The counselor's job is to support authentic living and to remind the patient that the world will forever remain one of paradox, with unresolvable polarities and inherent limitations, where both success and failure are possible and likely.

Of course, behavioral change and a finer appreciation and acceptance of emotions in all their depth and variety are both highly likely outcomes of successful existential counseling, simply because in becoming more true to himself, a client learns how to act more consistently with his personal values, and to value his emotions as existential guidelines for living. But none of these changes is imposed upon the client by the counselor, for in truth the existential counselor cannot know what is the best solution for her client's problems in living. All she can do is to engage her patients' sense of authorship for their own lives, supporting them to find the direction of their own destiny, helping them to discover who they are, while faithfully holding fast to the belief that they alone can figure out how best to live their lives with meaning and significance.

Project 8

Conducting the Initial Counseling Interview Using the BASIC I.D. Format for Assessment and for Developing the Treatment Protocol

Invent or present a psychosomatic case of your own: conduct a hypothetical initial counseling interview applying the BASIC I.D. formula to your real or hypothetical patient, both in terms of assessing the presenting dysfunction(s), and then to drawing up an appropriate treatment protocol. It is recommended that this be done comprehensively and in sufficient detail to give the case a realistic and plausible flavor.

Appendix A

List of Feeling or Emotion Words[18]

Feelings likely when wants are being satisfied:

absorbed	eager	gratification	pleasure
adventurous	ecstatic	groovy	proud
affection	effervescent	happy	quiet
affectionate	elated	helpful	radiant
alert	electrified	hopeful	rapturous
alive	encouraged	inquisitive	refreshed
amazed	energetic	inspired	relief
amused	engrossed	inspirited	relieved
animated	enjoyment	intense	satisfied
appreciation	enlivened	interested	satisfaction
aroused	enthusiastic	intrigued	secure
astonished	exalted	invigorated	serene
blissful	excited	involved	sensitive
breathless	exhilarated	joyful	spellbound
buoyant	expansive	joyous	sanguine
calm	expectant	jubilant	splendid
carefree	exuberant	keyed-up	stimulated
cheerful	fascinated	love	surprised
comfortable	free	loving	tender
complacent	friendly	mellow	tenderness
composed	fulfilled	merry	thankful
concerned	gay	mirthful	thrilled
confident	glad	moved	touched
contented	gleeful	optimism	tranquil
cool	glorious	overwhelmed	trust
curious	glowing	overjoyed	warm
dazzled	good humored	peaceful	warmth
delighted	grateful	pleasant	

Feelings likely when wants are <u>not</u> being satisfied:

afraid	disgusted	hurt	resentful
aggravated	disheartened	impatient	restless
agitation	disinterested	indifferent	sad
alarm	dislike	inert	scared
aloof	dismayed	infuriated	sensitive
angry	dispirited	inquisitive	shaky
anguish	displeased	insecure	shocked
animosity	disquieted	insensitive	skeptical
annoyance	distressed	intense	sleepy
anxious	disturbed	irate	sorrowful
aggressive	downcast	irked	sorry
apathetic	downheart'd	irritated	sour
apprehensive	dread	jealous	spiritless
aroused	dull	jittery	spiteful
aversion	edgy	keyed-up	startled
bad	embarrassed	lassitude	surprised
beat	embittered	lazy	suspicion
bitter	exasperated	let down	tepid
blah	exhausted	lethargy	terrified
blue	fatigued	listless	thwarted
bleak	fear	lonely	tired
bored	fearful	mad	troubled
breathless	fidgety	mean	tedium
brokenhearted	forlorn	melancholy	uncomfortable
chagrined	frightened	miserable	unconcerned
cold	frustrated	mopy	uneasy
concerned	furious	nervous	unglued
confused	gloomy	nettled	unhappy
cool	grief	overwhelmed	unnerved
cross	guilty	passive	unsteady
credulous	hate	perplexed	upset
dejected	heavy	pessimism	uptight
depressed	helpless	pessimistic	vexed
despair	hesitant	provoked	weary
despondent	horrified	puzzled	withdrawn
detached	horrible	rancorous	woeful
disappointed	hostile	reluctant	worried
discouraged	hot	reluctance	wretched
disgruntled	humdrum	repelled	

▰▰▰ Annotated Bibliography

Corey, Gerald. *Theory and Practice of Counseling and Psychotherapy.* Pacific Grove, CA: Brooks-Cole, 1991. A basic introduction to counseling and psychotherapy from the viewpoints of nine different schools of therapy. The chapter on ethics should be studied by anyone who is doing counseling on a regular basis. It is invaluable for alerting the practitioner to the current legal status of patients' rights and practitioners' obligations on issues of confidentiality and disclosure in mental health counseling.

Corsini, Raymond, and **Danny Wedding.** *Current Psychotherapies.* Itasca, IL: Peacock, 1989. This survey text treats in considerable detail the most popular current psychotherapies. Each chapter is written either by a distinguished disciple or the founder of the therapy school.

Gordon, Thomas. *P.E.T.: Parent Effectiveness Training.* Solana Beach, CA: Effectiveness Training Inc., 1976. This is the classic book on active listening, developed by Dr. Thomas Gordon, formerly a student of Carl Rogers. In addition to active listening, the book is excellent as an introduction to communication skills in general, including asserting your feelings through "I messages," with a useful section on conflict resolution. Although the examples are from child rearing, the principles are applicable to human relationships in general.

Hoffmann, David. *Successful Stress Control the Natural Way.* Wellingborough, Northamptonshire: Thorsons, 1986. Written by a contemporary medical herbalist, this book contains a brief section on counseling, as well as a useful introduction on using flower essences to work with emotional issues.

Rogers, Carl. *On Becoming a Person.* Boston: Houghton-Mifflin, 1961. The primer for understanding the roots of the humanistic view of psychology. In this perennial favorite, the founder of person-centered psychotherapy outlines the essence of its philosophy of living.

Wedding, Danny. *Case Studies in Psychotherapy.* Itasca, IL: Peacock, 1989. Case studies are essential to understand the subtleties of how counseling and psychotherapy are actually carried out in practice. Many of the cases in this book are classics, well worth detailed study. As there are no modern published case study collections where the presenting complaints are primarily physical illnesses, we have appended several in Chapter 14.

9

Psychosomatics:
Personality and Disease

*Sometimes it is more important to know what
kind of person has a disease than to know what
kind of disease a person has.*

—SIR WILLIAM OSLER

*T*HE FUNDAMENTAL IDEA OF psychosomatics—that bodily disease is influenced by emotions and temperament—is an ancient one indeed. As
we saw in Chapter 2, the four temperaments (called humors) of Greek medicine represent the oldest recorded attempt in Western medicine to associate personality characteristics with health and disease and were an important advance on all previous
supernatural views. In the first century, Galen developed Hippocrates' four-humor
theory and added grief, anger, lust and fear as a class of causes of disease which needed
to be diagnosed and treated. Galen's views had a lasting influence on Western medicine. Throughout the seventeenth, eighteenth and nineteenth centuries numerous
quotations can be found in European medical textbooks alluding to emotional causes
of disease.[1] J. Archer, a seventeenth-century English physician, wrote in 1673 of
"[g]reat discontent which results in sadness of mind" as the original cause of most
sickness. A century later the Dutch professor of medicine Gaubius described the
harmful effects on the body of terror, unrequited love and excessive joy, but also (significantly) of the deleterious effects of *suppressed* grief, which, when it "remains seated
firmly within, the body no less than the mind is eaten up and destroyed." In 1818 the
term *psychosomatic* was first used by the German psychiatrist Hienroth in describing
the origin of insomnia. In 1872 the English psychiatrist Daniel Hack Tuke compiled
the first manual of psychological medicine, an encyclopedic volume of clinical anec-
dotes attesting to the influence of the mind on the body in health and disease.

Psychogenesis

Compelling as they were, the anecdotal observations of doctors (as well as
Victorian novelists who wrote of illness and death from bereavement, unrequited

love, unfaithfulness and financial ruin) failed to provide a systematic theoretical framework from which effective, practical treatment could be derived. Ignorance of the psychophysiology of emotions made it difficult to integrate these observations with the new scientific medicine that was gathering momentum in the nineteenth century. Virchow's doctrine of cellular pathology, Pasteur's and Koch's germ theory of disease, and major developments in medicine's basic sciences—microbiology and biochemistry—led to a perception of disease as a reflection of malfunctioning bio-mechanisms, with attention focused on the faulty organ system.

Nevertheless, in the background of mainstream medicine very significant events were taking place that in time gave rise to a new approach to mind-body therapeutics. Part of that picture we have already discussed in Chapter 4, involving the work of Pavlov, Walter Canon, H. G. Wolff and Hans Selye in elucidating the autonomic and neuroendocrine mechanisms linking significant emotional events to body events. The other tributary begins, as do so many things in modern psychology, with Sigmund Freud. In 1893 Freud and Breuer published an account of a patient who "converted" an unconscious sexual conflict into symbolic body symptoms of hysterical paralysis. Freud himself did not elect to continue this promising direction, being more drawn to the study of psychoneurotic symptomatology. But his early observations proved seminal, for they were picked up and extended by other physicians and psychoanalysts. In 1917 Dr. Georg Groddeck in Baden-Baden reported cases of organic disease which were precipitated by psychological events, and which he treated successfully by psychoanalytic psychotherapy. Groddeck extrapolated Freud's "conversion" hypothesis to organic dysfunction, suggesting that disease symptoms had a symbolic, unconscious "meaning," the nature of which only the patient working deeply with the analyst/practitioner could ferret out. Groddeck maintained that when the patient achieved insight into this meaning the symptoms would disappear, as they were no longer necessary.

Beginning in the 1940s and continuing for nearly two decades at the Chicago Psychoanalytic Institute, Franz Alexander and his colleagues undertook a monumental study into the characterological bases of seven common illnesses whose organic causes were unknown: asthma, hypertension, rheumatic arthritis, duodenal ulcer, neurodermatitis, thyrotoxicosis and ulcerative colitis.[2] It was this work by Alexander's group in Chicago plus a growing body of laboratory studies of the psychophysiology of the emotions that came together under the rubric of *psychosomatic medicine.* Alexander initiated a concerted effort to test the hypothesis that the causal basis for these seven diseases, at least, was a specific, intra-psychic conflict derived from early childhood.

We have previously affirmed the importance of psychological factors such as stress and lifestyle to health and disease. Fig. 2.3 in Chapter 2 summarizes the multi-causal view of health and disease. According to that biopsychosocial conception, all disease must be seen as a complex product of influences ranging from inherited constitutional defects through environmental agents such as pollution, acid rain and radiation from the depleted ozone layer, to prolonged stressful life events and daily hassles. But Fig. 2.3 also depicts a personality layer which is significant for the etiology of disease. Whether an individual translates a potential stressor into actual stress or into a positive challenge depends on the person. Is there then a "disease-prone personality," and are particular diseases associated with certain pathogenic personality traits? Related to those questions is the search for "meaning" in symptoms. Do physical symptoms speak a kind of "body language" whose meaning, if we could decode it, would point unerringly to particular imbalances or conflicts about which the patient is unconscious?

We'll postpone an in-depth discussion of meaning in illness until Chapter 12, and focus here on the effects of personality in disease. For convenience of exposition, and to some extent following historical development, we have arbitrarily placed personality influences on disease under the heading of psychosomatics. In fact, psychosomatic medicine is nothing more nor less than holistic medicine itself,[3] and this entire text is actually a treatise in psychosomatics. Ignored for much of this century by medicine, psychogenic influences in disease remained the purview of an apparently specialized discipline called psychosomatic medicine. Now, in the last decade of the twentieth century, psychosomatics is being recognized by mainstream medicine for what it is: "the study of the interaction of the biological and psychosocial factors in maintaining health and causing disease."[4]

Before we discuss personality and illness in depth, we must dispense with certain common but quite misleading connotations of the term "psychosomatic." First of all, the word seems to imply a dualistic perspective in which psychic events cause bodily events.[5] As the influential, Polish-born psychiatrist and medical philosopher Z. G. Lipowski of Toronto's Clark Institute has so incisively noted, "It is meaningless to say that emotions cause disease; they cause nothing. It is equally incorrect to propose that any other psychological variable causes disease; it can only influence susceptibility to disease through the mediation of neuroendocrine processes controlled by the brain."[6] As the psychophysiological pathways linking emotionally significant life events to bodily organs gradually become clearer, so too does our understanding of the mediation between psychological factors and disease.

A second misconception about psychosomatics asserts that *certain* diseases (e.g., Alexander's "holy seven") are *ipso facto* psychosomatic, and these are to be distinguished from other (organic or "real") diseases. In fact, *all* disease is multifactorial in causation, and whether any particular illness is organic or psychosocial is rarely black or white (see Fig 9.1).

Doubtless there are diseases (e.g., congenital heart disease, birth defects, radiation sickness) in which psychosocial factors play a negligible role, but the diseases that the practitioner of natural medicine is likely to see are invariably multifactorial in causation. Yet to affirm that psychosocial factors and personality are important contributors to disease predisposition is not to deny the value of surgery, biomedicine, botanic medicine, physical medicine or any other modality which has shown its prac-

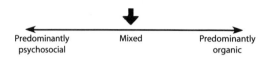

Fig. 9.1 Spectrum of Etiology

tical value. We really are in an era of true complementary medicine. As John Todd (1955) noted four decades ago, the discovery that a peptic ulcer has significant psychogenic aspects does not mean that treatment should be limited to psychotherapy. Once significant disease has developed in the body, medicines, diet and lifestyle changes are all indicated to return the patient to relative health, out of which personality changes aimed at correcting an imbalance in living are far more easily made.

Just as there are no distinctive psychosomatic diseases, it follows that the mere name of any given disease—whether it be asthma, hypertension, colitis, migraine or any other—cannot serve to locate it on the spectrum of Fig. 9.1. One patient's asthma may be largely stress-induced, while another's may be primarily allergenic. Yet another's may be the result of a childhood infectious respiratory disease which left the lungs weakened, and still a fourth the result of a rejecting mother. In every individual case there will be no substitute for the practitioner and the patient working together as an investigative team, digging into the possible contributions to the illness.

Psychosomatic disease is often mistakenly regarded as "imagined" disease. This is again part of our dualistic thinking whereby a *structural* defect in an organ is considered a biomechanical problem and outside our control, whereas a *functional* symptom (irritable bowel, chronic fatigue, headaches and certain skin diseases whose organic aspects remain obscure) is considered "all in the mind," hence "willpower" or a "good talking to" are the recommended remedies. In fact, a stress-induced or personality-related disease is a real disease. Whether or not an organic malfunction can be detected is largely a function of the resolving power of our current laboratory tests and the sophistication of our present conceptions of disease process. This is not to say that there are not secondary gains that may maintain an illness. Unlike psychopathic behavior, chronic anxiety and depression, or drug abuse, illness is a socially acceptable way of responding to problems in living. In our culture it evokes caring, attention and sympathy, as contrasted with accusation or the disdainful pity that addictions or psychoneurotic behavior evoke. The holistic practitioner is obliged to take into account all of these subtle aspects of illness, and to deal with every level—in effect to work multidimensionally. This requires the clinician to spend considerable time with each patient, delving deeply into the patient's current and past history, coming to see the patient not as a disturbed bowel or a chronic headache problem or constricted bronchi, but as a person embedded in a socio-cultural environment.

In *every* disease, then, there are three **P**s to be taken into account: the **P**redisposition factors, the **P**recipitating factors and the **P**erpetuating factors. The biopsychosocial model depicted in Fig. 2.3 from Chapter 2 is a way of gathering those multitudinous factors together in one picture. Fig. 9.2, on the other hand, is a way of illustrating the plausible pathway through which those factors operate. Any specific

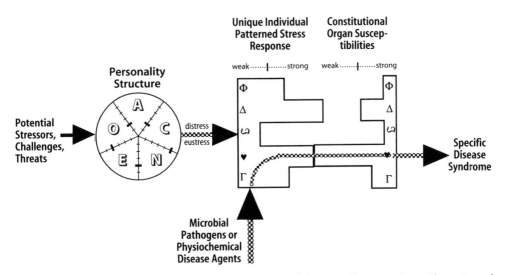

Fig. 9.2 Hypothetical mechanisms in the etiology of disease. The actual manifestation of disease is always multicausal and depends on the conjunction of precipitating psycho-social and pathogenic factors, along with constitutional susceptibilities in particular organ systems. Five sample somatic systems—respiratory (Γ), cardiovascular (♥), skeletal-muscular (Ϧ), digestive (Δ) and endocrine (Φ)—are represented above by symbolic characters. Aspects of personality (the five factors A, C, N, O and E explained in note 7) influence the conversion of potential stressors into actual stressors.

manifestation of a disease syndrome (e.g., asthma) is likely to involve a host of inter-linked processes and predispositions. Thus, looking at the left side of Fig. 9.2, challenges and threats are processed by the individual's particular personality structure.[7] The output of the potential stressors may be distress or eustress (Selye's term for positive, exhilarating effects of challenges) or some combination. The individual's uniquely patterned autonomic (physiological) stress response is represented in the hatched polygon as arousal in five sample organ systems. Coincidentally, external pathogenic influences in the form of germs, trauma, environmental hazards and so forth enter the system at the bottom right. The dotted polygon at the right represents this individual's constitutional organ susceptibilities. Disease takes place *only* when there is a physiochemical disease agent impacting on a chronically-aroused (stressed) system interacting with a constitutionally susceptible organ system (the point where the two polygons coincide). In the absence of any one of these conditions, disease will not develop.[8]

The Psychosomatic Specificity Hypothesis

Although now of interest primarily for its historical value, there is merit in beginning the examination of the relation of personality to disease with Alexander's psychoanalytic approach, which held sway in the early years of psychosomatic medicine. Such an examination shows up some of the pitfalls of trying to link personality, and especially early childhood influences, with somatic disease. Yet it also reveals a remarkably creative effort to achieve a comprehensive theoretical framework in which to set personality and illness. The central idea of the psychoanalysts was that for each of the seven diseases studied, a specific core intra-psychic conflict could be found. Alexander was not so naive as to suppose that the existence of the specific unresolved childhood conflict was in itself sufficient to bring about disease. Rather, he saw that

Disorder	Pathogenic childhood history	Blocks expression of:
Asthma	Rejecting mother. Child wants to cry out for mother's protection, but dares not for fear mother will reject.	Hurt feelings
Hypertension	Aggressive assertiveness must be inhibited for fear of loss of parents' love.	Hostile feelings
Rheumatoid arthritis	Tyrannical parents restricted muscular expression—a kind of "strait-jacket" situation.	Flexibility when later assertive domination fails
Peptic duodenal ulcer	Infant not allowed to be fully dependent, so grows up ashamed of dependency feelings and becomes excessively independent.	Feelings of weakness, dependency, asking for love
Certain skin disorders	Undemonstrative mother gave little physical intimacy, stroking or cuddling. Skin eruptions are a demand for this contact, while simultaneously regenerating mother's "keep away" message.	Physical contact
Hyperthyroid (thyrotoxicosis)	Exaggerated fear of death due to early exposure to death in family or severe threat to child's survival, leads to rapid maturation to grow up quickly and escape from the weakness of childhood. The adult may live dangerously to defy death.	Calmness, tranquility, attitude of "just being, doing nothing"
Ulcerative colitis	High parental expectations for the child to achieve that may exceed its capabilities or natural tendencies. Later, failure as adult to accomplish tasks leads to "giving up hope."	Accepting success and failure as normal parts of life

Table 9.1 Childhood patterns and their long-term emotional effects in seven diseases studied extensively by Alexander (1968) and his colleagues at the Chicago Institute of Psychoanalysis. (The original psychoanalytic terminology has been translated into everyday language.)

disease would only result if there also existed both a constitutional weakness in the organ system pertaining to that illness *and* some precipitating circumstance in adult life (we would call it stress) which reactivated the childhood conflict.

Table 9.1 lays out in non-psychoanalytic language the supposed nature of the pathogenic childhood history (as derived from patient interviews), and the kind of natural expression of feelings that such a history is believed to block. It is these blocked feelings that are increasingly seen as a cause of poor health.

The information in Table 9.1 is based on in-depth interviews that attempted to tap patients' ways of being in the world, and their habitual ways of solving interpersonal problems. Note carefully that the information is *not* based on any actual detailed investigation into the patient's childhood family situation. In some instances the patient might indeed have described such a childhood family situation as Table 9.1 reports, but generally the childhood history would have been inferred from the patient's current behavior. For that reason we have to be very cautious in interpreting the symbolic connections between the actual disease and the reconstructed pathogenic history. Thus, linking asthma to a childhood where crying was discouraged, certain skin disorders (neurodermatitis) to lack of contact in infancy, rheumatic arthritis with a strait-jacket childhood, and peptic ulcer to problems in childhood feeding has to be regarded as an intriguing, but unproven hypothesis.

In the face of this very plausible, almost seductive, formulation, we have to ask what went wrong, such that by the mid-1950s psychosomatic medicine was in danger of being relegated to medicine's graveyard along with other fads, like blood letting and mesmerism, that had once been fashionable only to fall by the wayside. Perhaps a principal problem was the one admitted by Alexander himself, namely that "it is easy to select psychological configurations from the immense variety of psychological events and discover in every patient just the pattern one wants to discover."[9] Although the Chicago group attempted to minimize this bias by independent assessment of interview material, the reliable identification of these patterns still required a trained analyst. In many ways this limited the generality of the work, since the general practitioner could not make use of it in daily work. And what was to be made of the fact that these "pathogenic" childhood histories were common in perfectly healthy people? Even in the psychoanalytic cases, too often a patient with a given disease would exhibit the personality patterns designated to a different disease, or worse, show none of the identified pathogenic patterns. Finally, since the psychoanalytic theory was derived exclusively from retrospective data (patients were already ill when they were studied) there was never any way to determine whether the personality patterns found were *causes* of the illness or *results* of it.

For temperament to be a useful piece of information, the general practitioner must be able to identify specific pathogenic personalities as easily and as reliably as he can identify low blood sugar, allergy to dairy products, a heart murmur or a vitamin deficiency. Even if that were possible, establishing etiology does not by itself provide unequivocal directions for treatment. Few patients will be drawn to a long, arduous and costly psychoanalysis with an uncertain result at the end. Probably the lesson to be learned is that in the end no amount of case history material, however suggestive, however it is worked up or theoretically massaged, can serve to establish a secure basis for specific personality factors in health and disease. Our twentieth century scientific minds demand the consistency and reliability that only repeated observations under replicable conditions of controlled investigation can bring. This is not to say that experimental rigor *per se* can substitute for inspired creative thinking: in the end the psychoanalytic approach withered on the vine for lack of predictive validity and practical utility, yet there lingers with us still a sense that in endeavoring to correlate early childhood experience with later adult illness the psychoanalysts were tapping an extremely important domain to which one day, with more sophisticated conceptual tools, medicine must yet return.

Type A Behavior and Coronary Heart Disease (CHD)[10]

In the late 1950s two cardiologists in San Francisco, Ray Rosenman and Meyer Friedman, introduced the term "type A behavior pattern" to refer to a constellation of behaviors—hard driving, competitive, hostile, aggressive and impatient—that seemed to characterize their patients with coronary heart disease (CHD).

> The type A individual has an intense and competitive drive for achievement and advancement; an exaggerated sense of the urgency of passing time, of the need to hurry; and considerable aggressiveness and hostility towards others. Type A persons are over-committed to their work, often attempt to carry on two activities at once, and believe that to get something done, they must do it themselves. They cannot abide waiting in queues and they play every game to win. Even when their opponents are children they are impatient and hostile. Fast-thinking, fast-talking, and abrupt in gesture, they often jiggle their knees, tap their fingers, and blink rapidly. Too busy to notice their surroundings or to be interested in things of beauty, they tabulate success in life in number of articles written, projects under way, and material goods acquired. The type B individual [those who are not type A] on the other hand, is less driven and relatively free of such pressures.[11]

Rosenman and Friedman devised a 15-minute structured interview consisting of a few dozen questions to try objectively to tap the existence of this pattern. Both the content of these questions and the way that the trained interviewer asks them are designed to elicit hostility, annoyance and irritation. For example, question 13 is delivered in a halting, hesitating manner, as though the interviewer has lost his place:

> Q13: Interviewer: Most people who work have to get up fairly early in the morning. In your particular case uh . . . what time . . . uh do you uh . . . ordinarily uh-uh-uh. . . get up?

The type A person typically cannot wait for the interviewer to finish the question and impatiently finishes it for him, sometimes adding the remark "Hell, let's get on with this damned interview!" The interviews are taped and assessed by independent judges who determine whether or not the patient is type A. The judgment is made primarily on the *way* questions are answered, whether with explosive, impatient, hostile voice tones, or mildly without sign of hostility (type B).

In a now-classic investigation, the structured interview was administered to over 3000 healthy men aged 39-59, and the subjects were followed for a period of eight-and-a-half years. Men who had been identified as type A were found to be more than twice as likely to develop coronary heart disease as type B men. In addition, the type A's who did develop CHD were five times more likely to have a *second* myocardial infarction than were the relatively few type B's who did develop CHD. This undeniably impressive result obtained under double-blind conditions initiated a torrent of research in the following two decades. Type A behavior was shown to be as great a risk factor in CHD as a family history of CHD, cigarette smoking, high blood levels of low density lipids and cholesterol, and sedentary lifestyle. Throughout the 1960s and 1970s further studies (including an important European one) collaborated the original report and found in addition that type A also predicted an increased likelihood of atherosclerosis and hypertension, known precursors of CHD. Hinting at the possible physiological mechanisms, type A individuals were also discovered to have relatively high levels of catecholamines, corticosteriods and testosterone, neurotransmitters and hormones that mobilize fats to the blood, thereby increasing the likelihood of plaque formation (arteriosclerosis).

The relation between type A and physical disease was perhaps the first incontrovertible evidence that psychological factors—specifically a measurable constellation of personality traits[12]—actually do constitute a serious health risk. Indeed it was in large part the discovery of the relation between type A and CHD that opened the doors for the rapid development of the disciplines of health psychology and behavioral medicine, placing modern psychology for the first time squarely in the medical mainstream.

Is type A an immutable personality characteristic, or can it somehow be modified, and if so will those individuals who do succeed in reducing their impatience, hostility and competetiveness and learn to go slow be less at risk for CHD? If low self-esteem underlies type A, as has been suggested,[13] a full treatment package must challenge typical beliefs such as:

• I must constantly prove myself worthy through successful, socially-recognized accomplishments.
• I do not believe that universal moral principles exist to ensure fairness, justice and goodness.
• I believe resources needed to be successful are scarce and insufficient.

Table 9.2 shows some of the elements of a typical treatment program using numerous behavioral medicine techniques (see Chapters 6 and 7) which was administered to 600 CHD patients in San Francisco over a three-year period. Compared with no treatment and medical counseling control groups, patients that participated in the

Behavioral Changes

Develop interpersonal skills
Develop active listening skills; practice being assertive without being aggressive; avoid letting anger build up to point of explosion.

Reduce freneticism
Avoid doing more than one thing at a time, such as eating dinner and watching t.v. or reading; avoid pretending to listen to others while preoccupied with business or personal matters.

Practice type B skills
Watch how type B's smile, speak, listen and react to frustrating situations and try to reproduce their type B behavior yourself.

Belief Modification

Re-examine achievement beliefs
Question view that I have to prove myself by my tangible achievements; that more is better; that type A behavior is required for my professional success.

Self-reinforcement
Reduce self-criticism when my behavior falls short of perfection; give myself encouragement for any actions that represent progress in reducing type A behavior.

Recycling of Emotions

Transforming hostility
Replace hostility with affection. Substitute compassion, understanding and forgiveness for anger and irritation. Try giving benefit of doubt. Consider what is a loving response to a difficult situation (e.g., when you have been offended).

Self-monitoring
Develop a type B self-monitor which alerts you when you are exhibiting type A behavior.

Restructuring of Environment

Personal and on the job
Modify work environment by delegating more authority, and abstaining from volunteering for everything because you think you do it best. Minimize time spent with people who arouse your hostility or whom you are with solely to impress.

Table 9.2 Elements from a Type A Treatment Program[14]

type A reduction program had significantly fewer cardiac recurrences over the three year period of the study. Moreover, those patients who self-reported the largest change in their type A behavior as assessed by questionnaire had only a quarter the recurrence rate of patients who reported little change in type A behavior. An interesting sidelight of this study was that a few of the participants in the medical information counseling control group (this group received information about CHD risk factors, including type A behavior) reduced type A on their own, and correspondingly the risk of recurrence. Thus, formal treatment programs can and do work and may be necessary for most, but not all, coronary patients.

Can the type A individual be identified by simpler, standardized paper and pencil self-report questionnaires that any general practitioner could utilize? The structured interview requires an interviewer who by temperament and special training must be adept at eliciting hostility from people. The structured interview is also inherently unreliable, since once a person finds out his type, he constrains his responses in further interviews. The concept of type A is now so well-known that it has accrued a social stigma. Unfortunately, the specialized paper and pencil self-report tests that have been designed to measure competitiveness, impatience and aggressive hostility have failed to yield consistent results in relation to disease outcomes. This problem has led behavioral scientists to attempt to break down the global concept of type A into well-known component traits that can be measured by standard personality tests. This strategy has indicated that of the various aspects of type A, only *hostility* and *freneticism* bear a measurable relation to increased CHD.

While the concept of type A has proven to be an undeniably powerful spur to the acceptance of psychological medicine, its relation to CHD is actually not so simple as originally believed. First, although type A's are at higher risk for CHD within the next eight-and-a-half years after being interviewed, if they *do* experience a coronary they die less often from it than do the type B's who experience coronaries. Second, the bulk of the positive research is almost exclusively with white middle-class American (very occasionally European) males under 50. Type A behavior may not be a coronary risk in minorities, women or older men. (After age 50, type B's have a greater risk than type A's.) Third, since something like 50 to 80 percent of the men tested fall into type A category, is the structured interview assessing anything more than the prevailing, culturally-sanctioned American masculine image? American culture has been characterized as one of "'rugged individualism,' a kind of fiercely autonomous, self-indulgent, and sometimes narcissistic perspective guided by economic, political and social self-interest."[15] In another culture, type A might have a very different meaning and origin and bear little or no relation to disease. Fourth, although the stereotype of a type B is "laid back and relaxed," the definition of type B as *not* type A actually provides no positive information about these individuals. A certain proportion of type B's are doubtless depressed or keeping their hostility inside, two traits that have themselves been related to increased health risk. Their confounded presence in the type B category may account for many studies that show no disease-prone differences between type A's and B's. Fifth, a serious difficulty with the global measurement of type A by the structured interview is that that measurement tool does not yield the *degree* of type A. Type A is a very blunt measurement instrument indeed. All of these considerations and complexities probably mean that future investigation will be focused on more fine-grained personality analyses, examining the health consequences of the discrete components of type A and the specific beliefs that underlie it.

Is There a Cancer Personality?

The observation that cancer patients suppress, repress and deny negative feelings such as anger, depression and guilt has long been suggested by folklore.

> There is an intuitive ring to the idea that giving vent to one's feelings and letting it all hang out is healthy. When someone has suffered a tragic loss he or she is encouraged to weep, and there is a suggestion that emotional weeping has the physically beneficial effect of ridding the body of toxins.[16]

Studies of lung cancer in the 1960s showed patients to have a diminished outlet for emotional discharge. The view has been advanced that the cancer itself is a kind of physical expression of the suppressed emotion.

The cancer-personality research illustrates in extreme form the difficulties in trying to assess whether personality is a cause of illness or a result of it. The diagnosis of cancer is a highly emotive event, and is bound to trigger powerful emotions that are only rarely experienced by healthy people or patients with less serious diseases. Suppression, repression and denial are natural initial reactions to such distressing news. Separating the emotional impact of a grave diagnosis from the causal role of emotion in the etiology of the disease is probably impossible.

Even studies that have administered personality tests prior to diagnosis do not guarantee to tease out psychogenic aspects of cancer. Women who were about to be examined for suspicious breast lumps were given personality tests prior to examination. Those women who were found to have breast cancer showed a heightened tendency to suppress feelings compared with women whose lumps proved on examination to be benign. However, it is not unlikely that the women who proved diseased may have sensed (consciously or unconsciously) that they were seriously ill and reacted accordingly. Practitioners of natural medicine are advised to take a conservative view and not assume that hypothetical psychological factors are operative in a life-threatening disease until established beyond the shadow of a doubt. To do otherwise is to risk the patient adding guilt to an already heavy emotional burden, or to deflect the patient from seeking other, perhaps more appropriate, therapies.

The Disease-Prone Personality

How can personality affect susceptibility to illness? Three primary possibilities are:

- Personality characteristics can modulate responses to significant life events (potential stressors). Type A personality both lowers the threshold for the stress response and increases its magnitude. But type A behavior also attracts conflict and strife. Conversely, there are indications that other kinds of "hardy" personalities are associated with low levels of reported illness.[17]

- Personality can predispose to disease when it fosters deleterious health behaviors such as imprudent diet, smoking, excessive alcohol consumption, overwork, insufficient rest and recreation, and sedentary lifestyle.

- Personality can exacerbate and perpetuate existing disease. The diagnosis of serious disease is itself a major challenge and the individual's response to the discovery of a life-threatening disease or a debilitating illness that will potentially limit future activities will affect the course of the illness itself.

All of these potential ways that personality can affect health, both for better and worse, are parts of each case that the practitioner must consider. The clinician must be sensitive to the potential contribution of each patient's personality to the presenting problem, and must be aware of the existing resources that can be brought to bear upon the problem to optimize personality factors in the direction of health rather than illness. When thinking about personality and whether it is relatively health-promoting or disease-prone, it helps to remember that personality is learned. And what is learned can be unlearned. Not that that may be easy. Indeed the difficulties in making such changes through the usual methods of social influence and persuasion are an important reason for making available here in a single reference source for practitioners and students of natural therapeutics a body of current knowledge about psychological medicine.

There are also some serious problems with personality research methodology that create conceptual difficulties for the practitioner desiring information of practical value. All too frequently the same trait is given an entirely different name: e.g., aggressive/dominance, hostility, antagonistic, angry. Thus, a supposedly new correlation with a disease may be nothing more than old wine in a new bottle. Perhaps even more confusing is the practice of giving different traits the *same* name, as when hostility, used by one group of researchers, means expressive anger, but another group uses it for the felt experience of anger which may never be expressed. Such erroneous equations are responsible for many of the contradictions found in investigations of personality and disease.

Ideally, the basic dimensions of personality would be based on some rational theory of personality, which would presumably end such arbitrary naming of traits. Unfortunately, the field of personality has to date resisted any such unified theory. In the absence of a systematic framework, psychologists have attempted to create some order out of this chaos by endeavoring to subsume personality as a set of independent points along the five personality dimensions shown in Fig. 9.3.[18] These five dimensions, while not based on a theory of personality, are not completely arbitrary. They are in fact the clusters that fall out when people sort the hundreds of different trait words of the English language into five categories.

The advantage of a model like Fig. 9.3 is that it allows us to place many of the various behavioral dispositions used in investigations of health and disease into a unified, coherent framework. It is not unreasonable, e.g., to consider type A as a composite of low A, high C, N and E. But it is still unclear whether a model like Fig. 9.3 can capture

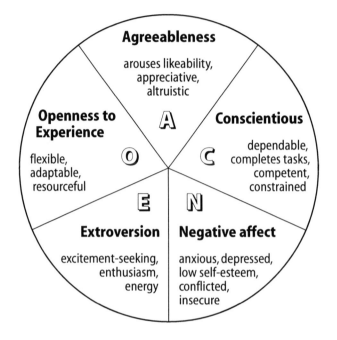

Fig. 9.3 The five-factor model of personality. (The traits shown here are the ends of five relatively independent continuua: agreeable↔antagonistic; conscientious↔unreliable; negative affect↔secure; extroverted↔introverted; open-to-experience↔closed/rigid.)

all the meaning implicit in such personality traits as hardiness, alexithymia (the inability to verbally express and identify emotion), optimism, sense-of-coherence, frustration-in-influencing-others, obsessive-compulsive, dependent—all of which boast at least one research study reporting them to be significantly related to disease outcomes. In particular, a number of studies show alexithymia to be related to an increased incidence of respiratory disorders, chronic pain and hypertension.

A survey of the medical and psychological literature from 1945-84 targeted on five personality traits (anger, hostility, aggression, depression or extroversion) that had been studied in relation to one or more of five target diseases (CHD, asthma, peptic ulcer, rheumatoid arthritis or headache). Only prospective or retrospective studies that used quantifiable variables (this excluded case studies and anecdotal reports) with large enough samples to yield reliable statistic tests were included. An attempt was made to see whether the bulk of the evidence over that 30-year period favored the view that personality variables do relate to health outcomes in either of two ways: (1) Is there evidence for a general disease-prone personality? and/or (2) Do specifically different personality traits cluster with different illnesses?

Such a survey and analysis across many research studies is called a *meta-analysis*. The results of this meta-analysis showed that two of the five personality variables, anxiety and depression, were related to all five disease categories. In addition, they showed that hostility was related to CHD and asthma. There was no evidence found that these personality traits define particular disease-prone personalities, e.g., an "arthritic personality" or a "coronary-prone personality." There was good evidence, however, for a *generic* disease-prone personality—all five diseases are associated with personalities prone to negative feelings. Overall the data seem much too consistent from 101 studies to warrant dismissing the link between personality and disease as folklore.[19] The truth seems much closer to the view that personality functions similarly to diet: imbalances and deficiencies in attitudes as well as in nutrition can predispose an individual to diseases of all sorts.[20]

Health-Promoting Personality Traits

In contrast to the long list of potentially toxic personality traits and psychological characteristics that have been examined in relation to their possible association to disease, relatively little research has been conducted on personalities that resist disease or are unusually healthy. There is at present information concerning a few such positive personality dimensions: the possibility of a "stress-hardy" personality that can in some way mitigate or resist stress, the optimistic personality, and a cluster of possible health-enhancing traits perhaps best described as "agreeableness."

The concept of stress-hardiness is based on the idea that psychogenic stress is in fact a personal response to challenges, threats and life changes. To the extent that this is so, we can well imagine people to differ in how easily they tend to generate a stress response to potential stressors. Thus, some individuals might be resistant to the potentially adverse health effects of threats, challenges and losses because they possess certain stress-resistant personality traits. Such traits could work either by modulating physiological stress responses, or by activating adaptive coping behaviors.

Psychologist Suzanne Kobasa and colleagues, working from an existential perspective, proposed that such persons would be stress-resistant or *stress-hardy* because they possessed a cluster of three personality traits: commitment, control and challenge.[21] Commitment refers to the belief in the meaningfulness of one's experiences and activities, and seems very similar, if not identical to, the sense of coherence discussed in Chapter 7. Control refers to the belief that one's actions are influential in the face of the varied contingencies of life. It contrasts with a sense of helplessness or victimization. Challenge refers to the ability to see change as normal and interesting, as opposed to a threat to one's security. Hardiness was conceived as a stress moderator or *buffer*. For the trait cluster to buffer the effects of a stressor, we would expect to find with a low frequency of stressors, little or no difference in health outcomes between hardy or non-hardy individuals. On the other hand, the buffering concept predicts that at high stress frequencies, hardiness should work to moderate the conversion of tension into the stress response with all its consequences for health.

Employing paper and pencil personality tests designed to measure commitment, challenge and perceived control, research was conducted with male executives working under potentially stressful circumstances. It was in fact found in this retrospective study that the tests did discriminate between those executives reporting high levels of illness and those reporting low levels. Further prospective studies demonstrated that the three-trait hardiness composite predicts both current and future health independent of constitutional predisposition, the existence of type A behavior pattern, prior illness or degree of social support.

Despite these suggestive results, the concept of hardiness as a unitary personality trait that buffers stress is not unequivocally established. One serious problem is that the hardiness research has used self-reported illness, not actual objective measure of disease. Thus it is possible that the three personality traits in the hardiness construct only predict the degree to which people take their bodily symptoms sufficiently serious to call them illnesses. Moreover, when the three components of hardiness are examined separately, only commitment and perceived control are significantly related to health, and even then not in the statistically interactive way with significant life events that the concept of a stress buffer predicts (see discussion above).

The notion that there is a hardy personality type that could help turn potential stressors into challenges and growth experiences is an attractive one. It probably incorporates an intuition that most practitioners of natural medicine share. The stress hardy personality may well possess a strong sense of coherence which Antonovsky conceives as having three components: (1) *comprehensibility,* a feeling that demands and life events have meaning; (2) *confidence,* a feeling that resources are available to meet demands as they arise; and (3) a tendency to frame demands as *challenges.*[22] Such a combination of skills, attitudes and dispositions gives us the makings of the possibility of a "health prone personality." How can we promote the development of such traits in our patients, children and society at large? Here the research laboratory would appear to be well placed to give the clinician practical information, but the literature is strangely silent on their development, either naturally or through a kind of hardiness training.[23] Doubtless as our emphasis begins to shift from a disease orientation to a preoccupation with wellness, we should begin to see research in this direction.

Turning to the notion that the optimistic personality is in general a healthy one, we may recall that this idea goes back to Galen, whose sanguine man was the one humoral type not associated with disease. Modern psychologists view the optimistic personality as one that tends to hold stable expectations that life situations are likely to have positive outcomes. Thus optimists—anticipating positive outcomes—are on the whole more likely to problem-solve or cope actively with challenges and potential stressors. This active, adaptive coping style of optimists should lessen the stress effects of life events, and therefore result in reduced incidence of disease and illness. Research studies in fact do show that high optimism scores on psychological tests are associated with reduced reports of physical illness. In addition, compared with their more pessimistic counterparts, expectant mothers with high optimism scores had a lower frequency of postpartum depression, and optimistic cardiac surgery patients demonstrated better post-operative recoveries and less likelihood of an intra-operative myocardial infarction.[24] Reduced cardiovascular reactivity to stress may be one physiological mechanism underlying the optimists' better health outcomes. One study investigated how a series of insoluble (and therefore potentially frustrating) problems might affect blood pressure. It was found that optimistic subjects exhibited a decrease in systolic blood pressure over time as they worked on these problems, whereas pessimistic subjects exhibited blood pressure increases. There is additional circumstantial evidence that optimism might also influence immune functioning positively, since optimism and depression are negatively correlated, and emotional depression is associated with poorer DNA repair in lymphocytes and other measures of immune impairment.[25]

A few studies found that individuals who are perceived as friendly, avoiding disagreement and enjoying time with others have fewer illnesses and exhibit better immune functioning.[26] This complex of traits appears to at least overlap, if not be identical to, the agreeableness dimension of the five-factor personality model in Fig. 9.3.

A useful way to summarize the evidence for health-enhancing effects of personality is via a mnemonic: the five "C's" of a health-promoting personality. The following traits or characteristics beginning with the letter "C" all show some evidence of reducing health risks or promoting health directly:

Control— the sense that one is able to influence the events in one's life.

Commitment — a tendency to involve oneself wholeheartedly in whatever one is doing.

Challenge — an ability to see or reframe threats and demands as challenges.

Coherence — the view that life makes sense, including the ability to generate meaning from the events in one's life.

Community — the ability to find a valued place in a group of like-minded individuals holding a shared vision.

To the degree that practitioners of natural medicine can support, sustain and encourage such traits in their patients, they may find that they are able to act as a positive force for health and the prevention of disease.

Project 9

Self-Monitoring One's Own Personality

Using your own personality as an example, examine it to see whether you are inclined towards type A or type B. Write a brief, balanced essay on the ways in which your personality is both health-fostering and potentially a risk factor for illness. What areas would you like to work on to make it even more of a health-enhancing asset?

Using the mind-body diary that was suggested earlier, describe some significant observations you have been able to make about the role of personality in your own health. Do you find self-monitoring (e.g., this diary) a useful way of gaining awareness about your own body and its relation to psychological factors?

Annotated Bibliography

Totman, Richard. *Social Causes of Illness.* London: Souvenir, 1987. The first two-thirds of this book are an excellent introduction to the field of psychosomatics and psychogenesis. The chapters on stress are notable for their conceptual clarity, and there is a useful discussion of personality and illness. The author's structural theory is perhaps of less value to the practitioner desiring practical clinical tools.

Wolman, Benjamin B. *Psychosomatic Disorder.* New York: Plenum, 1988. A brief historical introduction to the field, with chapters on many illnesses for which psychological factors have been found to play an important etiological role. The treatment is mildly psychoanalytic, but useful cases are provided.

10

Psychological Aspects of Common Syndromes (PART 1)

Patients turn their problems into illness, and . . .
the physician's task is to turn illnesses back into
problems.

—MICHAEL BALINT[1]

*P*REVIOUS CHAPTERS LOOKED at the role of personality and stress in illness in a general way that was independent of any particular disease state. But the multifaceted character of psychological aspects of disease and its treatment is best appreciated through concrete examples. Chapters 10 and 11 look at psychological aspects of a half dozen syndromes that will be familiar to every practitioner. Although organic lesions are present in some (skin disease, rheumatoid arthritis), only functional disturbances characterize others (asthma, irritable bowel syndrome). In still a third group (headache, chronic fatigue syndrome) somatic malfunction is generally undetected, although this may well be because of current limitations in medical diagnostic technology. In none of the six is either the etiology or the pathogenesis well understood; there are thus no curative treatments as such, and allopathic treatment is directed to management of symptomatology by drugs. These often have serious side effects and may make iatrogenic contributions to the illness itself.

In all six syndromes psychological aspects have traditionally been suggested as relevant, but the presumption of even partial psychogenesis must be tempered by the known fact that whenever a disease is poorly understood (as tuberculosis was a century ago) there is a tendency to fill the explanatory vacuum with psychological explanations.[2] A conservative stance is therefore prudent, imputing psychosocial factors in the disease process only where such are clearly demonstrated in the case, or where psychotherapy or behavioral therapy have been shown to have an ameliorating effect on the outcome of the disease. Only then can psychological treatment be viewed as a legitimate adjunct to the practitioner's natural therapeutics.

With these criteria in mind, each of the six syndromes shown in the left column

179

of Table 10.1 is discussed in the six-point framework shown in the top row of the table. This common descriptive framework promotes a comparison of features common to all syndromes. It also serves to illustrate the great diversity and uniqueness with which psychological factors can enter into the predisposition, precipitation and maintenance of disease states. In natural medicine we can no longer be content with the vague generality that in every illness mind and body interact reciprocally. Rather, we want to know in every case how, what, when and where psychological factors are relevant in the illness process. Thus, to anticipate, after first briefly describing the syndrome, its prevalence and usual course, as well as the conventional chemotherapies currently in vogue, we then ask: (1) By what psychophysiological mechanisms could personality characteristics or emotional distress conceivably be channeled into this symptomatology? (2) Is there a specific personality trait or traits that predispose for this particular syndrome? (3) Is either the onset of the syndrome or its exacerbations linked to stressful events in the individual's life? (4) Has either psychotherapy or behavioral therapy been shown to ameliorate the condition? (5) What special social or personal consequences, either reinforcing (gaining attention, care or avoiding responsibilities) or negative (stigmatizing, punitive, quality-of-life-reducing), are associated with the illness whose existence needs to be taken into account and addressed with behavioral medicine? (6) Do group psycho-educative therapies or patient support groups[3] have a value for patients with this condition? Table 10.1 illustrates the framework that will be followed in the discussion.

Psychological Dimension						
Syndrome	Psycho-physiology	Specific Personality	Link to Stress	Psycho-behavior Therapy	Special Illness Consequences	Value of Support Groups
Irritable Bowel	colon hyper-motility?	X	direction of causation unclear	stress inoculation	treats given in childhood when ill	group therapy may be useful
Asthma	reflex rebound bronchial spasm?	X	stress of attack creates positive feedback loop	breathing exercises	asthma attack leads to panic	serves educational function
Skin Disease		X	stress may exacerbate	biofeedback of value?	disfigurement leads to social ostracism	valuable to raise self-esteem
Rheumatoid Arthritis	suspected immune hyperactivity	?	suggestive in one type	pain management strategies	disability leads to depression	
Headache	muscle tension or arterial vasodilation	X	tension headaches	biofeedback and relaxation		educative and advocacy role
Chronic Fatigue	suspected immuno-suppression		burnout?	contra-indicated	viral depression confused with psychogenic depression	essential to combat alienation

Table 10.1 Six common illness syndromes and a six-point framework for analyzing relevant psychological parameters. (An empty cell means that there is no available data, or it is not applicable; a question mark means that the status is currently in question; and the letter "x" means that it is unsubstantiated.)

Irritable Bowel Syndrome[4]

About half the patients complaining of disordered gut function and subsequently referred to consultant gastroenterologists have no detectable organic disease (Thornton, 1989). A partial list of what these patients complain of includes dyspepsia, nausea, wind, abdominal pain, reflux, bloating, constipation and/or diarrhea (with or without pain). Although these are common symptoms experienced by everyone at some time or another, their presentation to a physician suggests that their frequency or severity has become unacceptable to the patient who is now soliciting expertise in abating the symptoms.

Although it is likely that such complaints are in reality a spectrum of disorders whose pathogenesis and etiology may be quite different, as reflected by such terms as spastic colon, irritable colon, mucomembraneous colitis and neurogenic mucous colitis, the general term *irritable bowel syndrome* (IBS) currently subsumes all these functional bowel disorders characterized by altered bowel habits with abdominal pain.[5] IBS is a chronic disorder, two to three times more common in women, with frequent remissions and relapses, but in many cases little progression. It is usually first diagnosed between ages 20 and 50, although a juvenile variation characterized by recurrent abdominal pain with nausea has been identified (Lask and Fosson, 1989). About a third of these children progress to IBS in adult life, another third develop recurrent headache or migraine, and the remainder "grow out of it."

The medical management of IBS involves bulking agents, antispasmodic drugs, antacids and minor tranquilizers, but evidence of the efficacy of these medications is weak. Patients on Valium may show less anxiety, but their bowel function remains unchanged.

Possible Physiological Mechanisms. Everyone knows the 'butterflies in the stomach', loose bowels and queasy stomach that can go along with anxiety. In fact, both constipation and painful diarrhea appear linked to increased segmental contractions of the colon. Nevertheless it is not certain whether these motility patterns seen in IBS patients are substantially different from the normal range of contractions (Thornton, 1989). However it does seem that IBS patients show a lower threshold for pain perception in the gut since patients with IBS report pain at lower volumes than control subjects when a balloon is inflated in the colon and rectum. Yet their pain thresholds for stimuli applied to the skin are the same as controls. IBS patients probably have a biological predisposition to respond to emotional stimuli with colonic hypermotility.

Personality. IBS patients show mildly elevated test scores on depression, anxiety and "neuroticism"[6] scales. Curiously, people with equivalent levels of IBS who do not bother to seek treatment show no such trends. In general, however, no specific personality or disturbed behavior patterns are found in patients. In particular the obsessive-compulsive personality traits predicted by psychoanalytic theory are no more frequent than in a normal population (Whitehead and Schuster, 1985). Somatization-of-affect scores are higher in IBS patients, indicating a preoccupation with physical symptoms, but whether this is the result of a long-term inability to obtain relief or a cause of the symptomatology remains moot.

Stress Links. Retrospective data show that about half of IBS patients notice a relationship between tension and exacerbations of their bowel symptoms. Half (not necessarily the same half) also recall psychological loss or threat of loss preceding the first episode of their symptoms. Patients also report more stressful life events than either non-patients or patients with organic gastrointestinal disease (e.g., Crohn's disease, ulcerative colitis). All of this information is, however, subject to the vicissitudes of retrospective self-report studies and can at best be considered suggestive. In fact, it is quite possible that the reported stress-induced exacerbations are the general result of having a chronic painful disorder rather than causing IBS.

Psychotherapy/Behavioral Therapy. If IBS is precipitated or maintained by emotional distress, psychological or behavioral treatments should reduce symptoms. A Swedish study compared medical treatment with and without three months of weekly sessions of individual psychotherapy.[7] Medical treatment consisted of standard IBS drugs plus advice about diet, smoking and drinking habits as well as reassurance that IBS is unrelated to bowel cancer. The psychotherapy focused on stress triggers and resources for coping with stress and for handling interpersonal conflicts positively. Pain severity and number of symptoms were reduced in both medical and medical-plus-psychotherapy groups after the three months of treatment, but much more so in the group that received psychotherapy. Moreover, and more significantly, the psychotherapy group continued to show even further improvement when examined a year later, whereas the medical group had relapsed back to their high level of pre-treatment symptomatology. There is also suggestive evidence that hypnotherapy directed to control of internal smooth muscle can give marked and durable symptomatic improvement. Relaxation training may also be effective for reducing pain and diarrhea. Biofeedback for the self-control of either bowel sounds or colonic mobility has proven inconclusive, and the absence of recent studies suggests that investigators have concluded that stress management and psychotherapy offer more therapeutic promise (Whitehead, 1992).

Distinctive Operant Aspects. The concept of IBS as a learned disorder via operant conditioning and vicarious modeling has recently been advanced. This idea is based on family history data and evidence that more people with IBS recall their parents giving them special treats during childhood illness than average.

> When reinforcing consequences frequently follow illness, these can condition an actual increase in the frequency of abnormal physiologic responses such as bowel motility, which give rise to the illness complaints. This is the same kind of learning involved in biofeedback training: people can be taught to alter physiologic responses, such as the rate of gastric acid secretion or the amount of gastric motility.

> Many patients with IBS have had early learning experiences in which illness in general and gastrointestinal complaints in particular were singled out for special attention.

Some grow up overly concerned with their health and likely to use illness complaints unintentionally to obtain attention or other social reinforcers from family members and friends.[8]

This novel view suggests that family therapy may be useful, with the patient contracting to talk about IBS symptoms only with his practitioner, and family members contracting to ignore any complaints in the home. It is suggested that the practitioner be sympathetic but not indulgent to IBS patients, following the model of reality therapy discussed in Chapter 8.

Group Therapy/Support Groups. Few IBS groups exist, although one therapy group that met for six 90-minute sessions reported a slight (30 percent) decrease in symptoms. Sessions combined formal lectures with a group discussion on such topics as the anatomy and physiology of IBS, dietary factors, life stressors and the relationship of personality to coping styles. Patients also learned progressive muscle relaxation, kept behavioral diaries, were encouraged to exercise dietary restraint, and remained on their drugs. The relatively short duration (only six sessions) and the absence of true group process in a rather didactic format may have limited its effectiveness. Future groups should incorporate more explicit group psychotherapeutic tools and continue for extended periods to test whether IBS patient/practitioner groups might indeed be of use in this syndrome.

Conclusions. IBS appears to be a heterogeneous class of disorders. Some cases may be learned illness behaviors, and if the patient is receptive to entertaining this possibility, behavioral modification programs and family therapy are indicated. A second class of patients may be those in whom symptoms occur via classical Pavlovian conditioning, as for instance when symptoms occur just as the patient is getting ready for (stressful) work on a Monday morning.

Many, but not all IBS patients may be predisposed to respond to stressors primarily in the gut, and for them stress reduction programs involving assertive training, stress inoculation, relaxation exercises and meditation are likely to prove of value. In general the practitioner of natural medicine will have to examine carefully each case to attempt to isolate the possible behavioral sources that contribute to the maintenance of the patient's symptomatology. A behavioral diary in which the patient charts times, frequency and severity of symptoms, any related stressor, relation to eating, etc., will give the practitioner further clues as to the relevant therapeutic measures.[9] Since many people perceive the possibility that psychological factors contribute to their illness as threatening or demeaning, patients must be reassured that the fact that stress could be playing a crucial role most emphatically does not mean either that the illness is "all in their head" or that they need psychiatric treatment.

Asthma[10]

Asthma is a reversible respiratory disorder characterized by acute narrowing of the airways (bronchoconstriction) with mucus plugging of the bronchial walls accompanied by dyspnea, wheezing, coughing and sputum. About 60 percent of sufferers are age 16 or less and as many as 5 percent of children may be asthmatic (Steptoe, 1984). Boys outnumber girls. A distinction is generally made between allergenic and non-allergenic asthma. The former, accounting for 60 percent of cases in children aged 5-14, is triggered by allergens such as house dust, pollen, high levels of air pollution and certain foods. The latter does not have allergenic precipitates and tends to occur later in life. These two classes correspond roughly to the two mechanisms thought to be involved in asthma. The first is allergic bronchial constriction with raised serum IgE and anaphylaxis. The second is bronchial hyper-reactivity. The airways of the asthmatic tend to respond with exaggerated constriction to challenge from various stimuli including sulfur dioxide, histamine, exercise, inhalation of cold air and stressful film presentations (Steptoe, 1984). The measurement of clinical severity in asthma requires a hand-held peak flow meter into which the subject takes deep breaths. In laboratory studies instruments that monitor the respiratory resistance of air passages provide more accurate indicators.

Asthma is managed in orthodox medicine by bronchodilating drugs. Beta-adrenergic drugs (epinephrine) are used for acute attacks, and hydrocortisone inhalation for chronic severe cases. These drugs have serious side effects and the development of the "aggressive" chemotherapies has been associated with increased morbidity and mortality from asthma in the developed world during the past decade.

Psychophysiology. There is a paradox in that the drugs used to treat asthma are the very chemicals (steroids and adrenaline) released in anger, anxiety and depression, typical concomitants of the emotional stress response. If stress has *dilatory* effects on bronchial tissue, how could it *cause* asthma? One possibility is that clinical asthma is a rebound effect. Another is that stress effects could be mediated by antagonistic (parasympathetic) reflex vagal nerve stimulation. There is circumstantial evidence for this in that coughing, crying, yelling and laughing all result in vagal stimulation, and these can all produce full-blown asthmatic attacks in susceptible individuals. Many examples of emotionally triggered asthma may be due therefore to such reflex bronchospasms. Anxiety, of course, can aggravate asthma directly via hyperventilation with its CO_2 reduction-induced bronchial constriction, rather than through emotional mechanisms.

Personality. On the basis of clinical impressions where the investigator was not blind to the diagnosis, or in flawed retrospective research studies which cannot discriminate cause from effect, asthmatics have been described with a bewildering and contradictory array of personality traits. Insecurity and dependency are traits commonly found, but given the frightening nature of juvenile asthmatic attacks and parents' natural concerns for the child, these almost certainly are the *result* of the disease, not its cause. When asthmatics are compared to those who suffer from other chronic diseases, no personality differences emerge. "Certainly no evidence suggests that unique personality factors contribute to the development of the disorder."[11]

There is a lesson here for alternative and complementary medicine in that impressionistic data that do not stand up to scientific scrutiny can be highly misleading and encourage misguided therapeutics. On the other hand, we must not allow scientific analysis to throw out the baby with the bath. Thus, the early hypothesis of the "asthma mother"—the parent who partly spoils and partly tyrannizes the child—has not really been given a scientific check. It is still possible that the child's asthma is a response to such a partly oppressive, partly caring, maternal environment.

Stress Links. The early literature (e.g., Bastiaans and Groen, 1955), based on anecdotal but detailed case histories, was replete with references to stress as both the precipitating factor for the first asthma attack, and its role as a trigger for later attacks. A landmark study[12] published in 1969 showed that beneficial effects of sending patients away to a new physical environment were not due to the changed location, but were due to changes in the psychological environment. When the investigators removed the *families* of asthmatic children to a hotel for several weeks while the child remained at home under the care of an adult child-care worker, asthma attacks were sharply reduced.

More recent studies have been less favorable on the role of emotional stress in asthma (cf. Alexander, 1982). This may be due partly to the more rigorous and reliable airways measurement of asthma available to us today, and to the fact that most recent scientific work is on *groups* of patients where the subtler features that the older clinical case reports claimed to find are obscured by grosser, if more objective, instruments for measuring and quantifying emotional stress and personality.

Psychotherapy/Behavioral Therapy. Various techniques have been used in the attempt to improve pulmonary function and decrease medication, since asthma drugs have dangerous side effects. Relaxation training has been reported to have a small beneficial effect. Biofeedback to decrease facial muscle tension or increase heart rate leads to improvement in pulmonary function. These systems were chosen for biofeedback because they are presumed to decrease vagal nerve tone via reflex pathways (Lehrer, Sargunaraj and Hochron, 1992). The training of diaphragmatic breathing is also beneficial. Despite these scattered positive results, the evidence to date for clinically significant behavioral modification of pulmonary function in asthma remains weak (exception: breathing exercises).

Distinctive Consequences. A full-blown asthma attack with a sense of one's inability to breathe is a terrifying event. Unless the individual (often a child) is aware that in itself an asthma attack is not a life-threatening situation, the dyspnea of asthma may incite a panic attack. The consequent hyperventilation as the sufferer struggles for breath is likely to deepen the attack as the lowered blood carbon dioxide concentration leads to further bronchoconstriction. Asthma sufferers need to know too that the respiratory vocal reflex mechanisms that accompany the responses of crying, laughing and yelling can induce an asthmatic attack. The principal therapeutic aid here is psychoeducative. It is vital that the practitioner ensures that the patient understands and learns that these positive feedback mechanisms that exacerbate attacks are under his control. Panic attacks can be avoided by well-practiced diaphragmatic breathing exercises that the patient can bring into play during an attack. The holistic practitioner should provide educative information to help the patient become an expert on his or her own disease, thus minimizing its effect on quality of life.

Patient Groups. Long ago, J. Bastiaans and J. Groen (1955), working in Amsterdam, described weekly asthma patient groups which served both an educative and thera-peutic role. Because the authors were working from the traditional psychosomatic view that asthma represents suppressed emotion, the group leaders (physician, psy-chologist, psychiatrist) aimed to create a safe space where patients could give vent to emotions. Patients also shared their experiences about the effects of various factors such as smoking, climate, food, dust and allergies, and drug side effects. The leader answered questions about medical and etiological aspects. As time went on and the group members became more comfortable with each other, deeper issues were ex-plored and strong feelings of frustration and resentment were expressed which in-cluded anger at the doctors for their inability to provide a cure. In some groups the theory that asthma attacks represent a choice of how to solve interpersonal conflicts was adopted as a principle: "We need not have attacks if we do not want to. But if we have them we can be sure that something must have been bothering us, however in-significant that something may seem."[13] Patients were encouraged to find out what it was and work it out with the person concerned; if this was not possible, it needed to be brought back to the group.

These were long-term groups and they are an early example of group therapy with a completely modern outlook. Although no patient was cured, the authors say that the groups were quite effective in reducing severity and frequency of attacks. Unfortunately, no objective measures were reported. There is little mention in the modern asthma literature of such groups. This is regrettable since the non-judgmen-tal and empowering format of such groups serves many educative and therapeutic purposes. The ideal leadership would appear to be a practitioner thoroughly familiar with all medical aspects of the disease as well as with the principles of psychotherapy, plus a patient co-leader. The latter would be an experienced group member who had brought about significant improvement in their own condition employing the tech-niques and viewpoints used in the group.

Skin Disease[14]

Three skin diseases—atopic eczema (neurodermatitis), hives (uticaria) and psoriasis—have traditionally been thought to be connected to psychological influ-ences. This review focuses on psoriasis and eczema. Psoriasis is a chronic, non-con-tagious, intractable, proliferative skin disease characterized by coalescing erythematous dry patches covered by graying-white plaques. The condition is associated with an abnormally increased rate of proliferation of the epidermal cells. Plaques are typically found on the extensor surfaces of the limbs, lower back and scalp. As psoriasis becomes more severe, plaques become painful as the skin grows dry and itches, forming heavy layers which crack and bleed. Psoriasis is estimated to affect about two percent of the population: "On a full double decker bus at least two people will have the condition" (Kaptein, 1990). A positive family history predisposes. Sixty percent of cases begin before the age of 30, and about that same percentage never experience complete remission. Medical treatment is via anxiolytics, and topical hydrocortisone ointments intended to control itching and scaling. Antidepressants, lithium and a number of other drugs must be avoided, for these can themselves produce dermatoses, thus exacerbating the original condition.

In atopic eczema the skin is chronically inflamed, itchy (pruritis) and irritable. As in psoriasis the condition is aggravated by scratching. Skin lesions are most common on the flexures of the arms and legs, and nape of the neck. About two percent of the population suffer from eczema, which generally begins in childhood. Allopathic treatment is by topical preparations (often containing steroids) plus anxiolytics. Minor tranquilizers may be prescribed if stress is considered a factor in the cause, or for the patient's anxiety stemming from the disfiguring nature of the lesions.

Psychophysiology. Although emotions are reflected in the skin (blushing in shame and humiliation, gooseflesh in anxiety, pallor in terror), the psychophysiological mechanisms are not well understood. A few studies have attempted to show that patients with dermatoses have lower thresholds to itch stimuli, or show more easily conditioned responses to tactile stimuli (as a theory of skin hypersensitivity might predict), but the results are inconclusive at this time.

Personality. The classic psychosomatic view was that skin lesions represented body language. Individuals who are unable to express their feelings, either because of conflicts or because they have not developed a language of emotion (alexithymic), somatize, since the verbal channel is blocked or deficient. The dermatological patient was thought to resort to expressing his or her feelings by skin lesions.[15] Unfortunately the evidence for this simplistic view is weak. A study of over 100 sufferers from psoriasis found no specific personality profiles to exist, nor any common emotional conflict situation (Musaph, 1976). There is no evidence of a specific personality picture for eczema, although the disease frequently goes along with personal or family histories of allergy, hay fever, migraine and irritable bowel (Folks and Kinney, 1991; Kaptein, 1990). It appears that the increases in anxiety, depression and negative affect often found in patients with eczema reflect the severity of skin involvement at the time of observation and are thus consequences of the disease, rather than causes of it (Wessely, 1990). The theme is beginning to sound familiar: what we thought was cause is just an effect.

Link to Stress. Authorities differ in their conclusions as to whether stress is or is not causally involved in the development of either psoriasis or eczema. The early "psychodermatology" literature indicated that separation experiences, severe emotional shock or upset within six months of onset was present in nearly half of eczema patients as compared with only 15 percent of a control group of dental patients. However, the clinical interviews used to elicit the information are not today considered a reliable methodology, since the investigator's bias toward his hypothesis may influence the results. There are individual case reports of psoriasis beginning with stress (unsuccessful change in employment, mounting family problems), but a summary of group studies (which are considered more reliable, although as we have seen, less sensitive) concluded that there is no consistent evidence for the *onset* of psoriasis being caused by stress or psychological factors (Gupta et al., 1987). Still, emotional distress can and does exacerbate episodes of eczema (Kaptein, 1990). As with asthma and IBS, attention is being turned from psychological factors in the *etiology* of skin conditions to the psychological and behavioral *consequences* of the illness.

Individual Psychotherapy/Behavioral Therapy. Very little work has been reported in this area with psoriasis. Does this mean that psychological interventions are not yet useful in ameliorating the condition, that clinicians have not taken time to collect systematic data, or that the topic has not found favor with research investigators? Skin temperature biofeedback was employed in one study[16] on the rationale that reduced heat production in the skin may, via vasoconstriction, decrease skin metabolic activity and slow down cell proliferation. Three psoriasis patients did succeed in lowering skin temperature on a plaque area about 1°C, and two of the patients showed clinical improvements in the lesions. Unfortunately, four months later lesions were returning to their original condition. Scattered reports hint that hand warming or frontalis muscle biofeedback, perhaps combined with progressive muscle relaxation, could be useful in attenuating eczematous lesions. Hypnosis has occasionally been used to treat eczema, but the results are not considered convincing due to lack of follow-up data and subjective evaluations of what constitutes improvement.

Distinctive Operant Effects. Disfiguring skin disease has negative social consequences, which in turn can lead to considerable emotional distress and low self-esteem. Patients with eczema say that the irritation, constant itching and actual marks on the skin are the worst aspects of the disease. Three-quarters of patients report shame and embarrassment, and anxiety and depression are frequent accompaniments of skin disease. Yet strangely, while patients find embarrassment over appearance the most serious factor of their disease, dermatologists rank this factor lowest in importance (Kaptein, 1990). The holistic practitioner would be wise to align herself with the patient's concerns, and to make use of psycho-behavioral therapeutics that can modulate the impact of the disease on the individual's self-esteem.

Eczema is almost always itchy, and since scratching provides short-term relief from itching, it is operantly reinforced. Unfortunately, because scratching, which often increases in stressful moments, aggravates the lesions, a vicious circle can be set up. Behavioral modification programs designed to reduce scratching have taught patients to recognize the trigger situations in which they are likely to begin to scratch unconsciously, and to replace scratching with incompatible behaviors (e.g., arm clenching, or making a diary entry in a pocket notebook). By breaking the vicious circle between itching and scratching, these techniques can significantly reduce dermatological symptoms, including itching itself.

Psoriasis has a very severe impact on the sufferer. Patients are sometimes sexually rejected by partners offended at the lesions, and ostracized in social situations. Although salt sea swimming and sunbathing are therapeutic, many patients are too embarrassed to reveal the lesions in public. Since nearly 90 percent of patients suffer from lack of confidence, anxiety and embarrassment, and another 50 percent from depression, health psychology needs to impart skills and attitudes that create inner self-esteem that is independent of other people's negative judgments based on superficial skin appearance. Yet just to emphasize the subtleties of disease consequences, the zealous but inexperienced practitioner needs reminding that some elderly patients with long-standing skin disease may know no other way than their lesions to gain emotional support and caring attention. It could be a serious medical mistake to cure such disease unless the patient has (or has the ability to create) healthier alternatives for recognition (Musaph, 1976).

Groups. Weekly groups providing mutual aid, education and emotional support for patients with psoriasis, co-led by a physician (trained in group process) and a patient, can bolster self-esteem and lead patients to dis-identify with their skin. Group format is conducive to discussions of the effects of diet, radiation, climate, new treatments and so forth. But emotional issues involved in embarrassment, sexual relationship difficulties and lack of understanding are also aired. One group follow-up assessment three months after the group ended showed reduction of medication, shame and shyness, and improvements in interpersonal skills and overall well-being.[17] The importance of the dual leadership is stressed. This format appears to be a useful model that practitioners of natural medicine could employ for a variety of patient sets where the social impact of the disease is a factor in overall well-being.

Rheumatoid Arthritis[18]

Rheumatoid arthritis (RhA) is a chronic inflammatory disorder characterized by swelling and stiffening of the joints, accompanied by moderate to severe pain. Some (about 15 percent) patients recover within two years after relatively mild symptomatology. A second group of patients (another 15 percent), despite medication, progress to destruction and deformity of joints. The remaining 70 percent experience unpredictable ups and downs in symptomatology with a slow, fluctuating progression to disability. Almost 60 percent of patients are obliged to quit working by 10 years after disease onset (Young, 1992). Although the most salient symptoms are in the joints, inflammation often extends to other bodily systems, indicating the systemic nature of RhA. The condition has no known cause nor cure at this time, although it is generally classed, along with a number of other chronic diseases (Crohn's disease, ulcerative colitis, multiple sclerosis, systemic lupus erythematosus, juvenile diabetes, Grave's disease and possibly polymyositis) as an auto-immune disease. RhA affects about 1 percent of the population, most commonly striking between ages 20-49, with women predominating 3 to 1 at the younger ages of onset, becoming equally common in men and women in older age.

Allopathic treatment typically begins initially with non-steroidal anti-inflammatory pain killers (aspirin, ibuprofen). At the same time slow-acting (2 to 6 mo.) agents (gold compounds, penicillinamine) are prescribed that do not affect pain or inflammation but in a sizable percentage of patients suppress the disease process. Corticosteroids (prednisone) are often administered for short-term relief, although they do not appear to affect the long-term course of this disease. All these and newer experimental drugs have serious side effects, and some (gold, penicillamine) are highly toxic. These side effects, along with the ineffectiveness of the drugs in many cases, may be one reason why patient adherence to drug therapy is poor (Young, 1992).

Psychophysiology. It has been suggested that chronically inhibited anger may lead, in individuals biologically so predisposed, to higher muscle tension at the joints. This increased joint pressure could in turn lead eventually to pain and inflammation (Solomon, 1970). In fact, RhA patients do have unusually high muscle tension in muscles traversing their affected joints, but quite possibly this is the *result* of the joint pain rather than its cause.

The fact that RhA is a systemic disease suggests a more central etiological mechanism, specifically a central immune deficiency. We know (see Chapter 4) that stress in the form of depression, anxiety and other prolonged negative emotions can lead to reductions in immune function, but the exact pathways between any possible stress input and manifestation of autoimmune activity at synovial tissue remains highly speculative. Again, we have the strange anomaly seen in asthma that the substances used to control symptoms (e.g., hydrocortisone) are the very ones released in stress which cause immuno-suppression, and should therefore exacerbate the disease if it is due to relative immunological incompetence.

Personality. Early work (Solomon, 1970) spoke of the arthritic as overtly calm and composed, rarely if ever expressing or feeling anger. Rorschach ink blot personality interpretations described arthritics as defective in emotional responsivity and with constricted personalities. The personality data are, however, complicated by the possibility that there might be two distinct classes of RhA patients.[19] In one type the onset is rapid, there is no hereditary predisposition, symptoms are associated with a psychological conflict, and there is a non-expressive constrictive personality. In a second type of RhA the onset is insidious, there is a positive family history, stress links are absent and the personality is healthy. In an ingenious attempt to circumvent the problem of interpretation associated with retrospective studies where the status of traits as causes or effects cannot be disentangled, Solomon (1976) obtained descriptions of RhA patients from their healthy siblings:

Siblings tended to utilize negatively toned descriptive phrases in describing what the patients were like as children, i.e., before the onset of arthritis. For example, phrases such as "poor little girl," "always felt inferior," "was told she was homely," was "sickly and inactive," "was shy, worried and lazy," etc., were generally used by the sibling in describing the patient as a child. [Such phrases] *were hardly ever used in the patient's description of what their siblings were like as children.*[20] [italics added]

Despite this suggestive early work, more recent studies with control groups and standardized personality trait tests have failed to find reliable evidence of an "arthritic personality." In one study, personality scores of patients with multiple sclerosis, gastric ulcers and lower back pain were compared with RhA. The four patient populations were essentially similar, suggesting that any personality traits seen in arthritis are indicative of a "chronic disease personality" probably induced by adapting *to* the disease rather than a causal factor in its onset. This is borne out by data showing, as you might expect, that the longer a person has arthritis, the more psychological disturbance in personality (Anderson et al., 1985).

Once again we are left with the feeling that either the older literature claiming specific personality traits resulted from investigator bias and projection, or that the modern standardized tests are simply not subtle enough to capture the features that the early impressionistic case studies alleged to find. Of course, these standardized psychological tests are far from flawless as measuring devices, sometimes indicating dysfunction when it may be absent. For instance, depression inventories that typically include questions concerning fatigue and sleep disruption are inadequate to measure a psychological depression in RhA, since such items merely indicate primary effects of joint pain, certainly not psychogenic depression.

Psychological Stress. Because most patients with RhA have a slow, insidious onset with fatigue and malaise months before noticing joint symptoms, it is often not easy for patients to associate significant recent life events with the illness. In two studies of juvenile RhA patients, significant life event scores were considerably greater than those of matched control subjects. Parental divorce, separation or death, and sibling birth were identified as key life events prior to onset of juvenile RhA (Anderson et al., 1985). There is some suggestion that stress (e.g., marital discord) may exacerbate symptoms in RhA patients, but on the whole the stress literature in relation to RhA is not robust. Indeed, consistent stress links would be hard to find if RhA is not a single disease entity, but rather reflects a similar phenotypic expression of several diseases with different etiologies.[21] Once again, *caveat docere:* view each case individually.

Psychotherapy/Behavioral Therapy. Since it is only relatively recently that health psychologists and clinicians in behavioral medicine have begun to liaise closely with rheumatologists, there are as yet few methodologically sound studies of psychologically-oriented treatment in the disease (Young, 1992). Rather, psychologists have focused on helping RhA patients to develop skills to cope with their pain, disability and discouragement. A variety of cognitive-behavior treatment packages involving stress inoculation techniques and pain management strategies has proven effective (Young, 1992) in producing beneficial changes in patients' pain levels, mood states and in countering feelings of helplessness. Occasionally, such packages can produce improvements in functional impairment along with positive changes in immune status.[22]

Special Operant Consequences. The principal consequences of chronic progressive RhA are increasing pain, disability, dependence on others, social isolation and economic deprivation. All these have the potential for seriously undermining the individual's quality of life. It's important for the practitioner of natural medicine to be aware that cognitive-behavioral programs for arthritics exist in many cities so that the question of concurrent treatment can be considered by the patient-practitioner team. Since disability is the main predictor for depression in this disease, psychological coping strategies that optimize the individual's ability to manage effectively should be considered.

Project 10

Designing a Patient Support Group

The reader is invited to design a patient support group for a specific chronic syndrome or disease. Assume yourself to be a practitioner with a number of such patients, and imagine yourself to be co-leading your group on a regular basis with one of your long-term patients who can openly share the challenges and management of this illness with other, newer patients.

The design of the group might include such considerations as the format (discussion, lecture-based, psycho-educative, etc.), how much group process would be encouraged, optimal time scheduling of meetings, what distinctive conceptual and practical tools might be used to work with the special problems inherent in that syndrome, and so forth.

It may also be helpful to note the expected benefits and limitations, what sort of patient is likely to find such a group of value, and for how long the average patient would attend.

11

Psychological Aspects of Common Syndromes (PART 2)

The name of the disease is of no concern to the physician.

—SAMUEL HAHNEMANN

Headache[1]

*M*IGRAINE AND MUSCLE contraction headaches are among the most common ailments known to humankind. Muscle contraction headaches have generally been regarded as the result of head and neck muscle tension. Pain occurs in forehead, temples or back of the head and neck. The pain is usually felt on both sides of the head and described as hat band-like, tight or vise-like. These tension headaches have a duration of hours or days and often disrupt sleep. Migraine headaches generally do not disturb sleep, show a positive family history and are thought to be of vascular origin. They are usually one-sided. Migraines are classified into three categories: classical (10%), common (85%) or cluster (5%). In classical migraine there is a sharply defined prodrome (aura) consisting of visual disturbances (e.g., scintillating zigzag lines, flashes of light, blurred vision), dizziness and transient aphasia in the hour before the onset of pain. The attack then follows with moderate to severe head pain of a throbbing quality, often accompanied by nausea and vomiting, confusion, tearing from one eye and extreme sensitivity to light and sound. Normal activities are disrupted in these attacks, which typically occur with a frequency of 1-4 attacks per month and last from 4-24 hours (7 hours average). In common migraine there is no prodrome, the average duration is longer and the pain may switch sides during the attack. The relatively rare cluster migraine also has no preceding aura; the severe pain is shorter (20-60 minutes) but occurs as often as 1-2 times a day, continuing over a period of 2-3 months. Then, as suddenly as they appeared, the cluster attacks inexplicably disappear for 1-2 years.

193

Migraine was clearly described in an Egyptian papyrus dated 1550 B.C. and its prevalence in Britain may be as high as 20 percent for women and somewhat less for men (Adams et al., 1980). By age 7 as many as one percent of school children may suffer from migraine that began as early as age four. Headache in general has a prevalence only exceeded by the common cold. About 35 percent of headache sufferers experience *both* migraine and muscle contraction headaches, and some people have difficulty telling which type they have, indicating that the diagnostic categories are not as neat as they might appear.

In a considerable proportion of migraine cases foods and additives (chocolate, cheese, oranges, onions, tea, pork, fats, monosodium glutamate, sodium nitrates), alcohol (especially red wine), flickering lights or television can elicit attacks. Migraines are also influenced (adversely) by oral contraceptives and in many women they bear a relation to the menstrual cycle. Pregnancy often temporarily abolishes migraine.

Ergot alkaloids administered promptly at onset of an attack can abort a migraine in many patients, but the drugs have no prophylactic use and are open to abuse. In cases that do not respond to ergotamine tartarate, beta blockers (usually for prevention) or amitriptyline are employed. Methylsergide, which inhibits brain serotonin, reduces frequency of attacks but can be quite toxic. Tension headaches are self-treated with over-the-counter analgesics or amitriptyline in severe cases. Habitual use of these analgesics (e.g., six or more aspirins a day) to relieve headache creates a vicious circle that actually increases the frequency of headaches.

Psychophysiology. Migraine headaches are associated with vascular changes in the intra- and extracranial arteries. During the prodrome phase these arteries constrict, instigating localized reductions of as much as 20 percent in cerebral blood flow to both hemispheres. At a certain point a reflex vasodilation rebound occurs in cerebral arteries, which is associated with the onset of the actual attack and pain. It has been suggested that this rebound is the result of the release of the neurochemical serotonin from blood platelets during the preceding vasoconstrictive phase. Migraineurs may exhibit greater reactivity in the vascular system, particularly in the temporal arteries. Since it is known that the response to aversive stimuli (physical and psychological) is vasoconstriction, the actual attacks would fit the concept of a stress rebound effect. Psychological factors, such as unexpressed anger, could create an over-reactive cephalic vasomotor system which eventually, in constitutionally susceptible individuals, could become dysfunctional. At present the contributions of such mechanisms is plausible but hypothetical. As for muscle contraction headaches, the usual cause is supposedly "tension," although it is generally not clear whether this is physical or emotional tension. In any case a search for increased tension in cephalic or neck muscles during these headaches has proven negative and a newer theory is that the pain is a delayed result of a build-up of fluid edema produced by frequent and intense use of these muscles.[2] This explains how a tension-filled day of work could produce a headache later that evening while the individual was relaxed at home.

Personality. As early as 1743 the cause of migraine was attributed to anger, especially when tacit and suppressed, and to this supposed cause the psychosomatic psychoanalysts added compulsive, rigid, perfectionistic, ambitious, competitive personality traits. By the 1970s it was becoming clear that many migraineurs could not be typed in this way and that the neuroticism often measured in headache patients was probably "a consequence of the risks of sudden intense pain or of adaptation to being a patient" (Packhard, 1987), with, it should be added, a condition highly refractory to the best that modern medicine had to offer. Muscle contraction headaches have been attributed to repressed hostility, tension anxiety, depression and sexual conflicts. In fact, modern research finds little if any personality differences distinguishing the two headache classes. Once again, the current conclusion is that there does not seem to be any clear personality type or profile associated with migraine.

Stress Links. A retrospective study of several hundred cases of unilateral headache found that in 67 percent of the cases, emotions (broadly defined) were implicated in instigating the onset of head pain. On the other hand it is still unclear how stress provokes migraine and why some attacks occur considerably after a period of prolonged stress, and not during the actual period of stress. The general consensus is that muscular contraction headaches are *ipso facto* stress headaches; indeed, that is another name for them. However their relation to experienced distress or significant life events is far from a simple one-to-one relation.

Psychotherapy/Behavioral Therapy. Due to limited effectiveness of drugs and the long-term property of analgesics to make headaches worse, headache patients are increasingly referred for psychological treatment. Behavior therapy in the form of progressive muscle relaxation, hypnotherapy, meditation and various forms of biofeedback plays a prominent role in psychological headache treatment, and these treatments are a typical part of the armamentarium of headache clinics. Conversely, client-centered or psychodynamic therapy seems less effective. Cognitive stress coping therapy, including assertive training, seems of value for tension headache, but perhaps of little or no value for migraine.[3]

Biofeedback for migraine headache is based on the theory that hand warming can result in peripheral vasomotor dilation. In contrast, biofeedback for muscle contraction headaches works by inducing reductions in frontalis forehead muscle tension, measured by decreases in electromyographic (EMG) resistance in this muscle.[4] Migraineurs who are able to learn to raise hand temperature to at least 95°F and patients with muscle contraction headaches who can reduce EMG tension in frontalis muscle show clinically significant reductions in severity and frequency of headache. The results are even better when these biofeedback techniques are supplemented with relaxation exercises. Follow-ups ranging up to five years show the majority of improved cases holding their therapeutic gains. These results are usefully contrasted to a control group of other headache sufferers who kept a headache diary but did not participate in biofeedback and showed essentially no improvement in symptomatology after three years (Blanchard, 1992). Overall the behavioral treatments are at least as effective as medications, and of course have no deleterious side effects.

Because the pain of headache is a purely subjective phenomenon and cannot be measured in the same way as airways resistance in asthma, degree of skin lesion in eczema, joint damage in RhA or even diarrhea in IBS, a daily headache diary monitoring self-reports of time, frequency, duration and intensity of pain is invaluable in work with headache patients. The diary allows both practitioner and patient to pick up the stress triggers (food, climate, situational, emotional) and to monitor the beneficial effects of the therapeutics.

The initial work with biofeedback in headache was carried out in clinics, but with the development of portable inexpensive electronic devices, patients today may have minimal contact with the clinic and may carry out their own biofeedback training at home with instructional audiotapes and training manuals. Provided that patient motivation can be sustained, the results from minimal therapist contact seem surprisingly good (Blanchard, 1992). The effectiveness of the two types of biofeedback described above, hypnotherapy and progressive muscle relaxation may well boil down to the common denominator that in each one the patient is learning how to relax. Yet another possibility is that all these procedures act to enhance endorphin production in the brain, known to be low at the time of an attack. However, there are two caveats to the generally impressive value of psycho- and behavioral therapy in headache. The first is that menstrual-related migraine may be more resistant to these behavioral interventions. The second is that there is *no* indication to date that *any* of these techniques has utility in cluster migraine, which remains refractory to all known psychobehavioral treatments.

Case Study. As there are no data related to the special consequences of headache, an illustrative case study is provided (see box).

Support Groups. The value of a support group for particular illnesses is increasingly being recognized. Every illness has its own special challenges and social impacts, and patients can learn from each other's experiences. Some of the benefits include (1) realizing that one is not alone; (2) discovering that there are others who care and understand their feelings; (3) learning new ways of coping; and (4) changing the power balance with physicians to gain the status of equal partners in the therapeutic enterprise. Many of these are the same functions that individual psychotherapy serves (see Chapter 8). In addition to these personal aspects, the group may also provide members with the latest medical/behavioral resources about their illness, bring them into contact with others experiencing the same ordeal, and increase public awareness of the distinctive problems undergone by sufferers in this condition.

Patient-led support groups for headache suffers have proven of considerable value.[6] These groups are typically led by lay members who first receive training by experienced support group leaders. A manual for facilitators has been developed and the leaders meet periodically to share problems and to receive further training. Groups

Case Study: Tension Headache Therapy[5]

Linda, a 10-year-old girl, is referred for behavior therapy by her family doctor because of headache complaints that have become much more serious during the past six months. The headache is felt like a tight band around the head, is of a pricking and stinging nature, and is almost permanently present, but in particular at the end of the afternoon. Once or twice a week the headache is so bad that Linda has to miss school. Apart from this headache, which has to be described as tension headache, Linda suffers from migraine accompanied by nausea and vomiting about once every six months. Linda also has problems going to sleep.

There are no apparent psychological problems. The therapy starts with relaxation and EMG biofeedback training of the facial muscles. Linda cooperates enthusiastically. After 10 sessions during a period of three months the headache has been reduced from some 21 to 10 mornings-afternoons-evenings per week. Linda does not have to miss school and hardly takes drugs anymore.

Meanwhile it has appeared from the headache diary, and from conversations with Linda and her parents, that there are some problems between Linda and her brother. In the following period various situations are gone through in the form of role playing, in which Linda learns to make clear to her brother calmly but resolutely what she wants, what she does not want, and what she finds annoying about him.

It appears also that Linda finds it hard to tolerate insecurity. To improve this situation, Linda undertakes cognitive therapy exercises, during which she is connected to an apparatus that measures the tension of the frontal facial muscle. She calls the particular situation into mind and replaces any insecure thoughts by positive self-affirmations. She reduces any increase in muscular tension by means of images she finds pleasant, like walking in a wood and feeding the squirrels.

From now on the headaches disappear completely. At follow-up one year after the therapy has ended, the improvement has been maintained.

meet monthly with typically about 15 members attending. Some of these groups produce self-funded newsletters containing articles by sufferers and professionals. Headache support organizations arose out of a desire to provide information, education and support to headache sufferers. But they also serve to increase public awareness about the impact of headaches on everyday functioning and to improve understanding among family, employees and—please take note—physicians. Thus, these grassroots groups serve an invaluable educative and advocacy role for their particular illness syndrome.

Chronic Fatigue Syndrome

Chronic fatigue syndrome (CFS) refers to a heterogeneous cluster of physical symptoms generally developing out of an acute viral illness (colds, influenza, glandular fever, infectious mononucleosis) that fails for unknown reasons to resolve normally.

Although the condition may not be new, its relatively recent appearance (or reappearance) in near-epidemic proportions, combined with no conclusive agreement as to either its etiology or pathogenesis, accounts for the wide variety of names currently given it: Icelandic disease, myalgic encephalomylitis (ME), chronic fatigue immune deficiency disease (CFIDS), Royal Free disease, post-viral fatigue, chronic Epstein-Barr infection and post-infective neurasthenia. The cardinal symptom is persisting or relapsing debilitating fatigue or easy fatiguability that has persisted for at least six months and does not resolve with bed rest, is aggravated by exercise and is severe enough to reduce average daily activity 50 percent or more.[7] In addition, and possibly pathogenomic, CFS sufferers feel sick with flu-like symptoms for months or even years.

The systemic nature of true CFS is suggested by the widespread effects seen throughout the body which vary from case to case but typically include muscle and joint pain and/or stiffness, disturbed sleep patterns, hypersensitivity to light, sound, heat and cold, impairment in short-term and associative memory and concentration. Naturally, the ability to perform tasks and make decisions based on these latter intellectual functions is also disrupted, sometimes severely. Impairment can be measured by the degree of deficit in the ability to perform mental arithmetic. Other common symptoms are chronic low grade fever, sore throat, lymph node pain, headaches, multiple allergies, cardiovascular disturbances (palpitations, low blood pressure) and digestive difficulties reminiscent of IBS. Depression is common. CFS ranges from relatively mild to severely disabling. Women predominate in a ratio of about 60/40. There is no known cause or cure at this writing. About 50 percent of patients spontaneously improve by two years, and a further 50 percent of the remainder are significantly better by four years after onset, leaving about 25 percent who drag on unimproved or with frequent relapses for years.[8] To date, despite the severity of many CFS cases, laboratory blood diagnostics are typically normal, muscle tests are negative and no somatic lesions are detectable that could account for the symptom picture. There is, however, a widespread belief that CFS is a viral disease and in fact a majority of patients do show an elevated titer of enteroviral protein VP1 factor, but the significance of this is not yet established. There are serious difficulties in attempting to separate out true CFS from other disorders in which fatigue is the prominent symptom. At any one time about one-fifth of the population consider themselves chronically fatigued,[9] but the causes are so variable that fatigue in itself can never be diagnostic. In particular hypoglycemia, candida and psychoneurotic depression can present with many of the symptoms of CFS.

Allopathic treatment is variable since as late as 1991 two-thirds of general practitioners stated that they did not believe there is any such syndrome,[10] reflecting their opinion that because laboratory tests have so far yielded no conclusive evidence of tissue pathology or infective agent, CFS is not an authentic disease. CFS patients are generally offered tricyclic anti-depressants, which in some cases can improve mood and insomnia without altering the course of the disease; in many others, however, anti-depressants can actually worsen the flu-like symptomatology. A large proportion of sufferers refuse psychotropic medication on the grounds that they do not consider themselves (rightfully, as we shall see) suffering from a psychiatric disorder. Prolonged rest seems to be the only well-documented treatment of consistent value,[11] although many doctors oppose it as habit-forming.

Psychophysiology. In its opportunistic attacking of many body systems the syndrome resembles a kind of "benign" AIDS; but unlike AIDS, the effects, although prolonged and debilitating, are usually reversible and self-limiting, and in any case do not have a terminal progression. Many of the symptoms would appear to be compatible with immunosuppression, while others imply hypothalamic and cortical dysfunction. Be that as it may, to date no definitive pathogenesis has been demonstrated. The most widely held hypothesis of those who see CFS as authentic disease is that it is viral based. The pathogen may, however, not be a new virus. Rather—for reasons that are currently unclear—common viruses that are normally confined to the upper respiratory tract may make their way to deeper places in the body (e.g., the gut) from which focus they resist attempts by the immune system to eliminate them.

To the extent that stress could play a role in the onset or maintenance of CFS, it presumably acts to predispose the constitutionally susceptible individual to colds, influenzas and mononucleosis. Thereafter, personality factors could be influential in those individuals who neglect the proper care of the primary viral infection by continuing to work in the face of obvious illness, neglecting diet and sufficient rest. Such injudicious behavior, hampering normal resolution, could eventually permit the viral agent to move from benign (upper respiratory) sites to central organs such as gut, liver, heart and brain. Central neural disturbances in the pituitary could compromise the adrenals, thereby impairing immune function itself. However, until the pathogenic pathways in CFS become clearer, this account must be taken as speculative.

Personality. In 1869 the American neurologist George Beard introduced the term *neurasthenia* (nerve weakness) to refer to a complex of symptoms, with fatiguability as its central defining element, that either closely resembles or is identical to CFS.[12] Reading Beard's descriptions of neurasthenia, a diagnosis that had virtually disappeared by mid-twentieth century, is like a *déjà vu* experience, so accurately did he describe the numerous weird and bizarre symptoms that have reappeared in recent literature as CFS/ME. Beard thought of neurasthenia as a "burn out" disease. When an individual "who is driven to think, to work, to strive for success presses himself and his life force to the limit, he eventually exhausts his circuits like an overloaded battery."[13] Over 100 years later this same personality pattern lurks behind the term of opprobrium, "yuppie flu." The CFS patient may be not so much an over-achiever as an individual with a strong sense of loyalty, dedication and commitment who remains over-long in taxing and highly responsible work situations without taking appropriate rest or periodic vacations to restore the body's vigor. Such a personality pattern would help explain why both in Victorian times and today this disease has a high prevalence amongst doctors, teachers, nurses and in general those with great responsibilities to others.

Just as neurasthenia originally represented a sharply specific syndrome with a presumed organic basis, but as time went on became a dumping ground for unexplained fatigue of any origin, so too CFS is in danger of being confused with fatigue states of all kinds and etiologies. If there are distinctive personality patterns associated with CFS they will be very difficult to extract if the syndrome is carelessly applied beyond its clearly-defined limits. Beard proposed neurasthenia as an organic disease whose neurophysiological pathogenesis would eventually be discovered. The failure of medical science to find the putative pathology meant that inevitably unexplained fatigue symptoms from a variety of causes got thrown into the wastebasket of neurasthenia, with a consequent degrading of the original diagnostic category. A similar muddying is likely to occur in CFS if the organic basis continues to elude virologists and immunologists, and if practitioners fail to distinguish fatigue symptomatology on the basis of its etiology. The holistic practitioner is less likely to do this, given his wide psychobiosocial focus, but there certainly are borderline cases where it is difficult to tell true CFS from psychogenic depression, candida or hypoglycemia. In doubtful cases it is best to err on the side of caution, since the failure to rest in the early stages of CFS is probably what contributes to its lengthy duration.

Considering the diagnostic difficulties, it is hardly surprising that at present there are no systematic studies of personality traits in CFS beyond reports showing that about half the patients are depressed.[14] As in the other disease syndromes considered in this chapter, cause and effect are muddled, but especially so in CFS, for not only is viral depression a primary symptom of the original influenza or mononucleosis, but the loss of mobility, income, personal relationships and overall quality of life in CFS creates the conditions for secondary illness-related depression. Craig noted in 1912 that depression was a common side effect of neurasthenia, but he was clear that the depression was phenomenologically different from the major psychiatric depressive disorders then called melancholia:

> The depression of neurasthenia is at times mistaken for that of melancholia, but this should not occur as the whole history is different and even the nature of the depression varies.[15]

Depression is a familiar direct and *primary* outcome of many organic disorders, including multiple sclerosis, Parkinson's disease and Cushing's syndrome. It also goes along with shingles, influenza, mononucleosis, hepatitis and many cases of hypothyroidism, resolving only when the disease resolves.[16] Moreover, the actual assessment of depression in CFS is fraught with methodological difficulties since the depression tests (e.g., Beck's Depression Inventory) use sleep disruption, loss of libido, anorexia—not to mention fatigue itself—as measures of depression. But these are all primary *effects* of CFS, not its cause.

Psychotherapy/Behavioral Therapy. The earliest effective behavioral therapy for neurasthenia was the "Rest Cure" developed by Beard's colleague, S. Weir Mitchell, which entailed several weeks of absolute bed rest.[17] For a time in the last century the rest cure was extremely popular and resulted in numerous cures. But eventually disillusionment set in as critics pointed to patients who rested months and even years but did not achieve beneficial results. Of course this would be quite what would be expected if, as was happening, neurasthenia was becoming a wastebasket diagnostic category for fatigue cases of varying etiologies. Rest would have been valuable only for those closely fitting Beard's original description of the disorder that includes not simply fatigue, but the etiology of "burn out." Conversely, rest would be contraindicated for cases where the fatigue was a consequence of other psychosocial causes such as disappointment in love, failed examinations, death of a spouse, financial ruin or unfulfilled creative potential.

When CFS (post-infectious neurasthenia) is viewed as a depressive disorder (e.g., Greenberg, 1990; Wessely, 1990), extraordinarily inappropriate behavioral therapy may be suggested in which patients are encouraged to get back into their normal daily activity despite symptomatology.[18] The CFS patient-support literature, as well as accounts written by practitioners suffering from the illness (Shepherd, 1989; MacIntyre, 1989; Millenson, 1992), make it very clear that pushing oneself is a prescription for delaying or perhaps preventing recovery. True CFS patients do not use rest to avoid responsibilities, neither today (Shepherd, 1989) nor 120 years ago (Craig, 1912).

Probably the most useful supportive counseling for sufferers is given by those who have had the illness and by caregivers who know its special characteristics extremely well. Education about the illness, its likely relation to overwork, and the provision of a safe, undemanding climate for the sufferer to rest without any traces of guilt or a sense that she must rush back to work at the first sign of improvement, is invaluable. On the other hand, psychotherapy that focuses on the depressive symptoms, failing to realize that these are the primary and secondary consequences of the illness and *not* its cause, can do more harm than good.

Special Consequences. Although half or more CFS patients associate a viral illness with the onset of their syndrome, there are others in whom the typical symptoms develop insidiously in the absence of any prior manifest infection. Because laboratory tests have so far not conclusively revealed the organic basis for CFS, this illness challenges our Western conceptions of the relation between disease and illness. In particular, CFS superficially fits the description of the psychiatric category of *somatization:* complaints of physical symptoms that either lack demonstrable organic basis or are judged to be grossly in excess of what would be expected on the grounds of objective medical findings.[19] Since depression—more accurately *demoralization* or *despondency*—is a frequent concomitant of CFS, an uncritical analysis by those who are not closely familiar with CFS can well conclude that CFS is nothing more than depressive psychiatric disorder.

Thus, one major consequence of this illness at this time is that patients are in serious danger of being misdiagnosed with psychiatric disease and treated (and stigmatized) inappropriately. The treatment for psychogenic depression consists of psychotropic drugs (antidepressants), minor and major tranquilizers, electro-convulsive shock and psychotherapy. These are highly inappropriate for CFS patients, whose principal current stressor, regardless of the original etiology, is a debilitating illness for which there is no cure, with an unknown course and uncertain prognosis, and which has radically disrupted every aspect of their lives. The end of the illness ends their depression. Many prominent sufferers have been physicians themselves, and they have spoken out forcefully against the psychiatric interpretation of CFS. Their publications, along with the strong political efforts of self-help support organizations world-wide, have been the major deterrents to turning CFS into the eighth holy psychosomatic disease with all the fallacious reasoning behind psychogenesis (see Chapter 9). Unfortunately, CFS sufferers are still subject to the skepticism of doctors, denial of disability benefits and lack of sympathy from employers and even family members.

Support Groups. Because mainstream medicine has been very slow to recognize CFS as an authentic disease, CFS support groups world-wide have been a major force in collecting information about the syndrome, encouraging research and evaluating treatments. These groups, similar in format to the headache support groups described above, have worked successfully, and against considerable resistance from establishment medicine, for patients' rights, e.g., disability status in severe cases and the recognition of CFS as an authentic disease. A few practitioners using specialized treatments (megavitamin therapies, colonic irrigation) have run their own patient groups. Since CFS patients have both physical weaknesses as well as mental confusion, and are still subject to suspicion and stigma, and because the uncertain recovery can be very long, punctuated by demoralizing relapses, practitioner-led support groups should be very valuable in this syndrome.

General Conclusions from the Six Syndromes

If we step back from our attempt at a detailed analysis of the psychological features of these six illness syndromes and try to assess common themes, pick out durable generalizations and catalog techniques for general use, we find a sketchy and confusing tapestry indeed. The scientific literature leaves the impression that this is a field still in a very rudimentary state of development. Our knowledge is limited in even the best-studied illnesses, valid generalization are few and far between, and there are many conflicting reports and contradictory theories. The few solid generalizations seem to be negative: older reports of specific personality profiles for these syndromes have *not* been confirmed, stress *cannot* be unequivocally pinpointed in the etiology of any of them, and personality differences that do exist between patients and healthy people *cannot* be disentangled from the effects of having a chronic disabling, painful, intractable, physically and socially limiting disease.

And yet, running through every syndrome, there appears therapeutic value in one or more psycho-behavioral therapies, broadly conceived. Thus, IBS can be considerably ameliorated by stress-reduction programs and psychotherapy; asthmatics showed beneficial effects from long-term group therapy and from behavioral techniques for managing behaviors that exacerbate attacks; headaches respond better to biofeedback with progressive muscle relaxation than to drugs. Arthritics respond positively to behavior modification pain programs; the anxiety, shame and embarrassment that eczema and psoriasis patients feel in relation to how others judge their disfiguring lesions can be alleviated by individual and group psychotherapy, which encourage self-esteem and independence from others' judgments. Patient support groups serve many of the functions of psychotherapy for CFS sufferers, buffering the severe social consequences of sudden, unexpected disability and promoting the one therapy of proven value for this condition: rest. Finally, simple monitoring devices such as patient self-report diaries have value in a variety of syndromes.

The difficulties in confirming the earlier psychosomatic psychoanalytic theories of personality in specific diseases have led researchers to move away from efforts to find psychological factors in illness etiology and towards identifying behavioral consequences of particular illnesses. This development, while commendable in that behavioral modification programs can indeed alleviate some of the worst aspects of a chronic debilitating illness, is probably not independent of the allopathic framework in which these chronic diseases are set, and in which their research takes place. Because these syndromes are regarded to be "of unknown etiology with no known cure," the focus of allopathic medicine is on their management, not cure. Complementary and alternative medicine takes a much more optimistic view of the six syndromes. Many patients with these disease syndromes respond to dietary and lifestyle changes, others to botanical medicine, still others to physical medicine, and others to a variety of other natural procedures. The evidence for the effectiveness of such natural therapeutics is not always laboratory science, but the patient records of individual practitioners and the handed-down wisdom of the generations embodied in the currently deprecated term, "folk lore." It is not, of course, merely the power of naturopathic techniques and remedies that inspire natural medicine's confidence. Rather it is the holistic medical philosophy that views most illness and disease as the direct consequence of imbalance in the individual's environment, habits and/or way of living (see Chapter 1) that is potentially correctable. Thus an important part of the practitioner's job is detective work: working in close collaboration with the patient in tracking down the pathogenic imbalance, and then with the aid of natural medicines and the patient's own commitment to change, trusting the healing power of nature, *vis medicatrix naturae*, to restore the balance we call health.

Because of the more optimistic view of natural medicine that these six syndromes and other chronic diseases are often in principle reversible, psychological factors in etiology still remain of crucial interest for practitioners in natural medicine. It is therefore very important to understand in what way the scientific evidence we have reviewed here can and cannot limit our perspective on how stress and personality play key roles in the predisposition, precipitation and perpetuation of somatic disease. As was frequently pointed out in the sections above, retrospective research, which looks at personality traits in people who already have an illness, simply lacks *in principle* the resolving power to assess the direction of causation between observed traits and somatic disorder. Similarly, severe methodological difficulties attend the correlating of stressful life events *after* a person has already fallen ill. As for the large scale group studies that have failed to find a specific personality for the specific syndrome, it is important to stress that such findings cannot, *in any individual case,* rule out that a morbid personality factor could have been a key factor in the onset of that particular person's illness. All that the negative group studies can ever show is that, within the limits of the personality tests being employed, no specific trends common to a majority of cases of this syndrome emerge.

The modern work does, on the other hand, go some way towards refuting the more speculative claims of the early psychosomaticists who thought that bowel disturbances were due to obsessive-compulsive personalities, asthma to dependence and insecurity, joint disease to a constrictive character, headaches to suppressed anger, and skin disease to alexithymia. Such views, of course, were the psychosomatic equivalent of the discredited concept of a single, unique cause in medicine for each single, unique disease.

To appreciate the limitations of group studies and the statistics that are used to summarize them, consider a hypothetical study of 20 cases of migraine. Suppose an investigator wants to know if migraine in women has a relation to menstrual cycle. So he makes a study of these 20 patients noting the frequency of headaches at various points in each woman's cycle, and after a few months carrying out repeated observations, discovers that migraines occur at every point in the cycle of this group of 20 women, no one point predominating. The investigator concludes therefore that migraine bears no relation to menstrual cycle and publishes the data and his conclusion in a peer-reviewed medical journal.

Individual women who know quite well that their personal migraines are related to their periods see a newspaper article describing this research and feel puzzled: how can science discover something that they themselves know quite well is wrong? In our twentieth-century Western world, science has the prestige of religion. Nevertheless, the investigator drew a faulty conclusion based on averaging the headaches of 20 different women together, the same kind of averaging that all group studies rely upon. Suppose, for example, that of these 20 women, half of them have headaches which indeed bear no relation to their menstrual cycle. But suppose in the other 10 women that their headaches *do* bear a relation to cycle, but in these 10 it is not the same relation. For some, their migraines tend to come on midcycle, others at the onset of the period, others at the end of the period. Now, although in these 10 women their migraines do definitely bear a relation to their menstrual cycle, the investigator, who did not look closely at the individual cases, failed to find it because he had added up all the data and then further confounded his results by averaging with another 10 cases which in fact had no relation at all to menstrual cycle, and might even represent a different disease with the common symptom of migraine headache.

Thus, stress and personality could be important etiological factors in many of the cases of the six syndromes reviewed, but because each disease category is heterogeneous and contains a family of diseases, related only by certain symptoms that they share in common, group studies will confound different kinds of diseases. Only an individual case-by-case analysis and treatment can reveal whether stress reduction and instilling more healthy personality traits and coping skills will be useful in the particular case under consideration. Primary symptomatology may not be the best predictor of the degree to which a given case is stress-related. The kind of evidence currently in vogue is both too gross (groups of cases lumped together for comparison, thereby obscuring individual differences) on the one hand, and tangential on the other (retrospective depression scores confounded with primary somatic symptomatology, for instance).

It is just this group statistical averaging and obscuring individual differences and combining heterogeneous diseases with similar symptoms (all six syndromes we examined above are prone to this confounding) that has led some scientists to urge that individual cases be studied intensively in the clinical setting. The methodology of studying a single case in great detail, trying different therapeutics selectively, and monitoring the results closely has been available for many years.[20] But medical science has been reluctant to use it extensively, perhaps because such studies would not be "cost-effective," might take much longer to carry out, and probably require considerable intuition and ingenuity. We have to remember that medical research after all is conducted in and supported by an industrialized consumer society that demands quick, cheap and universal solutions that can be standardized for mass production. In the medicine of such a society, practitioners are "providers" and patients are "consumers."

In this light, holistic medicine is far more than just an alternative and complementary set of therapeutics. It represents the holistic voice of dissent within medicine that seeks to redress the imbalances created by our culture's fragmentization and compartmentalization of life. Medical research will not be immune to the holistic critique. And in fact the kind of individual clinical case studies suggested ought to appeal to holistic practitioners who, if nothing else, go deeply into each case following each individual patient very closely, trying various therapeutic regimens until one or a combination or a sequence is found that is effective. Mainstream medicine has complained of the lack of research in alternative medicine, often stigmatizing it as "unscientific," but the funds to do large-scale statistical group studies are rarely available there. On the other hand, single-case research is very much open to the practitioner of natural medicine, requiring only that the symptomatology be measured accurately and reliably, the treatment protocol be described so that anyone else who so wishes can repeat it, and that accurate and complete records be kept of cases and their follow-ups. Unfortunately, practitioners in general often consider their case loads to be so heavy that they are not willing to devote the extra time to such precise symptom-monitoring, record-keeping and systematic follow-up that research requires.

If there is one generalization to take away from our review of six syndromes, it is the great complexity, heterogeneity and subtlety with which psychological factors can enter into somatic disease. It is very definitely time for holistic medicine to go beyond the simple-minded generalization that mind influences the body. Leaving aside the dubious dualism in that oft-repeated truism, let us agree by replying, "Quite so, but how?" Stress and personality can be factors in the etiology of a disease, after which the greatest stress is the dysfunction created by the illness itself. Some illnesses, like IBS, may actually be operantly reinforced. Others may have begun with a trauma or an infection, but then be exacerbated or maintained by personality factors that take over and perpetuate the illness long after the precipitating factor is gone. In other cases the initial factor might well have been stress, but the illness long outlives the initial predisposing stress condition due to new factors arising out of the consequences of being ill. Then too, the temporal relation between stress and illness is not necessarily a simple one. People sometimes get ill *after* the stressor has passed and gone. These are just a few illustrations of the many ways that emotional parameters can enter into the pathogenesis of a disease; in any particular case these psychological aspects could be combined, permuted or interactive.

What we know so far suggests that any given syndrome appears in conjunction with a particular individual's constitutional predisposition to respond to stress in a particular organ system, say with colonic hypermotility, skin hypersensitivity, cephalic artery vasomotor hyperactivity or whatever. Nevertheless, a particular syndrome or cluster of symptoms will always be the result of a variety of contributory factors, subtly different in every case. Clearly, the meaning of one person's asthma or eczema or arthritis may be radically different from another individual suffering from the same syndrome; hence the appropriate therapeutics will differ radically for each of these patients. If this is so, we would best avoid broad generalizations and concentrate on the individual case, being open to the possibility that any of the influences we have discussed in this chapter may be operating. Most of the information we have at present is at best suggestive, serving principally to alert the holistic practitioner to the possibility of subtle stress and personality aspects that must be considered with each syndrome and with each patient.

Project 11

Assessing the Psychological Dimensions of a Syndrome

Select a syndrome not discussed in Chapters 10 or 11, and, after briefly describing the condition, its epidemiology and its usual allopathic management, discuss it in terms of the six dimensions shown in Table 10.1.

This project is likely to benefit from a degree of library research, a skill that every modern practitioner of natural medicine must acquire. Medicine is, after all, an evolving art; new techniques are constantly being developed, and old points of view modified or discarded as their effectiveness is clinically evaluated. Specialized medical libraries have computerized data bases (MEDLINE and PSYCHLIT) that provide abstracts of dozens of articles on any diagnostic category or treatment mode selected. However, most of the articles surveyed are written from the allopathic viewpoint, and others are overly technical for the general practitioner's interests. Nevertheless, learning how to sift the wheat from the chaff, penetrating through medical jargon and bringing what is of value back to the patient is part of complementary medicine's social role of demystifying medicine.

12

The Language of Disease

*The meaning of illness is the warning—do not continue living
as you intend to.*
—GEORG GRODDECK, 1925

*Theories that diseases are caused by mental states and can be
cured by will power are always an index of how much is not
understood about the physical terrain of a disease.*
—SUSAN SONTAG, 1978

Illness has no inherent meaning, but I can make it meaningful.
—DONNA TALMAN, 1991

To SAY THAT disease speaks a language is to imply that disease has a meaning.
In traditional cultures, disease was always viewed meaningfully, usually
falling into one of three categories: (1) punishment for sin, (2) the result of a magic
spell cast by an enemy, or (3) the result of external agents and spirits. In addition,
many indigenous peoples believe that illness is caused by "loss of soul," and one of the
shaman's main tasks is to undertake a journey to the "other" world to search for the
soul of the sick person, and to bring it back. The shaman's training—through psychotropic drugs, sleep and food deprivation, dream analysis and hypnotic induction—
is designed to produce altered states of consciousness and out-of-body experiences
so that he becomes familiar with the geography, rules and dangers of the territory.[1]
Through ritual magic, spells and incantations the shaman exorcises evil spirits lodged
in the body, propitiates the gods demanding punishment who may require sacrifices,
and dispels the demons invoked by the jealousy and malice of an aggrieved third
party. Like the wise witches of medieval Europe, shamans are frequently skilled in the
use of medicinal plants, healing clay poultices, and are able to set bones and give hands-
on healing.

What are we to make of all of this? Our scientific world view relegates such tra-ditional notions of disease and healing to the realm of fantasy and superstition. Armed with the magic bullets of modern drugs, medical science sallies out to do battle with the forces of disease conceived of as invaders from without, alien bacteria, viruses and other microbes which, finding our weakest genetic organ, are bent on our destruction. This is not a medicine that seems to require meaning from our illnesses. Any mean-ing that is to be found for symptomatology is explained simply by the nature of the pathological process that creates the dysfunction we call the signs and symptoms of the disease. The disease itself is considered to be a random event, determined by the chance virulence of the infectious agent and our inherited constitution. This Western scientific view of disease, however, has been increasingly forced to give ground in the face of chronic degenerative and autoimmune disease which fit this model poorly, and by the overwhelming evidence summarized throughout this volume that stress, emotional factors and lifestyle are as much risk factors in disease as are the external infectious vectors.

Nevertheless, extending the causes of illness to the broader psychobiosocial framework of health and disease does not in itself imply that disease has any inherent meaning beyond that implicit in the wide-angled lens of holistic analysis. Even the shamanistic world view could be conceptualized in an expanded holistic framework. For instance, prolonged unresolved guilt arising out of a socially or morally disap-proved action is a powerful negative emotion, and as such a reliable indicator of stress, with all that that implies for the likelihood of a weakened immune system and the development of a psychophysiological disorder. The holistic practitioner, in employ-ing psychotherapeutic techniques of psychodrama, catharsis, hypnosis, active listen-ing, unconditional acceptance and so forth, might be said to be practicing something akin to some of the rituals used by shamans. Even the magic potions designed to root out demons find their equivalent in the doctor's placebo, well known to every practi-tioner. And the idea that illness can be a punishment for sin is taken for granted in minor complaints, for it is not just the child who makes itself sick from gorging on rich food or bingeing on chocolate cake and ice cream. We are accustomed to accept-ing a headcold or even the flu as possible consequences of going out into the rain without our umbrella, or letting ourselves get "run down." True, these are only minor peccadilloes, but the idea that more serious sins could bring on more serious illnesses is not foreign to a scientific framework that strips the word "sin" of its moral judg-ment and merely documents the empirical consequences to health that come from "violating the laws of nature."[2]

But meaning in illness goes deeper and is not exhausted by these attempts to reconcile it into the framework of cause and effect that we have, until now, relied upon. Meaning in illness cannot finally be divorced from the shaman's fourth great causal realm, "loss of soul." Loss of soul means to lose contact with the thread and purpose of our life, to stray from the path of inner harmony that is right and true for each one of us as individuals, to violate our own inherent nature. However complex, changeable and dimly illuminated that nature might be, ultimately its reality is sketched out by what proves harmonious or inharmonious to us in the day-to-day living of our lives. To delve into the meaning of an illness is to step inevitably into the realm of life's purpose, to question the existence and nature of a higher Self that somehow is trying to manifest through us.

Seen from this perspective, much disease represents a signal that we are off the trajectory of self-harmony, or that we as a collective species are off the path of harmony with the greater whole, which includes our social and physical environment, the planet Gaia herself. In exploring possible meanings of illness, and in examining attempts to decode the language of disease, we enter into a realm beyond science. This realm is not necessarily unscientific, for the philosophy of today is the source of the science of tomorrow. But this is certainly not an area where controlled experiments with double-blind groups testing meaning A, meaning B and no-meaning for diseases X and Y are going to have relevance. On the other hand, individual case histories frequently seem to reveal compelling psychospiritual disharmonies in patients' personal lives which, when addressed, prove beneficial in healing.[3] But because symbolic meanings discovered in patients' deep work remain unique and idiosyncratic, impossible to generalize across disease categories and different patients, we must not expect the development of a consistent dictionary of meanings for illnesses. The three quotations that open this chapter capture the spectrum of opinion about interpreting disease at a symbolic or psychospiritual level, and each quote is as valid as the other. Meaning is what you make of it.

But why should the practitioner of holistic medicine try to make anything of it? In fact there are three very good reasons to do so: (1) meaning is frequently valuable in the diagnosis and prognosis of a disease; (2) finding a meaning in an illness can prove to be an empowering source of hope and optimism for the patient; (3) interpretations in the form of possible life disharmonies suggest novel places to look for the causes of illness, namely in how some fundamental physical, emotional or spiritual needs of the patient are not being fulfilled.

Historical Precursors

Although one can find provocative hints of meaning attributed to illness in the writings of Hippocrates, Galen, the twelfth-century mystic physician Hildegaard of Bingen, Paracelsus, and in eighteenth-century European medicine, the modern history of meaning in illness begins, as do so many things in psychology, with Sigmund Freud. In the 1880s Freud, working in collaboration with Dr. Josef Breuer, began a systematic study of patients suffering from paralysis of limbs, anesthesias, disturbances of vision and speech, and other bodily symptoms for which no anatomical pathology could be found. Working with hypnosis and dreams, Breuer and Freud found that such unexplained *hysterical*[4] symptomatology was frequently associated with unacknowledged (unconsious) conflicts and forbidden desires, often of a highly sexual nature, and frequently originating in the patient's remote childhood. The cure of such patients proved to be via talking and emotional release (catharsis). To explain hysteria Freud conceived the idea that the symptoms represented a *conversion* of an unconscious conflict into a symbolic, physical symptom that bound and contained the anxiety of the forbidden desire.

The postulated lawfulness at the level of the unconscious, and the successful treatment based on a newly rationalized therapy, established this work as a landmark in a field hitherto regarded as beyond the pale of experimental science. Freud's conversion hypothesis brought into focus the possibility that many unexplained hysterical symptoms and behaviors could have a precisely-defined etiology whose elucidation would lie in bringing to light long-forgotten events from the patient's distant past. Additionally, the specificity implicit in the notion of conversion suggested that a natural catalogue of conversions and correspondences—something like the classification of animals and plants into genus and species—might be possible for psychic diseases. Of course, the notion of a sexual basis in disease opened up a veritable can of worms since it suggested that Victorian morality might be unhealthy and therefore should be brought under medical and scientific scrutiny. The implications of that aspect of their discovery so alarmed Breuer that he subsequently withdrew from further research with Freud, leaving the latter to blaze the trail of psychoanalysis alone.

Freud himself chose shortly to move his focus to the intellectual and affective ("mental") disorders arising out of unconscious conflicts and unresolved childhood needs, and left the conversion into physical symptomatology to others. The work was picked up by Georg Groddeck, a physician from Baden Baden, who published a series of cases in the 1920s in his classic, *The Meaning of Illness*. Groddeck's cases are significant because they went beyond the purely functional somatization characteristic of hysteric conversion to actual tissue pathology. In a famous case, Groddeck reported his treatment of a woman with generalized edema resulting from congestive heart failure. The swollen tissues subsided immediately upon the woman's disclosure to Dr. Groddeck during a consultation her tremendous guilt over having married after she had pledged herself to become a nun. It was this stored guilt, arising out of her belief that having broken a vow of celibacy she deserved punishment, that apparently precipitated the heart failure. Once she brought the feelings to light in the accepting relationship with her physician, she immediately began to improve, passing huge quantities of urine, and in a week had lost over 50 pounds. Groddeck's case remains, 65 years later, an excellent model of treatment through the revelation of symbolic meaning (in this case, 'conflict of the heart').

In a series of letters to Freud, Groddeck reported on numerous cases of organic pathology in various body systems where he was able to find a symbolic component which seemed logically to clarify the disease process and which, when consciously acknowledged and embraced, expedited the treatment. Although Groddeck's method was psychoanalytic and the symbols he explored tended to be Freudian and sexual, he actually raised virtually all of the questions that modern work on meaning in illness is now exploring. In Groddeck, we find the following seminal ideas:

- While we can work with universal meanings for particular illnesses through a variety of symbolic systems such as mythology, psychoanalysis or the language of emotional metaphor, ultimately only the patient himself can validate the meaning of his own illness.
- The search for meaning is a human universal: we seem to have an inherent need to find and validate meanings for puzzling events (such as our diseases) that occur around us or to us. Just as nature abhors a vacuum, so human nature abhors meaninglessness.
- Whatever the particular meaning of an illness, the invariable message is always the same warning: "Do not continue living as you intend to" (or have been doing).
- Illness does not come from the outside; it is not an enemy, but a creation of the organism.[5]

In this medical philosophy illness is a creation of some vital force in us that can be known only by its effects. This vital force is expressed through symptoms whose aim is to correct some imbalance.[6] Groddeck called this mysterious vital force the "IT," but Groddeck's IT is nothing more than what is elsewhere called the soul, the higher Self, the real Self, the vital force, spirit, God, and when it is linked to our dreams, the Dreambody. Whatever we call it, however we conceive of it, if diseases are to be given symbolic interpretations, some kind of transcendental force must be postulated as the source of the messages that symptoms carry.

The psychoanalytic psychosomaticists of the 1950s saw in the threads of these original insights the tantalizing possibility for discovering specific dysfunctional personality traits that might be played out symbolically in the body, thereby explaining anomalous chronic illnesses that continued to elude the growing mechanistic and pathologically-oriented framework of mainstream Western medicine. However, as Chapter 9 emphasized, despite meticulous explorations of the psychogenic origins of disease, this grand enterprise failed to prove its thesis of specific psychological cause-effect etiologies. Disease remains generally multidimensional, both in its causes and in its meanings. In endeavoring to reduce the particular to a general law, the psychosomaticists aspired to create a science of psychogenesis. But had they heeded Groddeck's warning that there is no universal meaning in a particular symptom or syndrome, they might have guessed that the problem of symbolic meaning could not be easily resolved in a set of consistent personality traits correlated with each disease. Today we applaud them for their efforts; they taught us to respect the complexity of the disease process. But we have abandoned their heroic hypothesis of a generic lexicon of universally applicable meanings. It would have been easier if meaning in illness had proved to be as simple as they hoped.

The collapse of the psychoanalytic psychosomatic enterprise left an unfilled vacuum in the study of the meaning of illness. Once the field was abandoned by those most marginal of medical professionals (psychiatrists), few if any researchers dared to re-enter the radioactive waters of meaning in illness. But the lack of a method of investigation hardly dispels the fundamental questions and issues that the early psychoanalysts raised, especially their hints that illness could often be a spiritual sickness. Alternative medicines such as homeopathy, herbalism and naturopathy have always pledged an allegiance to vitalism; and others, such as acupuncture, polarity and reflexology, are derived from energetic conceptions that go beyond mechanistic notions of the body. The increased strength and vigor of these traditional therapeutics in the past two decades, plus increasing evidence for substantial influences of our feelings, attitudes and beliefs in disease, served to open the door for New-Age conceptions of meaning in illness.

The Meaning of Meaning

A systematic exploration of how meaning and illness may be related begins with basic definitions. There is a deceptive simplicity in the phrase "meaning of illness" that belies the complexity of these concepts—"illness" and "meaning." Illness is often casually regarded as synonymous with disease, a common error that confounds psychological levels with biological ones.[7] Disease is expressed at the somatic level in physiological or biochemical pathology of body function or structure. My temperature is 105°, sedimentation rate of 44, white blood cell count of 50,000, unusual calcium deposits in the joints, circulating antibody complex to antigens produced by salmonella brucellosis, retinal nerve degeneration, systolic heart murmur, absence of insulin in response to sugar challenge, enlarged liver, CAT and MRI scans that deviate in some measurable way from the normal, bone mass loss, and so forth. While the instruments of science have extended and greatly refined our powers of observation, allowing us to discern a great variety of otherwise unobservable disease processes, bodily pathology hardly depends on modern science. Hippocrates, for instance, was able to describe dozens of somatic abnormalities including very precise descriptions of malignant tumors.

Illness, in contrast to disease pathology, is our *experience* of dysfunction—the aches and pains in their myriad combinations and dimensions, burning sensations inside and on the surface of our bodies, discomfort localized and general, the terror of waking and finding we cannot move a limb, exhausting fatigue, nausea, heartburn, dizziness, the panic of feeling our body out of control, the fear that we may die from the disease, and simply feeling sick, off, not our usual selves.

Canadian physician David Jennings maintains that the doctor's job is to attend to the somatic pathology, and to leave any further work that needs to be done for the illness to others who might be qualified: clergy, psychotherapists, spiritual healers, friends and family. But that is to confirm the physician as a medical mechanic, to authorize the great abyss into which modern medicine has plunged, that of trying to treat the person as a highly complex machine that has developed a defect or broken down. In the holistic philosophy of medicine (which coincides closely with the philosophy of classical homeopathy) there are simply a variety of *levels* at which disease is expressed. The level called "illness" is emotional (affective) and cognitive (mental), but it is just as significant as the somatic and it would be an error to fragment the person by confining each level of disease to its own specialist.

The distinction between disease pathology and illness experience is, however, valuable because it helps us remember that while health and illness are polarities, health and disease need not necessarily be so. Our bodies routinely harbor some of the major infectious disease pathogens, yet only rarely do we succumb to them. Dossey (1991) has observed that some of the greatest saints and sages succumbed to malignant diseases that we generally associate with severe illness, yet throughout the course of their disease they retained their poise, equanimity and balance—in a word, their health, their wholeness—accepting bodily degeneration with tranquility. In general, it is the illness that drives us to the doctor and it is the illness we want to lose. It is only because of our medicine's focus on disease that we are persuaded that the two must invariably go together.

"Meaning" in reference to disease and illness is essentially an exploration into the teleology of symptomatology. When we ask about what a symptom means we are basically inquiring as to its possible purpose. Why would we ever be inclined to ask such a question? It is because the biopsychosocial framework, being a *general* model of cause and effect in medicine, cannot always precisely explain particular occurrences of disease. For instance, while we may understand generally that a certain disease results from a maladaptive lifestyle interacting with a constitutional (inherited) organ weakness, we still may remain mystified as to what in that lifestyle is maladaptive and we may also be puzzled as to "why me, why now?" Our general laws are not sufficiently detailed for us to understand why I developed chronic fatigue syndrome and you did not; or why Donna Talman developed systemic lupus and Treya Wilber breast cancer. When disease is inexplicable by our science, we seek its meaning elsewhere, often in symbolic terms.

Transpersonal philosopher Ken Wilber has identified some of the major types of meaning traditionally given to disease by various religions and philosophies:[8]

Christian Fundamentalist: Illness is basically a punishment from God for some sort of sin. The worse the illness, the more unspeakable the sin.

New Age: Illness is a lesson. You are giving yourself this disease because there is something important you have to learn from it to continue your spiritual growth and evolution. Mind causes illness and mind cures it.

Biomedical/Scientific: Illness is a biophysical disorder caused by one or a cluster of biophysical factors ranging from viruses to trauma to genetic predisposition to environmental triggers. Meaning would be referring the disease to its causal vectors, which in any given case may or may not be verifiable.

Karma: Illness is the result of some non-virtuous past actions now coming to fruition in the form of a disease. The disease process represents the purification of the past misdeed.

Pop-Psychology: As Woody Allen put it, "I don't get angry, I grow tumors." In other words, repressed or suppressed emotions cause illness.

Holistic: Illness is a product of physical, emotional, mental and spiritual factors, none of which can be ignored. Treatment and meaning may involve any or all of these dimensions.

Existential: Illness, like life itself, is without meaning. Accordingly, it can take any personal meaning I choose to give it as my authentic response to accepting it as part of my finitude.

To complete Wilber's list we should add:

Family Therapy: Symptoms exhibited by one member of a family, while personally dysfunctional, serve the function of holding the entire family system intact. Treatment must focus on the whole family, never the individual sick person.

While we may be inclined to reject some of the meanings suggested above as either unverifiable in principle or little more than moral judgments, others invite us to enter new domains over and above the established risk factors of disease, beyond even the expanded psychological, environmental or genetic ones of holistic medicine. How shall we regard the occurrence of a disease whose cause we cannot exactly pinpoint in the biopsychosocial field? Should we view it as a fortuitous event, containing no more meaning than the afflictions of Job, something that chanced to come to us at this time due to random combinations of genetics and/or environmental events over which we have no control? Or is it *useful* to ask questions about the symbolic meaning of this disease/illness? That is, does it suggest something about a life (or our collective lives) which is out of harmony with nature? Could this sickness be an urgent message, delivered in the form of a somatic symptom, from some part of me that knows better than I what I need?

These are *teleological* questions, the kind we habitually ask when seeking the meaning of everyday, purposive human actions. And their answers there are invariably found in *motives*: what we are seeking and what we are avoiding. But how can we apply that teleological principle to a disease symptom? Nobody consciously seeks disease and avoids health. What possibly could be the purpose in producing the terrible suffering and tragic disruption of our lives that disease and illness bring? Even if disease had such a bizarre purpose, who or what exactly could be said to be producing it? Language fails us. We are forced to imagine ourselves split into multiple selves, one self punishing another with symptoms.

How are we going to answer teleological questions about meaning that seem to demand some purpose or goal? It's true that we sometimes see people acting self-destructively, but when somebody invites pain we recognize it as a perversion of a normal process and give it a name (masochism), explaining it by reference to a history in which love and attention were received only by injuring the self. Both our intuitions and our experience tell us that nobody is intentionally going to bring on even the relatively mild aches and pains of a minor ailment, much less the immense agony and suffering of a serious life-threatening disease. What is going on here? To imagine that "we" have some role in purposefully bringing on an illness suggests that one part of us knows best what the rest of us needs. Despite our aversion toward disease, this allknowing part of us introduces symptomatology in an attempt to oblige us to restore some lost balance and return to harmonious living. In these terms, disease is a message from one part of us to another and its meaning must be about self-transformation.

The New Age in Medicine

Where the angels of science feared to tread, the New-Age trainers and gurus boldly stepped in. Beginning in the decade of the 1980s there has been an information explosion in books on the relationship between mind and body in disease and illness. Many of these are very superficial restatements of positive thinking—what you believe, you can make happen—a viewpoint that Ken Wilber (1991) has rightly called misguided and dangerous. The workshops, for instance, that teach that cancer is caused by resentment, that poverty is your own choice and that oppression is brought on by yourself, divert attention away from the actual physical, environmental, legal, political and socioeconomic levels where work is urgently needed to change these conditions that create and maintain them. This extreme, New Age "you create your own reality" fantasy is actually an apologia for our inequitable society, its hyperindividuality and its arrogant imperialism that is devouring the planet's resources. These beliefs "have all the hallmarks of the infantile and magical worldview of the narcissistic personality disorders, including grandiosity, omnipotence, and narcissism."[9] The idea that thoughts don't just influence reality but create reality is the direct result of a failure to separate thought from object, the basic principle of magic and a romantization of the way that very young children think.

In trying to extract what is of value in New-Age concepts we have to keep in mind that the complexity of the human condition cannot be reduced to any simple formula. We also have to distinguish carefully the very useful idea that we do have some personal responsibility for what we attract in life from the moralistic judgments and blame that our culture gratuitously adds to this responsibility. Adding blame to the already present suffering of illness will not be helpful to healing. Unconditional caring acceptance is as important as any other natural therapeutic. Let us remember too Groddeck's warning that only the patient can verify the true meaning of his illness. By respecting both the multidimensional character of disease as well as the complexity of the human condition we can capture what is valuable in the transpersonal insights of the New-Age approach, while still remaining grounded in the biopsychosocial framework.

Symbolic Anatomy

Figure 12.1 looks vaguely like an illustration from an anatomy textbook, but look closer. It depicts symbolic meanings of many organs and structures according to Louise

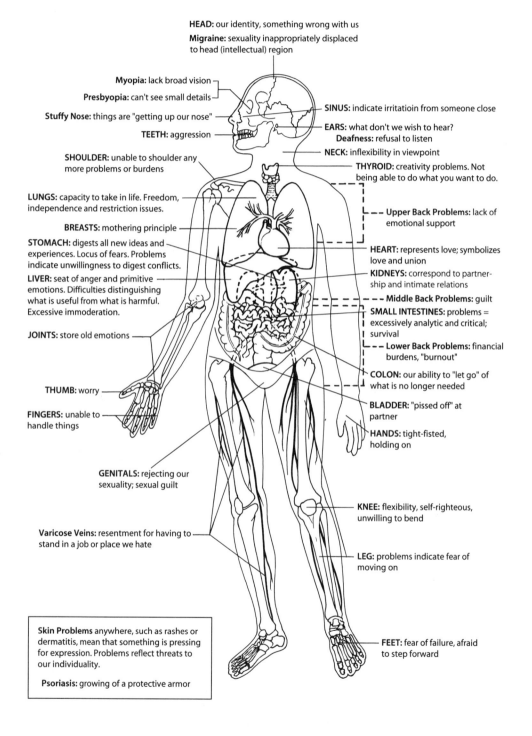

HEAD: our identity, something wrong with us
Migraine: sexuality inappropriately displaced to head (intellectual) region

Myopia: lack broad vision
Presbyopia: can't see small details
Stuffy Nose: things are "getting up our nose"
TEETH: aggression

SINUS: indicate irritatioin from someone close
EARS: what don't we wish to hear?
Deafness: refusal to listen
NECK: inflexibility in viewpoint
THYROID: creativity problems. Not being able to do what you want to do.

SHOULDER: unable to shoulder any more problems or burdens

LUNGS: capacity to take in life. Freedom, independence and restriction issues.

BREASTS: mothering principle

STOMACH: digests all new ideas and experiences. Locus of fears. Problems indicate unwillingness to digest conflicts.

LIVER: seat of anger and primitive emotions. Difficulties distinguishing what is useful from what is harmful. Excessive immoderation.

JOINTS: store old emotions

THUMB: worry

FINGERS: unable to handle things

Upper Back Problems: lack of emotional support

HEART: represents love; symbolizes love and union

KIDNEYS: correspond to partnership and intimate relations

Middle Back Problems: guilt

SMALL INTESTINES: problems = excessively analytic and critical; survival

Lower Back Problems: financial burdens, "burnout"

COLON: our ability to "let go" of what is no longer needed

BLADDER: "pissed off" at partner

HANDS: tight-fisted, holding on

GENITALS: rejecting our sexuality; sexual guilt

Varicose Veins: resentment for having to stand in a job or place we hate

KNEE: flexibility, self-righteous, unwilling to bend

LEG: problems indicate fear of moving on

Skin Problems anywhere, such as rashes or dermatitis, mean that something is pressing for expression. Problems reflect threats to our individuality.

Psoriasis: growing of a protective armor

FEET: fear of failure, afraid to step forward

Fig. 12.1 Symbolic Anatomy Chart[10]

Hay and German spiritual psychologist Thorwald Dethlefsen. If you examine these correspondences closely you can see that there are basically three sorts of statements, each progressively more abstract and tenuous. In one, a body part or organ is assigned a symbolic meaning that is closely related to metaphorical and idiomatic speech usage. Thus the legs are associated with *moving on* (and leg problems hint at problems in moving on to the next phase of development); the back is a symbolic as well as an actual physical *support system,* and back problems accordingly have both meanings; the stomach is the organ of both food digestion and *experience digestion,* and problems there may reflect both levels.

There is some intriguing evidence that much of our language actually has developed from the experience of our corporeality; that is, we first acquired names for body parts and functions and then began metaphorically to apply them to more abstract events and concepts.

> Our whole language is psychosomatic. Virtually all the words and expressions with which we describe psychological conditions and processes are borrowed from what we have experienced with our bodies. We can never understand or grasp anything that we cannot physically grasp with our hands or stand on with our feet.[11]

A second kind of statement is much more tenuous and entails the assignment of emotional states to body systems, e.g., guilt to the middle back, fear to the stomach and small intestine, anger to the liver and throat, and love to the heart. The rationale for these assignments is almost wholly intuitive, for the psychophysiological evidence reveals surprisingly few differences in the autonomic activation patterns of different emotions. That is, if you only look at the bodily changes, anger, fear and joy are remarkably similar.

Fig. 12.1 contains another, even more complex kind of meaning derived from clinical impressions. The illustration shows that some systems are believed to be associated with relationship difficulties (kidneys), threats to our individuality and concept of self (skin), and others to creativity difficulties (thyroid). The rationale for these linkings is largely based on analogy and not always easy to trace. The three levels of symbolic meanings might be aptly called *metaphorical, emotional* and *analogical.* What value is such a symbolic anatomy and physiology chart? Certainly none of these impressionistic observations have been validated by scientific studies, nor are they likely to be. The correspondences pictured in Fig. 12.1 are best viewed as *suggestions* for how the practitioner might go about beginning to open up the full picture of an illness. They help to break the physician's habitual gaze at the disease as something totally fortuitous, a purely mechanical, bodily dysfunction. Thus, bearing in mind that the patient ultimately must be the final arbiter, the chart provides hints as to where to begin to look for meaning. There is rarely a single ultimate, fixed symbolic correspondence to be found, because meaning in illness is ephemeral, multidimensional, individual. As former Jungian analyst Arnold Mindell noted, one day a pain in your stomach may be telling you about a problem with your mother, and the next day that same pain may be telling you about a problem with your father. On the third day its

AIDS Response to the massive collective victimization of life in this century: political oppression, destruction of rain forests and animal species, killing the life in lakes & rivers, nuclear testing, acid rain. *(Myss, 1988)*

Increased interpersonal isolation due to electronic communication. In promiscuity and sexuality divorced from love, the person becomes merely an object of stimulation. The immune system attempts to compensate for this failure to let down our boundaries (as occurs in true intimacy), with disastrous results. *(Dethlefsen & Dahlke, 1983).*

CANCER (17.2%) Inability to move on to the next phase of our lives, to grow spiritually due to excessive fears, guilt, self-denial. Prolonged interference with natural self-growth leads to abnormal cell growth. *(Myss, 1988)*

Cancer is a perverted form of love, love for the small self. Failing to see that we are part of the whole and refusing to restrain our growth and egocentricity, we are over-populating and suicidally destroying our planet, our environment. In deadly sympathy, the cancerous cell too thinks only of itself and its own growth, and so destroys the whole organism. *(Dethlefsen & Dahlke, 1983)*

ALZHEIMER'S Related to the breakdown of the family unit and the dissolving of familial bonds of security that once extended naturally from birth to death. A society that has little value for the wisdom of its elders introduces an entirely new dimension of stress to the process of aging. Fear of rejection, of having to prove one's self-worth in the golden years when such should be a given, is the root cause of the need to become unconscious and dependent. *(Myss, 1988)*

A desire to leave the planet. The inability to face life as it is. *(Hay, 1984)*

CORONARY HEART DISEASE (38.3%) Blockages of our needs to give and receive love. Bottling up fears and anger of failure. Inability to meet emotional demands or to process disappointments in personal relationships may lead to coronary explosion. *(Myss, 1988)*

Failure to follow our hearts, to balance our feelings and intellect; hard-hearted. Holding aggression in; not allowing ourselves to feel or express our emotions. Eventually the hardened heart "breaks" out in an "attack" that obliges us at last to feel it. *(Dethlefsen & Dahlke, 1983)*

STROKE (10.8%) Dominant, excessive need to control the physical environment or others. Cumulative distrust of others leads to fears of material security and need to always be in charge. This accumulated, undischarged stress eventually produces eruption and brain shutdown. *(Myss, 1988)*

Giving up, resistance. Rather die than change. Rejection of life. *(Hay, 1984)*

DIABETES (2%) Resentment over having to be responsible for another person (often a parent in juvenile diabetes) or oneself. Preventing or abetting another from developing their own responsibility. These extraneous energy demands drain the body's storage tank (the pancreas) of energy. *(Myss, 1988)*

Unsatisfied desire for love, along with an inability to accept and absorb it unreservedly. Not having learnt to love oneself. *(Dethlefsen and Dahlke, 1983)*

Table 12.1 Symbolic table of diseases. In the interests of space I have abridged and edited some of the authors' interpretations. The percentages refer to death rates in the USA during 1983.

message may be that you should eat prunes (organic, of course).

The concept of symbolic anatomy is extended to teleological explanations for actual diseases in Table 12.1, which shows some sample symbolic interpretations that have been assigned to six syndromes. These six include the four diseases in the developed world that account for 70% of deaths. AIDS and Alzheimer's syndrome, the focus of much current concern, are included as well.

The material in Table 12.1 is the product of three different theorists, each one of whom has a different general principle guiding their therapeutic approach to disease. For intuitive diagnostician Carolyne Myss, the goal of the work is to use interpretative material to find and release the specific stresses that are causing the destruction of the physical body. German psychologist Thorwald Dethlefsen's aim in introducing interpretations into therapeutics is to know one's shadow and embrace it, for that will render the symptom superfluous. For Louise Hay, the root of all illness is the failure to adore oneself sufficiently, so that learning to love oneself is the key to healing.

Once again it is extraordinarily important for the practitioner to take the interpretations offered in Table 12.1 as suggested guidelines only, useful principally in opening one's awareness to possibilities that might go beyond the usual questions asked in taking the case. It is unlikely that any particular case will fit exactly the interpretations of Table 12.1, and many may be radically different. (Please note that the three theorists themselves generally do not agree on a common interpretation for these diseases.) Individuality in expression remains a far more powerful principle than these generalized pictures: a tumor in my knee almost certainly means something very different from the one in your knee. Shealy and Myss (1988) put it well:

> Understanding the emotional, psychological and spiritual stresses that underlie the creation of illness is a complex process. It is not like a game of connecting the dots in which eye problems connect to a desire not to see clearly, ear problems connect to a desire to tune something or someone out of a person's life, and leg problems signify difficulty in standing on one's own. Symbolic analysis is not that simple and not that obvious. *People are complicated and their personal histories and emotional patterns are highly individual and complex.*[12] [italics added]

Dethlefsen and Dahlke, who have provided some of the most intriguing correspondences between illness and its symbolic meanings, regard the stock illustrations as only a means of teaching a new way of seeing which will enable one to develop one's own interpretations:

> A given theme or problem can express itself via a whole variety of organs and systems. There is no fixed scheme of allocation whereby a given theme has to choose any one particular symptom as its em-body-ment.[13]

For all their limitations, Fig 12.1 and Table 12.1 can serve to open new dimensions of understanding illness we might not have been inclined to consider, such as global or collective aspects of disease that go beyond our usual focus on the person— my body, my problem. The interpretations given for AIDS and Alzheimer's by Myss, and for cancer by Dethlefsen and Dahlke, suggest correspondences between personal somatic responses and collective ills. Even though we may not yet understand how an individual organism could reflect some of these collective imbalances in the wider field, the extension to social and ecological imbalance is very significant, for it forces the practitioner to face the possibility that healing a particular physical disease may require social change. We want to practice holistic medicine; how holistic do we dare to be?

Symbolic Meaning: Substitute, Complement or Catalyst for Treatment

Patients visit their doctors to get rid of unwanted symptoms—that persistent backache, those recurrent bellyaches and nausea, this disturbing growth, the inconvenient and frightening asthma attacks, the growing stiffness in an arthritic finger, the pains in the chest halfway up the stairs. To search for symbolic meanings for our infirmities is to enter a realm of transformation and responsibility where our physical disease is regarded as carrying information about another (psychospiritual) domain. Certainly not everyone, and perhaps only a small percentage of our patients are at a place in their lives where they are ready to embark on such a problematic search. Patients who come to alternative practitioners do so mainly because they have not been helped by orthodox doctors. Helped almost always means "helped to eradicate their symptoms." It is true that by the time they come, they may be ready to become more involved in their own healing, more open to the idea that stress, attitudes and lifestyle could be health-risk factors. But it is a further step still to take a patient into the realm of personal transformation, which is so closely tied to explorations of the symbolic meaning of illness.

We do know, however, that a purely problem-oriented approach with natural medicines often initiates a personal transformation without any explicit focus on symbolic interpretations of the symptoms. "Some rise from the acupuncture table with fresh insights: 'I'm only staying sick,' one depressed woman announced, 'so I can make my husband take care of me.'"[14] When a homeopath finds the remedy that matches her patient's symptoms (the simulium), the disease process is likely to unfold naturally with or without the cognitive component that an explicit focus on the meaning of the illness might produce. Healing may proceed through emotional discharge brought on by the remedy. This discharge can lead to the rebalancing of vital energy that explicit psychotherapy or a conscious descent into symbolic meaning can eventually bring. Nevertheless, although catalyzed by the simulium, even the homeopathic patient eventually has to do the work.

> A person has to participate in the emotions as the remedies release them, but she doesn't necessarily get immediate insight into the origin of these emotions. The experience, of course, has practical results in that her life is changed, she recovers and probably lives and thinks differently.[15]

Indeed, if the patient fails to integrate the process initiated by the remedy, fails to understand the issues and make the transformation that is demanded, the symptoms are likely to reoccur.

Although rarely mentioned, it seems clear that herbal remedies in material doses, aromatherapy massage, acupuncture and acupressure, and certainly the flower essences and the affirmations generally given with them, are all capable of initiating profound transformations at emotional and spiritual levels. Even a change in diet to more fresh vegetables, less red meat, avoiding foods with preservatives, coloring and additives, and seeking out whole grains as opposed to processed, devitalized ones initiates a change in consciousness. One begins to think about where the food came from and what it underwent before it arrived on our plates. Many practitioners elect to stay out of the process and allow their natural medicines and therapeutics to bring about changes at various levels. A search for symbolic meaning, especially in a serious chronic illness, can be a lifetime journey and require deep inner work.[16] Yet symbolic or psychological meaning often emerges naturally in the process of the work done together if both practitioner and patient are receptive to the idea that illness can carry a message. Even so, meaning must never be pushed on a patient.

> I no longer advocate transformation to everyone. I have realized that there is a natural inner timing and that people can be helped to go only as far as that allows. All judgment or coercion to go further must be released. It is natural for me now to accept and honor people as they are. People who are not ready cannot be brought forward into the fuller transformative energies even if it is clear that doing so could possibly release them from the forces configurating their illness.[17]

Notwithstanding such cautions and considerations, it is in fact often possible to suggest meanings for relatively minor complaints and take advantage of the subsequent healing process that may accompany such explorations. Acne patients tend to 'pick at' their skin lesions, and according to counselor Barbara Levine, these are people who frequently feel 'picked on' in life. In one study patients were encouraged, through psychotherapy, to eliminate this victim consciousness, to learn how their very belief was a self-fulfilling prophecy that actually encouraged others to treat them exactly as they anticipated. The results of the therapy were very encouraging: 30 of the 38 patients in this sample were significantly improved within eight weeks, and skin lesions cleared completely over the long term for half of the participants, the remainder exhibiting 80-90% improvement.[18]

When we work with symbolic meaning it is important to realize that we are in effect working with just another aspect or *channel* of the illness process. We can work with the meaning of a symptom while simultaneously working in a problem-oriented way with our other natural therapeutics. Even if we are convinced that our skin disease has something to do with a side of ourselves that we are afraid to show the world; or that our chronic fatigue is partly about our body's need, after many years of achieving and goal orientation, for rest and our need to just be; or that our autoimmune disease is reflecting a part of ourselves that hates and blames ourselves for being the way we are, we are still going to "treat" these disease pictures with the appropriate natural therapeutics.

Responsibility, Blame and Punishment in Medicine

Conjuring up a symbolic meaning behind physical symptoms implies that we are, at least in part, the author of our own diseases. But if we are responsible for them, then aren't we also to *blame* for them? The suffering that results from a life-threatening disease is grim enough, and the last thing a patient needs is to be blamed for it as well. Our cultural tendency to associate responsibility with blame is a strong reason why psychological meaning must never, never be forced down anyone's throat, be they family, friend, acquaintance or patient. Aside from the fact that the person with the symptom is the final authority on its meaning, an individual must be open to the idea that there *is* some meaning in their illness. Many are not open to this idea, and they have strong support from distinguished professionals and commentators. Jungian analysts Guggenbühl-Craig and Micklem, for instance, regard the search for meaning in illness as little more than a futile pursuit of psychosomatic fantasies, in principle unverifiable by the methods of science. And they go further in their criticism:

> The disturbing feature is not the fantasy aspect . . . but its all pervasive moralism. All these beautiful modern symbolic explanations are harmful in their very moralism. Sick people . . . not only have to suffer, but are made to feel guilty as well: their diseases are entirely their own fault; they have failed to develop psychologically; they have suppressed their feelings or have not suppressed them enough; they have been too friendly, or not friendly enough.[19]

Susan Sontag has argued strongly that illness should never be viewed metaphorically, and has reminded us how easy it is to give a disease a psychological interpretation when we do not understand its functional causal antecedents. "Nothing is more punitive than to give disease a meaning—that meaning being invariably a moralistic one. Any disease whose causality is murky, and for which treatment is ineffective tends to be awash in significance."[20] The diseases in Table 12.1 are exactly the sort that Sontag has in mind; the causality of most of them is indeed murky, and their current treatment protocols much less effective than we'd like.

Thus the search for meaning in illness should be treated as a *supplement,* not an alternative to a functional analysis of the internal and external biopsychosocial causes. And certainly it must never be moralistic. Although our culture tends to link responsibility with blame, this is a wholly gratuitous association. To say that we have some responsibility in the occurrence of a phenomenon is to acknowledge that our input, large or small, was a crucial component to the occurrence of the event. To then blame ourselves for our role in the causal process is to add the extraneous moral judgment "and that was bad, and should be judged and treated accordingly."

The practitioner of natural medicine must go beyond such conventional judgments and remain impeccably non-judgmental. Whatever material she and her patient turn up has to be viewed with exactly the same mixture of detachment and keen interest that a botanist experiences in observing the process of osmosis in a plant membrane, or a physicist feels in observing cloud tracks in a particle chamber. Treya Wilber, in searching for the meaning of the breast cancer that ultimately killed her, coined the term *passionate equanimity* to capture the spirit one needs in pursuing symbolic meaning in illness. In three moving autobiographies of journeys into illness and meaning,[21] the common theme that emerges is that the *search for meaning* is as important if not more so than its ultimate discovery. Contrast this to the opposing view that illness is inherently without meaning, that it is a "meaningless onslaught, a disaster of major or minor proportions inflicted apparently on an unsuspecting and undeserving victim."[22]

Yet even this belief that illness has *no* meaning is itself a way of making the experience meaningful. Wilber never did discover "the meaning" of her cancer, but the process of searching for it at all levels—physical, emotional, spiritual—was the healing force in her process. Embracing the "negative meaning"—that, as mere particles of matter and consciousness in the vast cosmos, with limited personal control over most of the events that are taking place in and around us, this disease is not our fault—can be extraordinarily consoling.

Ultimately, we reach a kind of bottom line—that the tendency to seek meaning out of the chaos of events is an inherent part of our human nature. Meaning turns out to be one of those intrinsic human motives high up in Maslow's pyramid of human motives that foster well-being and self-actualization. In the face of the stress of a serious unexplained illness, *the sense of coherence*—that the world is somehow meaningful and that one can make sense of one's existence in it—remains a remarkably comforting, inspiring and healing resource. Based on his experience with thousands of patients, Dr. Larry Dossey contends that

> [a]nyone who is seriously sick will find or create a meaning to explain what is happening. It is simply our nature to do so, and *I have never seen an exception to this generalization.*[23] [italics added]

Yet we are not always going to find a meaning behind an illness. We may find one meaning that somehow puts it all into focus for us, a meaning that may or may not have a psychological import; we may find no meaning; or we may find a kaleidoscope of changing meanings, emerging level after level like the skin of an onion. It is finally the process of searching for meaning and the resulting self-discovery that justifies our introducing it here in a text concerned with rationalizing practical psychological tools for healing.

Process-Oriented Psychology

Those of us who do feel drawn to working with symbolic meaning in illness need some practical tools for how to do it. We want some techniques and orienting attitudes that are likely to yield, if not universal meanings, specific ways of working that can be useful adjuncts to classical natural therapeutics. One simple technique is to ask our patient questions about what he can no longer do in life because of the disease, and what it now obliges him to do. This strategy (described more fully in Project 12) is based on the premise that our disease somehow knows for the moment more than we do about what we need, and has commandeered our body to make it comply.

This approach, pioneered by Dethlefsen and Dahlke (1990), views diseases as friendly allies to be welcomed for what they might have to teach, and contrasts markedly with our usual strategy of trying to eradicate the disease as quickly as possible and asking questions later. It has the virtue of galvanizing our interest in learning as much as possible about ourselves and our disease, which can restore a valuable sense of perceived control for the patient. But we can go deeper still with the practical tools, techniques and therapeutic attitudes called *process-oriented psychology* (POP), developed by former Jungian analyst and physicist Arnold Mindell and his research group that has been active for over 15 years in Zurich and, more recently, in Portland, Oregon.[24]

In treating physical symptoms as entry points to underlying psychological processes, process-oriented psychology stands as a bridge between psychotherapeutic and somatic healing schools. However, the symptom is not considered to be the problem, the cause of which needs rooting out, or the effect of which needs releasing. On the contrary, the symptom is respectfully addressed as a friend and carrier of wise messages from the real Self, some of whose needs have been overlooked. The symptom itself is revered as the expert, em–body–ing the wisdom as to what is trying to express itself in a person's "process."

The concept of mind-body interaction in medicine represents an attempt to bring these two aspects—the psychological and the somatic—back together again after being split off into different schools of caring. However, the retention of the very terms body and mind suggest a separation which POP does not recognize. In POP terms, there is only an ongoing process which seeks to express itself through various representational systems. These systems include our fantasies and dreams, our everyday behavior, our relationships, our role as a member of a social collective, and of course our bodies. These independent systems are known as *channels*. The concept of healing or restoring the body or mind is also not one that POP embraces. Rather, a person's process is likened to a traveling train:

> Healing and disease are train stops on the train line. You can get off at these stops, or you can get back on the train. . . . If you do process work you are interested in the total life process and this means you are not interested in just one train station. You want to go the whole line. Your process can bring you everything you need in time. If you learn to follow your process without aiming at one station, or goal, then you become an individuated person. Your life becomes richer and you learn to reduce your projections and integrate your pain.[25]

Here we can see that in POP, integrating the states (the experiences at train stations) is more important than arriving at any particular destination.

The ever-changing flow of a river or stream, never exactly repeated, is an apt metaphor for the process paradigm. Looking at the stream we conceptualize, by means of our perceptual apparatus and memory, patterns of vortices, waves, ripples and splashes. Actually these states have no independent existence of their own. Rather, they are our constructions by which we endeavor to capture repetitive patterns in the ever-changing process, abstracted out of the flowing movement as it arises and vanishes in the total process of the flow.

Human behavior and experience also flow like a river. There too we abstract out for purposes of convenience, states—personality traits, moods, attitudes, beliefs— to which we give name and form. This tendency to conceptualize the world of events, including sickness and health, in terms of static states (disease entities, syndromes, neurotic and psychotic states) makes possible the identification of recurrent patterns. That identification in turn permits us to relate past and present unique events to each other, the basis both of diagnosis and effective treatment, not to mention ordinary communication. Nonetheless, such categorization must by definition omit the bulk of the details that are individual and unique to each patient's overall behavioral and ex- periential flow. Process-oriented psychology endeavors to focus through the habitual categories and states onto the moment to moment events occurring in the experiential flow. The rationale for this focus on process is simply that allowing behavioral and experiential events to flow and unfold relatively unencumbered by the conventional judgments that categorization, conceptualization and interpretation impose has significant therapeutic effects.

The therapeutic tools of process work are the familiar ones used by many schools of psychotherapy, some of which have been described in Chapter 8. They are the tech- niques and tricks used by gestalt therapists, bioenergetic therapists, Jungian analysts, Reichian body therapists, hypnotherapists, art therapists, and yet with a distinctly different slant. The process worker is using these methods not to get rid of a symptom or problem, but to *amplify* it. There is an important principle of unconditional accep- tance behind this which has been described as "what happens is right and should be encouraged."[26] This stance contrasts rather markedly with our conventional position about symptomatology, namely that it constitutes pathology and needs to be changed. In a word, the process-oriented therapist, even though constantly using intuitions as to how to draw out the client's process, must studiously avoid imposing any goals upon the client, other than the goal of bringing as much of the process to the surface so that its energy can be observed and integrated. Yet as we see in the material to come, the therapist's work is far from that of a passive, detached observer.

Finding Meaning in a Symptom. Recently my lower backache returned again, having subsided into a background warning system for the last six months. I could not locate where I had ignored its warnings, or lifted something too heavy, or pushed myself into doing too much, as I have so often done in the past. I complained for a day or two about the unfairness of having the ache return when I had been so much more careful recently. Eventually I realized that in complaining this way I was trapping myself into the role of powerless victim, when in fact my body might have a powerful message for me, if only I was prepared to listen to it. From POP's point of view, pain is the beginning of a great deal of awareness. Despite the fact that I was certain I had heard all its messages before, I decided to work with it and listen to what it was trying to make me aware of. I asked my partner Anne to help me.

As we will see from the detailed analysis of the transcripts set forth below, the message was that I should make more demands of people, which was hard to accept, because I have a great investment in not being a demanding person. After I got that insight, I decided to experiment by making more demands of Anne. She found it a great relief and in turn felt empowered to say either yes or no to my demands. In receiving some definite information about my needs and desires to which she could choose how to respond, she experienced a distinct feeling of liberation. I have been helped to move on to another step in my own personal process by recognizing that there is benefit in becoming more aware of myself also as a demanding person. I now realize that while I had been splitting off 'demandingness' from my self-identity, I had nevertheless been insisting that Anne and others intuit my demands. And when they failed to do so, I often felt irritated. Thus the work, prompted by my backache, has also helped a relationship process.

How to Process Physical Symptoms. The main method for decoding a symptom is *amplification*. The experience of the symptom is amplified so that more of its hidden meaning can be discovered. A physical symptom is usually experienced in the feeling or proprioceptive channel, so it must be amplified in this channel. Before it can be amplified it must be known as fully as possible as a sensory-based experience.

> When I stop trying to avoid my discomfort and become very still in order to experience it more closely, what I had loosely described as a lower backache is in fact a sensation centered on one particular place just below my hip bone high up on the buttock, where I feel a focused sensation of continuously persistent pressure.

Once fully experienced proprioceptively, the sensation is amplified until it is almost impossible to bear. At this point a spontaneous channel change usually occurs, releasing more information from the symptom.

> Having amplified the feeling of persistent localized pressure, I then demonstrate with my finger the feeling of someone pressing a finger into my body at precisely that point. The act of demonstrating with my finger is evidence of my having switched quite spontaneously into the movement sensation or kinesthetic channel.

An important aspect of this work is to be able to identify with the *symptom-maker.*

> In order to have the experience of the pain-maker, I press my finger into Anne's buttock in the same place and with just the quality of pressure and persistence that I felt victim of. Now I have a chance to feel what this energy and information that have become split off from my awareness and thus manifest in the symptom is actually like. Switching into the relationship channel, I poke her with my finger and allow myself still more identification with the pain-maker. I find myself telling her that I am only trying to warn her. We then swap roles. Anne becomes the pain-maker and picking up my words, tells me she is only trying to warn me. I, as the victim again, insist that I don't need any more warnings. I am already protecting myself sufficiently—physically anyway! We swap roles again. When Anne complains, as the victim, that she doesn't need warning, I find that I lack energy for further poking.

Process work always assumes that what is happening is exactly right just the way it is happening. What bears investigating, however, is *exactly how or in just what way it is right.*

> In some way it must be right that I lack energy now for further body prodding. We acknowledge that we may need to be on another track. Anne, now in the role of ther- apist, guesses that the pointing itself is important. To find out precisely how it might be important, she encourages me to amplify again, putting emphasis on the finger pointing this time. I become the finger-pointer and as this figure, I find myself mak- ing demands of her about all sorts of issues within our relationship. We have now re- leased the energetic information previously hidden within my symptom. Both my personal and our relationship processes have moved on. My symptom is no longer needed in its latest role and my backache subsides within 24 hours.

Illness as the Beginning of Healing. The example of processing a physical symptom as described above illustrates the value of treating illness as the beginning of a healing or balancing process. Note that there was no question of following a set formula or table of meanings (such as those presented in the earlier sections of the chapter) that might have imposed an outward, and false, interpretation onto the process that was unfold- ing. In a way the backache was not so much a metaphor of what was out of balance, as the key to the energy needed in that moment for integration and rebalancing.

Opening up the symptom opened up a door to a part that was until then hidden, a shadowy side wanting expression, but hitherto lying at the *boundaries* of my being. At any particular moment we are consciously aware of only certain aspects, motives, attitudes, ways of being about ourselves. POP calls this information with which we identify most closely and which we can easily access verbally, our *primary process.* Aspects of ourselves which remain further from our awareness, yet which neverthe- less are pressing to express themselves, are referred to as information operating in a *secondary process.* Most of these secondary processes, even if we were to be appraised of them, generally contradict our current notion of our self-identity and so we tend to disown them. For this reason, the sum of these secondary processes is usually equated to C. G. Jung's concept of our *shadow.* In the work on my lower backache, my primary process is to be undemanding. That is how I identify myself. My backache is a signal from a secondary process that needs me to be more demanding, a quality far from my self-awareness, although in fact I am likely to be perceived as demanding by oth- ers at times.

In order to integrate the message(s) of symptoms we have to find a way to turn their energy from a passive into an active force. But the moment we are brought face to face with a secondary shadow process, we find ourselves standing at the very limits or the *edge* of what we are prepared to do or be in our relationships and in the world. This edge that exists between the primary and secondary process challenges our very self-identity, and dares us to expand to include it. In this sense, all symptoms attempt to increase our boundaries. I did not know or want to even think of myself as a de- manding person. I was more comfortable splitting off that polarity by leaving it unconscious, until doing so created a disturbance to the status quo, waking me up to new potential. Much of process work takes place around these edges—becoming aware of them, discovering through the various techniques illustrated above what keeps us on the familiar side of them, and then when we are ready, going over them. Sometimes it is a long time before an explored edge can actually be crossed. Often the edge has to be crossed and re-crossed time and time again before the energy of the symptom is sufficiently integrated.

The Chronic Symptom. According to Mindell a chronic disease is often a lifelong problem, a part of someone's individuation process that can take the form of changing messages that the soul expresses through the disease. A chronic symptom often serves as a metaphor for a lifelong problem. Working with my lower backache, I have become accustomed to this aching pressure as a friend warning me not to push myself into doing too much or lifting something too heavy. However, in my most recent encounter with it the message changed (as we have seen) to "Make more demands of people!" Of course the two messages may well be linked: The suggested link here might be my not having to always see myself as the person who has to do everything. In general, a chronic body problem may contain changing information about various psychological problems, so that one season issues with your mother can be found in your stomach, while in the next your father appears there. The dynamic nature of meaning makes it easier to avoid the dangers of one-dimensional psychosomatic approaches which try to relate particular personality types to specific symptoms. Allowing chronic symptoms to express here-and-now information from the depths of a person's ongoing process will not necessarily remove the discomfort, or if it does, it may not do so forever. The important thing that does seem to happen is that

> if you really get to the root of a process, then your projections can be integrated and the experience of your disease changes radically. If you are lucky, healing may occur. If you are even luckier, you will begin to grow. Even if your chronic symptoms do not disappear, they become friendly allies ushering you into a new phase of existence in which you behave as a whole and congruent person in the midst of a rich and meaningful life.[27]

Conclusion
From the ancient religio-magical origins of our medicines to Groddeck and Mindell in this century, meaning in illness remains elusive, intensely personal, controversial and transcendental. As a complementary teleological perspective to our generally scientific practices, symbolism in disease expands our vistas beyond not just the frontiers, but also the accepted ground-rules of our science. Rejected as fantasy by some, condemned as a substitute for knowledge by others, and extolled as the ultimate ground of understanding by a few, meaning in illness is likely to remain an ever-fertile ground for both idle speculation and brilliant insight. Caveat emptor.

Project 12

Decoding the Messages of the Body

In this project we will be focusing on one body symptom and inquiring into its current meaning. We'll use four rules suggested by Dethlefsen and Dahlke (1983) to probe for and expand the meaning of our symptom.

Begin by selecting an ache or pain, stiffness or some more durable symptom or syndrome that you are experiencing at this time. If you are unable to conjure up a symptom of your own you may decide to select one from a friend, acquaintance or patient, but if you work with someone else you must be sure that you have their permission and active interest in searching for a meaning of their symptom. It is especially important that you do not go searching for meaning of symptoms in a person who is not receptive to the basic idea that a symbolic meaning may underlie their physical symptom.

You have to remember that your average friends and neighbors are not the least bit interested in psychology. Aside from the fact that they stigmatize neurotic behavior as an unacceptable, weak and morally distasteful way of responding to problems of living, they also suspect psychologists and psychotherapists of being a bit "off" themselves. And, as Arnold Mindell observes, there is a germ of truth in their judgments:

> Not all psychologists are trustworthy, psychology is not yet a perfected science, and it does depend on teamwork in order to function properly. [Nonetheless] the most fascinating thing about [these average friends and neighbors] is that they begin to show interest in their inner life when they are troubled by diseases.[28]

So be cautious in working with meaning with others, and "on no account should you foist on other people your interpretations of their symptoms."[29]

Rule 1. Once having chosen the symptom, ignore all apparent causal functional relationships that may be known or suspected. The symptom might have originated with trauma, or you might be sure it's related to diet or lifestyle, or be an infection—it doesn't matter. The functional analysis is not a substitute for symptom-interpretation; all that is relevant is that it exists.

Rule 2. Work out the exact time at which each symptom appeared (if it is a series you are examining). Inquire into the life situation, thoughts, fantasies, dreams, events and items of news that make up the symptom's temporal framework.

What kind of mood were we in? Was there some change occurring in our life? We have to be careful not to overlook something that on the surface seemed quite trivial at the time, but in fact could have been very significant. Since the symptom itself is assumed to be a manifestation of something not obvious, the significance of its surrounding context is also not likely to be obvious. And in doing this exploration, pay special attention to the first thing that comes to you—don't immediately dismiss it as irrelevant or trivial. Also don't be in a hurry to lay a prejudged theory on the symptom. Be open to subtle and surprising new meaning that may be lying below the surface.

Rule 3. Consider the metaphorical significance of the symptom. See Fig 12.1 (Symbolic Anatomy Chart) for hints. If you are working with a partner, listen for the psychosomatic and metaphorical correspondences in language. Remember that words often have double meanings: heartless, fed-up, sick and tired, "he gives me a pain," thick-skinned, and so forth.

Then try to abstract the principle from the symptomatology, and apply this pattern on the psychological level. If you are on target you may get a sense of recognition, a kind of 'aha!' reaction.

Rule 4. Ask the twin questions and try to go quite deeply into them:
  (i) What does the symptom stop me (you) from doing?
  (ii) What is the symptom obliging me (you) to do?

Any enforced behavior is an obligatory change in our life and is therefore to be taken seriously. The symptom stops us from doing something we should like to do, and on the other hand obliges us to do things we never intended to do. If there were a mysterious force—the symptom-maker—outside of us who wished to pull our strings like this, what would that force be wanting from us? What could its purpose possibly be?

Having applied the four rules, now try to integrate the message that the symptom is embodying into your conscious awareness. Did you discover anything new? Would you be willing to bring the new knowledge which might be about your shadow— that side of you that you do not totally accept—into your life and allow it to manifest? Would you dare to express this side of yourself in action and ways of being to allow it out of the dark shadow of your being?

Take time to write this work up in your mind-body journal, and add a brief discussion on the theme, "Illness is a path to self-knowledge and wholeness."

▬▬ Annotated Bibliography

Borysenko, Joan. *Minding the Body, Mending the Mind.* Reading, MA: Addison-Wesley, 1987. Important corrective to oversimplistic positive thinking. Many practical tools for increasing one's personal control and emotional balance. Useful section on the myth of negative emotions.

Dethlefsen, Thorwald and **Rüdiger Dahlke.** *The Healing Power of Illness.* Translated by Peter Lemesurier. Shaftsbury, Dorset: Element, 1990. The meaning of symptoms and how to interpret them. Physical disease is viewed as messages and signals from the unexpressed shadow, whose purpose is to propel us towards wholeness in body, mind and spirit.

Dossey, Larry. *Meaning and Medicine.* New York: Bantam, 1991. Useful case histories illustrating the healing power of finding uniquely personal meaning in disease.

Duff, Kat. *The Alchemy of Illness.* New York: Pantheon, 1993; **Donna Talman,** *Heartsearch.* Berkeley: North Atlantic, 1991; **Ken Wilber,** *Grace and Grit.* Boston: Shambhala, 1991. These magnificent autobiographical case histories are required reading for anyone embarking in the helping professions. Chronicling three different illnesses (chronic fatigue syndrome, systemic lupus erythematosus, breast cancer), each one illustrates the immense complexity and subtlety of disease, and how the search for meaning ultimately yields a spiritual transformation forged from suffering.

Groddeck, Georg. *The Meaning of Illness.* New York: International Universities Press, 1977. This reprinted volume brings together Groddeck's classic papers from the 1920s.

Hay, Louise. *You Can Heal Your Life.* London: Eden Grove, 1984. A catalogue of thought patterns and the emotional states that they lead to are coordinated to some 400 physical ailments. The general panacea for them all is "learn to love yourself."

Kidel, Mark and **Stephen Rowe-Leete.** *The Meaning of Illness.* London: Routledge, 1988. A collection of articles from a Dartington conference on this topic. The contributions cover a wide spectrum of points of view and are valuable for illustrating the basic issues arising out of attributing meaning to disease.

Levine, Barbara H. *Your Body Believes Every Word You Say.* Lower Lake, CA: Aslan, 1991. Some interesting instances of metaphorical body symptoms, and valuable ways (visualization, affirmations) of working on them.

Mindell, Arnold. *Dreambody.* New York: Arkana, 1982; **Arnold Mindell,** *Working with the Dreaming Body.* New York: Arkana, 1986; **Joseph Goodbread,** *The Dreambody Toolkit.* London: Routledge & Kegan Paul, 1987. A trio of books introducing process-oriented psychology. They discuss the body's role in revealing the self, techniques for amplifying body symptoms as signals from the higher self, and the philosophy, goals and practices of this psychology, which draws its roots from Jungian analysis and Taoism.

Shealy, C. Norman, and **Carolyn M. Myss.** *The Creation of Health.* Walpole, NH: Stillpoint, 1988. Investigating and transforming the emotional patterns behind illness using psychotherapeutic tools and spiritual guidelines. Detailed case histories illustrating the connections between symbolic causes and the development of illness are given, along with discussion of intuitive diagnoses.

Sontag, Susan. *Illness as Metaphor.* New York: Farrar, Straus and Giroux, 1977. Important illustrations of the dangers in attempting to attribute simplistic psychological meaning to disease.

Webster, Lynn. *Dream-work.* London: Dryad, 1987. Useful primer for how to use dreams to produce integration of all one's diverse aspects.

13

Patient/Practitioner Partnership: The Therapeutic Alliance

The physician has always been the man between two worlds. Caring for the physical body while attending to the inner man . . . he is master of both the mechanical and the conscious side of life. The authentic physician is both a healer and a man of knowledge.

—JOSEPH NEEDLEMAN[1]

Roots of the Patient/Physician Relationship[2]

*P*LATO CALLED MEDICINE 'the science that pertains to the love of the body.' Evidently technique and caring are inextricably combined in the person of the ideal physician. Although the modern physician—orthodox or alternative—is able to call upon an impressive array of high-tech instruments, equipment and gadgetry for diagnosis and therapy, the age-old elements that go into the compassionate, caring side of the equation remain the same. Indeed, it is actually the overshadowing of the caring function by the scientification of Western medicine in this century that is primarily responsible for the renaissance of the traditional medicines. Herbalism, naturopathy and various forms of energy medicines which stem from Chinese, Tibetan and Indian roots are enjoying a vigorous revival. In addition, many relatively new therapies such as applied kinesiology, osteopathy, chiropractic, homeopathy, reflexology and aromatherapy continue to attract practitioners, students and patients. In emphasizing the body as machine and focusing on disease pathology, orthodox medicine has tended to relegate the caring function to a minor supporting role, more or less delegating it to nurses and paraprofessionals. Lacking the physician's authority, both that vested in him by the culture and his own inherent authority as an expert on disease and the body, these individuals, no matter how well-intentioned, cannot exercise the complete function of a fully developed patient/practitioner relationship.

It is clear that throughout the recorded history of medicine with its fads and fashions in treatments, what consistently heals is this relationship established between the patient and the practitioner. From our modern vantage point we can look back on medicine prior to the nineteenth-century clarification of asepsis and hygiene, the formulation of the cellular pathology theory of disease and the discovery of germs, and wonder how throughout history the practice of medicine not only endured, but actually flourished with few effective therapeutics. No doubt the fact that the majority of illnesses are self-limiting and resolve on their own untreated has something to do with the profession's durability. But this cannot account for it all, since many professions have come and gone over the course of centuries as the need for them waxed and then waned. The physician-priest, the shaman and the witch doctor remained prominent figures in traditional cultures because in time of body crisis and sickness we turn to another for help. A crucial consequence of identification with the body means that when the body sickens inexplicably, we are likely to panic as our very identity is threatened. In disease we lose the familiar feeling of control of the body, our physical and mental powers are diminished and we are thrown into uncertainty about our ability to regain our autonomy and personal control. And so we seek out another who is familiar with such states to reassure us, explain and give a name tag to what is happening to us, and hopefully to guide us through the uncertainty and the existential darkness.

The patient/physician relationship is a Jungian archetype—prevalent in all cultures, changing its forms to fit the particular socio-cultural nexus of the society in which it is embedded, but invariably containing certain enduring elements: one who knows and is well, attending one who does not know and is ill. The first physicians we know about were in fact priests, and the modern practitioner too has inherited the priestly vestments of aloofness, special powers and access to a world only vaguely known to others. The patient's ignorance of the reasons for her distress and the belief that the physician has the knowledge and power to give relief have always been associated with a dependency of the patient on the one who supposedly knows and can explain. Moreover, as Dr. Thomas Preston has so eloquently pointed out, this archetype is instilled into each of us in our formative childhood years. The awe of the parents for the physician is transferred to the child:

> The alacrity with which the doctor's commands are carried out gives them precedence over those of the parents. The physician is the only one who is allowed to violate the rules and taboos of the home, entering the bedroom and physically handling the child's body in an atmosphere in which everything is subordinated to his wishes. The physician is above family law in ordering the Mother to get this, or do that, while other household activities cease in deference to his presence.[3]

Thus we grow up viewing the physician as all-powerful, and somehow through his magical ability to heal, elevated to larger than life status. Since we associate the recovery from our childhood illnesses with this exalted figure, we have all learned to connect recovery from illness with his ministrations. These associations, spurious or genuine as the case may be, strengthen and perpetuate the relationship of the helpless child to the all-powerful healer, the relationship to which we are likely to regress as adults at the onset of disease.

Yet as we approach the twenty-first century, this relationship between all-powerful physician and dependent patient is breaking down. The doctor's scientification and preoccupation with the physiology and biochemistry of body pathology, valuable as it may be for infectious disease and traumatic injury, is far less appropriate and useful for the chronic diseases that now increasingly dominate an aging population. The doctor as sophisticated body mechanic is also unable to offer much of value to the stress-related complaints and functional symptomatology which make up anywhere from one-third to perhaps as much as 90 percent of the cases that a family general practitioner sees.[4]

The allopathic biomedical model of illness and disease is based on the premise that curing the disease—i.e., eliminating the body pathology—should also heal the illness. It was the very success of this model in providing a framework to treat the infectious diseases that were the primary cause of death in the last century that began to relegate the caring function—the relationship between doctor and patient—to the sidelines. If the therapeutics do the work, then the relationship becomes merely a way to ensure the patient's cooperation and "compliance" with the treatment, be it antibiotics, steroid or insulin injections, or surgical operations.

As that model begins to reveal its limitations, the elements that are entailed in the caring function of the relationship begin again to assume major importance. And this is not simply because if we can't fix the disease with modern medicine, at least we would like to have a caring, compassionate relationship as a substitute. The fact is that the patient/practitioner relationship is actually itself a very powerful 'drug,' but one whose pharmacology, side effects and dosage remain virtually unexplored. Even the manufacture of this drug is not consistent in its quality control, some believing it to be nothing more than common sense and good-natured reassurance, while others suggest that it entails special learnable skills and attitudes. It is exactly those illnesses for which the biomedical procedures, technologically sophisticated though they may be, are impotent that the patient/practitioner relationship seems to have the power to influence in beneficial ways.

This chapter is intended to elucidate for the practitioner some of the properties of the drug 'physician,' and to try to establish its appropriateness and its general relationship to healing. Along the way we shall be obliged again to examine in more depth than hitherto our core concepts of a humanistic medicine, the differences between healing and curing, what it means to 'treat the person' not just the disease, and how once again that relates to our views of human nature. Because the interview is both the means of establishing the psychobiosocial diagnosis as well as the beginnings of a rational therapy that incorporates psychosocial elements, we shall be looking in detail at the communication skills involved in the practitioner's interviewing techniques. Practically speaking, the quality of the patient/practitioner relationship is of special importance to us in natural medicine because such an important part of our therapeutics centers around lifestyle changes (dietary, exercise, stress reduction) that require self-responsibility on the part of the patient. Such changes are powerfully assisted by a strong patient/practitioner partnership. Lastly, because the placebo, long a strange medical anomaly, has sometimes been taken as the basis for whatever virtue alternative medicine has, we must take a serious look at the placebo to decide whether it is (as allopathic medicine usually views it) a nuisance, or whether it is a genuine token of the patient/practitioner relationship, and therefore something to be enhanced and consciously applied wherever possible.

Current Dissatisfactions with Mainstream Medicine

The archetype of the all-knowing doctor and the helpless patient is actually only one of three principal patient/physician (P/P) modes. A fuller schemata appears in Table 13.1.

Patient/Physician mode	Physician's role	Patient's role	Family analogue	Appropriate for
Active-Passive	'Treat' the patient	Relatively inert	Parent/infant	Acute trauma, coma, delirium, emergencies
Guidance-Cooperative	Advise the patient what to do	Cooperate, or 'comply'	Parent/adolescent	Infections, congenital or deficiency disease
Egalitarian Partnership	Assist the patient to help herself	Participate as an equal partner	Adult/adult	Most chronic illnesses, those with substantial psychogenic components

Table 13.1 Three Modes of the Patient/Physician Relationship[5]

I believe that it is fair to say that in alternative medicine we tend, on the whole, to encourage a more egalitarian partnership, and that is why in fact I chose the word in the title of this chapter. However, I think it important to understand that the majority of patients who come to complementary medicine do so because they seek a more egalitarian relationship in the first place. This implies, in fact, that no one of these three modes is *the* right one for all patients and all situations. Pediatrician and professor of behavioral medicine Dr. Naomi Remen reminds us that in the deep distress of a sudden incapacitating disease, and in certain phases of an illness, we *want* and need to be taken care of. A temporary dependence on "the expert who knows" is not unhealthy at those times, provided it is not prolonged longer than necessary. Just as an adolescent still needs parents to guide, encourage and even occasionally confront her, so too the patient with an acute infectious disease probably is best served by an expert who fully understands the etiology and prognosis of that disease and can effectively advise what should be done to maximize full recovery. And indeed what such a relationship does demand *is* cooperation and compliance with the doctor's orders. The difficulty arises—once again, chronic illness and psychosomatics are the instructive prototypes—when such a mode is no longer appropriate. The physician so used to playing active or guidance role models may have grave difficulty shifting gears and assuming the role of an equal partner with the patient. But patients too, accustomed to expecting the doctor to provide the answer, are bewildered when the physician says "there's nothing more we can do for you."

Holistic medicine is going to have to move out of these rigid, two-dimensional models. Probably both patient and physician are best served by a new medicine that invites the patient to play as great a role in her illness as she is prepared to assume. Doctors often say that patients don't want to know about their illnesses, but the evidence is actually in the other direction: in general patients do want to know more. Once again, because of natural medicine's inherent interest in lifestyle changes, which after all do require increased self-responsibility and that the patient to do much of the work, our patient/practitioner relationships must provide effective vehicles for assisting patients to develop skills and self-confidence in becoming experts on their own disease. The practitioner, then, needs to be skilled in helping a patient to look deeply into causes—lifestyle and psychosocial—and he also needs to act as a support for the difficult work of making the necessary changes that are likely to be called for. Indeed this is a new medicine, although no doubt the patient/practitioner relationship has at times worked exactly this way throughout history, without the variables having been explicitly identified. We have simply arrived at a point where we need to be able to describe the drug 'physician' in sufficient detail so as to be able to use it more explicitly and with greater reliability in a variety of illness situations.

There is little doubt that the patient/practitioner relationship is a major source of discontent in the modern health care system. Various North American studies have found estimates as high as 65 percent of patients dissatisfied with their physician.[6] The following reasons for dissatisfaction were cited:

- Physician's lack of warmth and friendliness
- Failure to consider the patient's concerns and expectations
- Use of unfamiliar terms
- Lack of adequate explanations concerning the diagnosis and cause of illness.

I have not been able to find any studies on the relative satisfaction with alternative practitioners, but it seems clear that the rapid growth of complementary medicine in the past decade must be due in part to these reported dissatisfactions with mainstream medicine. On the other hand, not all alternative practitioners are immune from the implied criticism of these findings, since we too often use unfamiliar terms (chi energy, foods classified into yin and yang, auric healing, toxic theories of clogged intestines, iris diagnosis, chakra analysis, balancing of subtle energies) that we do not always explain adequately to our patients. I suspect, however, that the majority of alternative practitioners do address seriously the first two of the above four complaints, an important reason for our currently thriving practices. For instance, it is common for many practitioners of natural medicine to provide comprehensive handouts on treatments as well as detailed literature on syndromes, and some recommend homework.

There is a considerable literature[7] that shows consistently that the young medical student enters training as idealistically and as full of humanistic values and the desire to relieve human suffering as the alternative practitioner. However, as the emphasis in medical schools is pre-eminently science—biochemistry, anatomy and physiology, microbiology—at the expense of ethics, psychology, medical anthropology and medical philosophy, his original values gradually become submerged in the training in disease pathology. Even if psychosocial influences are given lip service, the curriculum emphasis is "hard science," and there are few courses in training the young doctor in communication skills and how to impart humanistic values in his practice. Overworked and frequently oppressed by superiors during his internship, he is given little support for taking time to "talk with patients."

The Physician's Job

What actually is the medical practitioner's job? On the surface it appears simply to restore health, or if this is impossible, to assist the patient to retain as high a quality of life as possible. But this statement is deceptive. In the first place, as many have noted, health is not, as is so commonly assumed, the absence of disease. Indeed as we emphasized in the last chapter, health and disease can be independent of each other. Remen (1980) has even titled one of her chapters, "How to Have a Disease in a Healthy Way." The roots of "health" come from the old German verb *haelen*, meaning hale or whole. Health has something to do with a feeling of aliveness, zest, a sense of wholeness. Evidently it is an experience, and its opposite is not disease, but illness. Since some doctors have actually taken the position that their job is simply to treat disease, they have effectively opted out of the business of attending another's illness. Again, we can see why in this vacuum, alternative medicine flourishes. People wish to have their physicians take their illnesses seriously, but to do that the physician must treat the whole person, since it is the whole person, and not the liver, gallbladder, joints or any other part of the body, that has the illness.

Nevertheless, it is very easy to use glib phrases such as "treat the whole person" without actually clarifying just what this means for medical practice. Medical philosopher Joseph Needleman (1985) has put his finger on the complementary skills entailed in his plea for the physician to be a person of knowledge *and* skilled in the art of healing. To treat the whole person we need to know just what a person is. True, we all know intuitively what we mean by a person, and we all have some sense of what it would mean to treat the person holistically. However, the business of science is in part to refine our intuitions and to create systematic bodies of knowledge and conceptual formulations that we can apply to particular cases, and to teach the knowledge to others. In condemning the over-scientification of modern medicine I do not mean to condemn science at large, for I believe, along with Drs. Needleman and Cassell, and medical ethnobotanist Andrew Weil, that true medicine is a subtle blend of art and science. The fact is, however, that modern mainstream medicine is hamstrung not so much by its overemphasis on science, but by the fact that its scientific philosophy, in contrast to its state of the art technology, is tied to the outdated mechanistic model of the last century. That mechanical view of matter fails to acknowledge the more relativistic advances of this century, the discovery that the subject matter being observed is not independent of the observer even in physics, much less in medicine, and the holistic and teleological perspectives of the life sciences. Moreover, the practice of medicine continues to ignore the considerable advances in the social sciences—in particular in the psychological and behavioral sciences—showing that behavior and experience have their own independent laws which, while consistent with neurophysiology and neurochemistry, will nevertheless have to be discovered and elaborated at their own (holistic) level of analysis.

Having said that, what does it mean for a practitioner to treat the person? One thing it certainly means is to see the patient in the wide framework of the biopsychosocial etiologic framework which we have been emphasizing throughout this text. Tissue pathology simply is an insufficient and myopic view of disease and illness causation. But apart from etiology, person-centered medicine means that treatment also must take into account an individual's idiosyncratic needs and values, his locus within a community, and his relationships to significant others. If unfulfilled needs can predispose to disease, how can the practitioner remain aloof from understanding a patient's unique needs and values? And that certainly cannot be done by treating the sick person purely as a diseased object.

Evidently we need to understand as much about personhood as we do about anatomy and physiology. It is well known that we do not give the same objective analysis and treatment to a patient who says, "I can't seem to stop smoking," as we do to a pancreas that says, "I can't seem to generate as much insulin as the body needs." For the latter we bring to bear all the scientific knowledge of blood sugar mechanisms and metabolic dysfunction that current biochemistry and neuroendocrinology permit. For the former we are likely simply to chide our patient, or worse, vent our own frustration upon him. Yet such aspects of personhood as the hierarchy of motives discussed in Chapter 3, certain unique moral values, a desire to be creative, have fulfilling relationships, and to exhibit conflicts between self needs and the desire to please others, to be inhibited from what one wants by fears and anxieties, are as much a part of the anatomy of a person as the gallbladder is part of the anatomy of the body. In Dr. Eric Cassell's words,

> a sense of responsibility, the ability to form relationships, curiosity, the need for control, the need to be loved and to be needed, embarrassment, shame, dignity, honor and many other attributes are all universally found among persons to a varying degree and in varying manifestations.[8]

If these complex aspects of a person are indeed related to their health, as shown throughout this text, then they must be taken into account by the physician. Cassell's quotation above reminds us that these qualities of persons are as much a part of a person as are their anatomical characteristics, and I think he is right when he implies that the biopsychosocial framework, valuable as it is for widening our perspective on causality, does not actually give us sufficient information to take all these aspects of "person" into account in our therapeutics. Ultimately we have to go into each case and make a diagnosis that involves distinctly human factors and personal qualities that are applicable in that person's life. Unfortunately, such a detailed diagnosis is going to differ quite radically from the sorts of diagnoses we are accustomed to in medicine, be they based on tissue pathology or the diagnostic categories of psychiatry. What is needed is no less than a science of the person. Progress in holistic medicine not only depends upon the evolution of that science, but it actually will be a substantial contributor to it.

Diagnosing Illness vs. Diagnosing Disease

For the patient, illness is frequently an uncanny experience. Something seems to have gone wrong with the body: it is no longer the familiar servant functioning automatically without requiring awareness or attention. The sense that in illness the body is no longer under our control underlies the belief in traditional cultures that in disease the body is possessed. But even in our modern era, illness demands an explanation: we want to know what has gone wrong, find a name for the disruption of function so as to relieve our anxiety and return to the land of the known.

Naming the disease is an important function of diagnosis, for it reduces the unfamiliar to the familiar. Furthermore, diagnosis is as reassuring to the physician as it is for the patient, since a treatment protocol generally cannot be implemented until the disease has been identified. This is all very well if the diagnosis really does describe the pathological process, that is to say, if it really does provide patient and practitioner alike with something more than just a name.

Diagnosis is, of course, approached rather differently in complementary medicine. Firstly, Ayurvedic physicians or practitioners of various Eastern systems of medicine diagnose within completely different conceptual frameworks, using signs derived from the tongue or the pulse. The homeopath has a unique system for diagnosing. Additionally, there are various other diagnostic devices such as muscle testing, allergy tests, iridology, reflexology, hair analysis, radionics, pendulums and others. Some of these diagnostic aids point to anatomy and physiology, whereas others locate dysfunction and imbalance within different conceptual frameworks altogether. Another large group of practitioners of natural medicine avoids altogether giving a name to the patient's disharmony. Since they regard their treatments as assisting to rebalance the organism as a whole, they are not interested in the particular pathological anatomy or physiology. Working as a clinical herbalist, I personally rely on the patient's allopathic diagnosis that he generally brings with him. I know that the medical doctor's training in physical diagnosis is far more extensive than my own, and unless I have reason to doubt the patient's family physician and the various specialists he usually has seen prior to arriving at my consulting rooms, I generally work from the allopathic diagnosis as a point of departure.

Part of every doctor's job in fact is to try to make a four-part diagnosis of the patient's physical problem. Consider the patient coming with certain symptoms: epigastric abdominal pain, indigestion, belching, reflux and an uncomfortable full feeling in the chest. After physical examination designed to rule out by exclusion various alternatives, a diagnosis of *hiatus hernia* is arrived at. This is the first step, the naming, which brings the patient and physician a certain degree of relief, for it brings the problem into the realm of the known.

The second part of the diagnosis is the *mechanical (body) explanation.* Part of the stomach has been pushed up into the hole of the diaphragm through which the esophagus passes to join the stomach.

Thirdly, hiatus hernia, having occurred frequently enough in the past and the effects of various rational treatments studied, has both an established treatment (a set of possibilities) and a statistical prognosis.

Often these three aspects are all that are given in a typical diagnosis, but in fact a fourth causal element is always implicit. Did this disease develop out of overwork, poor diet, trauma or strain, aging, hereditary influences or what? As Cassell (1976) points out, these four aspects—naming, anatomical/physiological explanation, treatment and cause—are always in the air with every diagnosis, even if implicit. Even in the physician's simple statement, "You have a virus," our shared socio-cultural background allows us to fill in the missing ingredients, the usual course, refractoriness to antibiotics, and so forth.

Given the various advantages—and there are many—to such a straightforward physical diagnosis, it is understandable that medicine has endeavored to extend this simple four-point model to all illness. Thus, psychiatry has created name tags for extreme mental states—catatonic, hebephrenic and paranoid schizophrenia, manic depressive psychosis, hysteria, obsessive-compulsive neurosis, depression, character disorder, anxiety neurosis and so forth. Furthermore, search continues for possible neurophysiological correlates of these name tags, again in an attempt to find bodily explanations. Unfortunately, the psychiatric categories are little more than names for symptoms, and thus just labels. Moreover, these psychiatric labels have accrued considerable stigma and thus, in contrast to the diagnosis of hiatus hernia or gallstones, have become terms of opprobrium which dehumanize the patient. They are, therefore, of limited help to the general practitioner of natural medicine, save perhaps as a way of identifying very difficult patients that the clinician may, lacking expertise with extreme states, choose to refer to a specialist in psychotherapy.

If it is true, however, that a considerable portion of patients—perhaps as many as a third or more presenting with physical complaints to general practitioners—actually do have stress components in the predisposition or maintenance of the condition, and if another considerable proportion are converting problems of living into physical complaints as their "tickets of admission" to professional help, then it is a strong presumption that many patients coming to a practitioner of natural medicine are likely to require a diagnosis that takes the psychogenic factors into account.

But if no useful diagnostic categories exist, what is the practitioner to do? How can he create a rational treatment protocol in the absence of a valid diagnosis? Fortunately the situation is not inherently insoluble. Through a comprehensive holistic interview, the practitioner can gradually bring a case into focus. He does this, however, not by pigeonholing his patient's illness into familiar categories that can then be looked up in a handbook for the effective treatment and prognosis, but by piecing together, in partnership with the patient, the story behind the illness.

Let me give three brief examples taken from Balint (1964) of the kind of diagnoses that are likely to be discovered. In Case 2, a child presented with frequent tonsillitis, colds, influenzas, coughs, bronchitis and screaming fits over a year period. In consultation with the mother, the physician eventually was able to discover that "the real cause of the illness lay not in the boy, but in the mother-child relationship which could not develop freely because, in her anxious insecurity, the mother overburdened it by restricting the boy's freedom more than was tolerable for a healthy child."

Case 11, man of 54, with abdominal pains, diarrhea, giddiness, fear of crowds, afraid of going to the cinema or the barber. Surgery for gallstones was performed with only temporary remission of symptoms. The full diagnosis took some years to get, principally because the doctor continued to focus fruitlessly on a physical diagnosis. It turned out that the patient "never liked his job, though he is not certain what he would have liked to do instead." One clue to the possible treatment direction was: "Born musician and played the fiddle without being able to read music."

Case 13, a woman suffering severe backache, suspected slipped disk, unconfirmed by physical examination and X-rays. Headache and insomnia after bumping head in minor jolt on a bus. All physical exams negative. Here the diagnosis turned out to entail guilt feelings about divorcing her husband on the (dubious) grounds that he had become psychotic, and then marrying her lover. A subsidiary causal element was anger at the daughter for living with a man the patient disliked.

Notice that in these three cases there is no attempt to give any empty verbal labels such as neurotic, hysteric, depressive or the like. Rather the physician was encouraged to try to piece together the central threads of each patient's problems in living that were being expressed as physical symptoms. This took much work over considerable time on the part of the physicians.[9] And the result in each case was a diagnosis consisting of a plain language statement, devoid of any "psychological" interpretations. What these physicians discovered were only three out of an immense possibility of themes and variations.

If we now ask what kinds of treatments these patients need, the general answer must be some kind of psychological, not biochemical, medicine. In mainstream medicine the general practitioner often feels very limited in the kinds of psychological medicine he is willing to offer. The general fare is sympathy, reassurance, advice, confronting with reality, and interpretations. In general these "common sense" remedies are ineffectual, and worse, often detrimental to the patient/practitioner relationship. Doctors are generally surprised and dismayed when the reassurance that nothing physical can be found to explain a patient's symptoms is not followed by relief and satisfaction. Sympathy and advice in how to live can be had from friends and neighbors, and the patient is right to expect something better from her physician. Interpretations too are rarely of therapeutic use unless discovered independently by the patient. Confrontations are occasionally valuable if the ground has been adequately prepared, but even then the real work is in "preparing the ground," that is to say, employing the techniques of counseling and psychotherapy discussed in Chapter 8.

The poverty of the typical general practitioner's repertoire of psychological medicine is in part due to his emphasis on finding a physical pathology for every illness. If he can do that, he has a rational therapeutic plan. But in those cases where he cannot, he often has very little to offer. These patients certainly form a large proportion of those who eventually give up on their allopathic physicians and turn to complementary medicine.

The alternative practitioner is likely to help them in two ways. By being willing to take the time to listen carefully to the history and to be open to psychosocial elements in the etiology, we shall discover that the actual interview itself can be not only diagnostic but also therapeutic. Then, by bringing dedicated, caring, close attention to the person, the practitioner establishes his concentrated presence and attention as the basis for a strong patient/practitioner relationship out of which the healing power of nature, Hippocrates' *vis medicatrix naturae*, can begin to work.

The practitioner's dedicated attention or presence has been cited by some[10] as the actual basis for healing. It certainly is a common factor to all successful therapies and is worthy of greater study. Certainly, every practitioner of natural medicine will of course employ the specialized techniques and therapeutics of his discipline, and may be somewhat surprised to learn that the patient/practitioner relationship itself may be of equal power to his therapeutics. Indeed, the therapeutics themselves may derive much of their very strength from the patient/practitioner relationship. To understand that statement better, however, we must turn to the illuminating phenomenon of the placebo, or what should more accurately be called the token or symbol of the patient/practitioner relationship.

The Placebo: Enduring Token of the Therapeutic Alliance

The term *placebo* is derived from the Latin "I shall please." The word entered the English language designating a particular vesper service which had overtones of flattery, hence was not genuine. By the early nineteenth century the word was in common use in medicine to denote substances given more to please than to benefit the patient.[11]

In the classical sense, then, a placebo is an imitation medicine—a sugar pill dressed up to look like a pharmacologically active drug. This might be given to placate a patient when the physician suspects that the disease is purely functional and doesn't want to continue giving drugs with dangerous side effects or addictive potential. With the rise of scientific medicine and the medical-industrial complex, the placebo has found use in research studies to provide a baseline against which new medicines or experimental treatments can be compared. Although the classical placebo is supposedly inert, it nonetheless exerts a considerable therapeutic effect. Thus a new drug or treatment has to have an effect consistently over and above the placebo effect to be judged of clinical value.

In fact, the classical placebo pill is merely a special case of the power of the patient/practitioner relationship to influence the patient's well-being. It is the patient's belief that she is receiving genuine medicine that brings about the placebo response. And that belief arises partly out of the personal relationship established between the doctor and patient, and partly out of the socio-cultural authority vested in the physician and his remedies. The placebo pill is our equivalent of the witch doctor's healing dance and the shaman's incantations.

That the placebo effect goes well beyond sugar pills is attested by the vast number of formerly accepted therapeutic procedures, substances and "treatments" that once enjoyed great popularity, but which now lie abandoned and discredited in the dusty annals of the history of medicine. Indeed, there are those who regard the history of medicine as merely the history of the placebo effect.[12] Certainly the so-called "cures" of the past seem bizarre to us today. A partial list includes purges, bloodletting, lancing and cupping, blistering, arsenic, mercury, cow dung, urine, crab eyes and mummy dust. Various operations now known to be utterly worthless include internal mammary artery ligation for angina, and glomectomy for asthma. Most tonsillectomies, appendectomies and hysterectomies performed "electively" are probably placebo surgery at best, and the sources of iatrogenic disease at worst. All of the obsolete and discredited procedures and "medicines" were at one time enthusiastically recommended, endorsed by authority and, for a time at least, seemingly effective. Yet whatever beneficial effects followed were surely placebo effects.

What underlies the placebo, gives it potency? Dr. Andrew Weil regards it as the product of three interlocking beliefs: (1) the patient's belief in the method, (2) the practitioner's belief in the method, and (3) the patient and practitioner's belief in each other, i.e., the strength of their relationship.[13] I propose to show in the remainder of this section that the placebo effect is a pure instance of the power of the patient/practitioner relationship undiluted by treatment-specific factors. But first some of the myths and fallacies surrounding the placebo must be dispelled. Five common misconceptions are: (1) placebo effects are not as strong or as widely applicable as "objective" effects of treatments; (2) whatever effects placebos have are due to "non-specific" factors; (3) the placebo operates mainly with very suggestible individuals or those with low intelligence; (4) the placebo is restricted to imitation pills; and (5) the placebo can only work for functional disorders, and hence is a way to "prove" that a disorder is functional or imaginary.

Placebos have strong and widespread effects. Although there is some controversy about their ability to affect disease pathology (Spiro, 1986), most commentators agree that they can, under optimal circumstances, affect both the disease process and its symptomatology, that is to say, both disease and illness. Placebos have been shown to

> relieve severe postoperative pain, induce sleep or mental alertness, bring about drastic remission in both symptoms and objective signs of chronic diseases, initiate the rejection of warts and other abnormal growths, and so forth.[14]

Other conditions shown to be affected by placebo include seasickness, headaches and coughs. Pathological processes that have been affected include rheumatoid and degenerative arthritis, blood cell count, respiratory rates, vasomotor function, peptic ulcers, hay fever and hypertension.[15] In the form of pills, placebos also elicit many of the usual undesirable side effects of medication including nausea, headaches, skin rashes, allergic reactions and even addiction.

These undesirable side effects of placebos are a special case of the reverse placebo effect, called *nocebo*, meaning noxious rather than pleasing. Voodoo death spells and various anecdotal evidence of patients believing (mistakenly) that they were told their case was hopeless, and dying soon after, are testimonials to the nocebo effect. A physician presenting a grim prognosis to a patient in a pessimistic way that fails to balance the diagnosis with an emphasis on the patient's unique strengths and resources as a spiritual being, is likely to exert a strong, potentially damaging, nocebo effect on the patient. The nocebo can be seen clearly in experimental studies where the normal effects of potent drugs are sharply diminished when patients are misled to believe that they are receiving placebos.[16]

There is no special personality type susceptible to placebo, and the effect does not correlate with hypnotic suggestibility. If anything, the placebo response is slightly enhanced with intelligence rather than the other way around.[17]

Until quite recently the percentage of cases of severe pain substantially alleviated by placebo was taken to be about one-third of patients, a modest value, leaving considerable room for direct treatment effects to operate on the remaining two-thirds. But newer research, evaluating not only pain relief but improvement in a variety of other symptoms, indicates that the figure is closer to 70 percent.[18] These studies include treatments originally believed to be effective for asthma, herpes simplex and duodenal ulcer, but later discarded as worthless. Evidently treatments which the physician believed were effective, even though they were not, maximize the placebo effect, a result which is consistent with the three-part belief system that empowers the placebo in the first place.

These experimental findings not only attest to the power of the belief system arising out of the patient/practitioner relationship to heal, they also make it clear that the notion that the placebo is due to "nonspecific" factors is at best misleading. So-called nonspecifics include physician attention, interest and concern in a healing setting, patient and physician expectation of treatment effects, and the reputation, expense and impressiveness of the treatment.[19] These are all, of course, important variables that have from time immemorial, over a spectrum of cultures, contributed to the potency of the patient/practitioner relationship. A good patient/practitioner relationship is quite specific: anyone can recognize it, and the skills and attitudes that characterize it can be taught, as the next section on interviewing shows.

In general, placebos are enhanced if they are active substances, or entail operations with direct anatomical and physiological consequences. Such is the case for all the discredited treatments and repugnant medicines of history. Their direct, usually disagreeable effects can be perceived, and operations leave scars and damage. Treatments and drugs that have these noticeable direct effects are termed *active placebos*, as opposed to the classic, relatively inert sugar-pill placebo. When the contributing beliefs are optimal, and combined with active treatment-induced features, we discover that the placebo effect is truly impressive. Indeed, since it arises out of the patient/ practitioner relationship and all the psychosocial trappings in which that relationship is embedded, we can conclude that there is nothing non-specific about it at all. The inert pill, or the sham treatment, known to be a fake by the physician who gives it, probably exerts the least placebo effect, yet even these, because of the patient's trust and the doctor's authority, are effective in 33 percent of cases. Thus, far from being a medical curiosity, a nuisance or a fake, the placebo is indeed a symbol of the therapeutic alliance between patient and practitioner.

The great power of the physician/patient relationship to heal forces us to consider closely how much of the power of our alternative therapies might indeed be due to the power of the strong patient/practitioner relationship that, because of their focus on the person and not just the disease, many holistic practitioners establish. Mainstream allopathic medicine has been reluctant, as we know, to acknowledge alternative procedures and methods as anything more than placebos.[20] Part of the skepticism towards alternative medicine is due to the lack of *double blind* controlled studies that might establish statistically reliable specific treatment effects that exceed the effects due to relationship variables. In double blind studies patients with a given condition are typically divided into two groups, equally matched for socio-economic status, age and any other variables expected to contribute towards the treatment outcome. The patients from both groups are given identical professional examinations, explanations, instructions and so forth, but those in the experimental group get the actual treatment or medicine, while those in the control group get a sham treatment or a placebo pill. The procedure is called double blind because ideally neither the doctor nor the patient knows whether a particular individual has received the sham/placebo or the actual treatment/medicine under investigation. The great virtue of such a technique is that, in principle, it enables one to discern any treatment effects above and beyond those of the doctor/patient relationship itself.

Why have so few natural therapeutics been subjected to the scrutiny of the double blind methodology? First of all, scientific research requires money, and until very recently government funding for alternative medicine has been virtually nonexistent.

And the sums involved are not trivial. To subject an herb (e.g., feverfew for migraine or garlic for hypertension) to the kinds of extensive tests and studies demanded of a new chemical drug costs a few million dollars. But there are other difficulties. How could colonics be evaluated by a double blind study? What exactly could serve as a "sham colonic" that neither the practitioner nor the patient could discern from a real colonic? Could a Bach Flower practitioner or a homeopath give the same kind of consultation knowing that his patient has a 50/50 chance of receiving a placebo instead of his prescribed remedy? Complementary medicine will doubtless have to evolve its own strategies and methodologies to evaluate its procedures and therapeutics following the pattern of other new sciences.[21]

Normally the skepticism of orthodox medicine towards alternative medicine is meant and taken as a disdainful commentary on the worthlessness of our therapeutics. But if we realize that the placebo, far from being an imitation of the real thing, is actually a token of the power of relationship to heal, we might then withdraw some of our defensiveness and take pride in the judgment. Clearly, the effects of relationship interact synergistically with the effects of active treatment to influence positive patient outcomes. It therefore follows that the practitioner should do everything possible to enhance the relationship effect, known otherwise as placebo. Suppose for a moment (to take an extreme devil's advocate position) that a considerable proportion of our therapeutics proved in the long run to be mainly vehicles for organizing our beliefs about sickness and health in a positive way, for directing our focused attention towards the patient's problems of living, and for engendering caring and presence towards a suffering patient. How important is it whether our procedures work via the patient/practitioner relationship or via some more biological mediator? The physician's first and foremost obligation is to relieve human suffering. If he does it by lending strength, helping the ill person bring meaning to her life, serving as a witness to another's pain and deepest fears, being with another in their journey, so be it. Such a practitioner will have served the healing profession well.[22]

The Biopsychosocial Interview

The diagnostic interview is the pivot of every form of physical or psychosocial therapy. Influenced by the mechanistic philosophy of nineteenth-century science, the strictly medical interview, as we know it, has made a virtue out of objectivity. Such an interview consists of a search for signs and symptoms in order to reach a decisive disease diagnosis by exclusion. The interview is conducted not unlike the way a geologist examines a rock sample for mineral content, or a botanist examines a flower to place the plant within its proper genus and species. It is true that the patient in a clinical examination is required to be conscious in order to answer questions, but beyond that her participation is minimal. Indeed, the "cooperative" patient is the one who does nothing more than respond to a standardized routine series of physician-initiated questions.

This kind of objective medical interview, however valuable it may be for eliciting the facts of physical disease, will not do for grasping the full nature of illness with its multifaceted, biopsychosocial dimensions. Aside from the power dynamics which put the person-patient in the dependent, dehumanizing role of an object, such an interview inhibits the development of an authentic patient/practitioner relationship, the very ingredient necessary for a biopsychosocial diagnosis. It is only in the context of relationship that the illness story can emerge in such a way that the practitioner can begin to grasp its nature and therefore propose a rational treatment plan.

The classical medical examination is almost entirely a physiological and anatomical examination appropriate to the person as a biological organism. However, a full biopsychosocial examination is, as Balint and Balint (1961) have put it so well, essentially the examination of a human relationship. In contrast to a biological or other scientific examination, its success depends on the substantial contributions of both participants.

One consequence of this need for two-way communication is that any hope of a "routine medical examination" must be ruled out from the onset, since the "examination" is actually an interaction, the direction of which will be set in part by the patient. The two kinds of examinations that we are discussing are actually best regarded as the two ends of a the continuum shown graphically in Fig. 13.1.

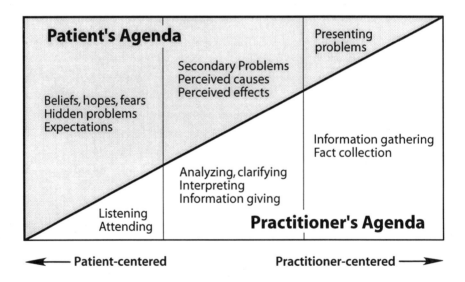

Fig. 13.1 The Continuum of Interview Styles [23]

In the illustration the extreme right sector, marked practitioner-centered, represents the standard medical interview where nearly all the initiative activity is on the part of the physician (corresponding to a large white area below the diagonal line, and a very small area for the patient above the diagonal). As the interview becomes more and more patient-centered (looking leftward), the interaction becomes more equal until eventually, when the patient is sharing her story of the illness and initiating most of the dialogue, the practitioner is mainly listening and commenting empathically. Fig. 13.1 suggests that the practitioner can choose to move back and forth along this continuum, depending on the needs of the session or the stage of the treatment process.

Once again we should emphasize that the psychosocial aspects of the interview are not going to yield name tags that will point to standard treatments. Rather, what emerges is a holistic picture or story, best described in plain language statements. These will describe in non-theoretical terms the patient's problems of living, likely including such things as conflicts experienced by the patient between meeting her own needs and those of others in her life, degree of personal fulfillment in areas of work, creativity, family and relationships, interpersonal skills or lack thereof, as well as anxieties and insecurities that keep the patient from doing what she would like to do. Along the way, of course, the practitioner remains alert to picking up possible sources of imbalance and potential health hazards deriving from the wider biopsychosocial field. Notice that disease pathology is not ignored in such a patient-centered interview and diagnosis. Aside from serving as the "ticket of admission" to the practitioner's consulting room, physical symptoms becomes one of a myriad of facets to the illness which must be addressed and evaluated. In the biopsychosocial interview, body pathology is simply no longer the sole focus.

The complexity of such an interview means that no standardized routine can be suggested that will be useful for all practitioners in all situations. (Project 13 suggests guidelines that direct the practitioner's attention to skills, knowledge, orienting attitudes and the personal work he must do on himself to acquire the ability to create a strong patient/practitioner relationship that will expedite both diagnosis and therapeutics.) The interview is going to be a deeply searching contact with another fellow human being, and the practitioner must be ready and willing to enter into such an encounter.

> The sincere opening up of a patient's intimate life, with all its miseries, petty and profound fears, frustrated hopes, few and often very precarious joys, is a deeply moving experience. Moreover the help that can be thought of or offered is often hopelessly inadequate to the real need.[24]

The practitioner who is inexperienced in life or the intricacies of a professional helping relationship (or both), faced with a patient's profound existential and practical problems, may find his own feelings of impotence, futility or injustice aroused. No doubt fears of such feelings keep many practitioners from offering the open-ended interviews that are likely to expose the patient fully, preferring to remain within the bounds of their therapeutic modality.

> Fostering greater intimacy with patients brings us more deeply into their experiences. We cannot listen empathically to their descriptions of pain without feeling it ourselves. Moreover, the issues that they bring to us often resonate with our own unresolved griefs or remind us of our own unhealed wounds. Without some source of strong grounding and support, we could easily become engulfed in or overwhelmed by the suffering we encounter and our inability to fix it.[25]

Psychological medicine is not for all. But the practitioner who is inclined to go deeper with attentive caring, patience and a firm grasp on his own spiritual resources will be surprised at how *vis medicatrix naturae*—the healing power of nature—operates in the psychological as well as the physical realm. Sometimes the simple recital of problems to a caring, compassionate listener is enough to engage the patient's underlying personal strengths, spiritual reserves and healing resources. This potential power of mere listening is why communication skills that enhance respect, caring, regard, genuine encounter and empathy are emphasized in the training of those who wish to facilitate whole-person wellness.

In the classical medical examination it is the practitioner who does the examining (the extreme right side of Fig. 13.1), but in the full biopsychosocial examination, the practitioner must conduct the examination with the patient in such a way that he must strive to have the *symptoms examined by the patient*.[26] This is a revolutionary departure from standard medical practice. Yet failure of the patient to see the full picture of her illness—which may and often does involve a series of physical complaints extending over a period of years—can perpetuate it indefinitely. Patients must be brought to the same general understanding of their symptomatology as this text has been striving to impart to students and practitioners. It is inadequate in this kind of medicine for the physician alone to understand the patient; unprepared interpretations handed out to patients like tranquilizer prescriptions are rarely effective.

In the wide-ranging interview, which is simultaneously diagnostic *and* therapeutic, the practitioner is really cast in the archetypal role of teacher, *docere*. Every practitioner imparts his view of disease and illness to his patients. Whether he does so explicitly with diagrams, explanations and bibliotherapy, or whether by omission, he will still teach. The practitioner of natural medicine, exploring the full biopsychosocial field, does it by the nature of his concerns and interests, what he looks for, and finally in his recommendations for treatment, which so often involve lifestyle changes in the areas of diet, exercise and stress management. All these considerations mean that psychological medicine is generally best practiced from the patient/practitioner mode of equal partnership, out of which negotiated treatment plans are created in close consultation with the patient. The practitioner is, or should be, an expert on healthy living and prevention of disease. If his expertise extends to an understanding of the psychosocial dimensions that also contribute to disease and health, he is then in an optimum position to serve as an effective, all-round wellness consultant to his patients. Yet in spite of the practitioner's knowledge and skills, ultimately it is the patient who knows the most about herself, her life concerns, constraints, limits and assets. The patient with physical symptoms has come perhaps out of puzzlement, uncertainty, anxiety. Out of the interactive interview with the patient, the practitioner will offer information, diagnosis and recommend a treatment protocol. Nevertheless, it is the patient, finally, who must make the decision whether or not to engage the practitioner. This is the full partnership mode which I believe general practice in holistic medicine must endeavor to cultivate.

Communication Skills for Enhancing Relationship and Optimizing Treatment Adherence

Chapter 8 introduced some basic helping attitudes derived from several different approaches to psychotherapy and counseling. Now we describe a core of basic communication skills that can be used by the practitioner no matter what psychotherapeutic mode he chooses. In large part, these derive from a psychoeducative approach to learning skills termed microcounseling or *microtraining*, pioneered by Professor Allen E. Ivey and colleagues at the University of Massachusetts.

What microtraining attempts to do is break down the verbal and non-verbal skills used by successful counselors and therapists into simple component units that can then be taught to anyone who has a professional (or other) reason to be a helper. The microcounseling model identifies the basic skills underlying a wide variety of therapeutic orientations as *attending and listening*. Microcounseling explains precisely what is involved in each, then typically arranges for the student to (1) read about the skills, and (2) practice them in a brief five-minute simulated interview with a client, which is videotaped. Then (3) the student and supervisor review the video looking for instances where the skills were used effectively, after which (4) a second short client-student therapist interview takes place.

An appropriate introduction to microcounseling's beginning communication skills starts with the common observation that novice interviewers make many communication errors. They frequently cut off interactions with their clients by asking closed-ended questions,[27] making long awkward speeches, sending the roadblocks to communication identified in Chapter 8, and exhibiting noticeable discomfort with periods of silence. Most of these problems stem simply from the fact that novices do not know what to do to facilitate communication, and do not have a beginning behavioral repertoire of skills to rely on when awkward moments arise or hiatuses appear.

Microcounseling identifies *attending* as the beginning skill that underlies many dimensions of counseling. Attending is the basis of listening, which itself is the dooropener that creates a climate of caring interest, thereby encouraging the client to express her concerns. Attending behavior is in fact simply listening thoughtfully to another person. It is primarily made up of the following three identifiable skills: (1) eye contact with the speaker, (2) a relaxed posture indicating interest, and (3) the ability to verbally follow the speaker with active listening, paraphrasing or summarizing of what has just been said.

In microtraining each of the three beginning skills in attentive listening is taught separately and rehearsed in five-minute videotaped interviews, after which trainee and supervisor review the tape giving positive feedback for the trainee's use of the skill. Eye contact is quite self-evident. The relaxed listening posture too requires little comment.

Perhaps the best way to show some of the alternatives for verbal following is to take a small passage from a statement of a patient who is explaining difficulties she has been having in keeping to a healthy eating plan to which she and her practitioner had previously agreed. Table 13.2 gives the patient's explanation on the left, and five different ways that the therapist/counselor could "follow" the patient's statement on the right, thereby demonstrating listening.

Patient's Statement

Well, it's been very difficult to keep to the dietary plan we made. I've had to work late at the office nearly every night for the past few weeks. When I get home, I'm usually so tired and hungry I can't get into preparing new food I'm not used to cooking. So I just heat up some left-overs or make a cheese sandwich or microwave a frozen pizza. Sometimes I've even been too tired to do that, and then I've stopped at a fast-food junk restaurant on the way home. I know I oughtn't to do this, but I really just don't seem to have the energy to get into cooking a healthy meal after I've worked all day.

Alternative "Following" Responses

Paraphrase: If I understand you, when you've been working all day until quite late at the office, you simply feel too tired to prepare a healthy meal for yourself.

Reflection of feelings: You seem a bit frustrated and a little guilty too that you haven't been able to keep to the healthy diet plan we worked out.

Invitation to expand: Working late just now because. . . New food recipes, kind of unfamiliar and . . . Just so much energy and then . . .

Non-verbal flow maintainers:[28] Nod of the head = "go on, you're on the right track." Rotational movement of head = "continue, that seems interesting." Puzzled, quizzical look with furrowed brow = "I don't understand, please elaborate." Um hum = "continue, I'm interested."

Direct questions: Just what time do you get back home? How often do you find yourself working late? Is there any way you can reduce the late nights?

Table 13.2 Alternative "Following" Responses that a Physician Might Make to a Patient's Statement[29]

As Table 13.2 illustrates, the practitioner could paraphrase back to the patient the *content* of her communication. Or he could *reflect the feelings* that are lying just behind the patient's words, and which in part will be communicated by various non-verbal cues, including the patient's tone of voice, gestures and posture. Sometimes merely repeating a fragment of the patient's sentence is helpful in encouraging the patient to expand and go deeper. A simple nod of the head, movement of the hands, an upraised eyebrow also communicate interest to go on. And lastly, the practitioner may fall back on direct questions, open-ended if possible.

All of these communication skills of attentive listening are straightforward, and can be learned by anyone interested in getting to know another better. Some may question the artificiality of breaking down a complex human interaction into a set of stylized responses or exercises drawn from a "kit bag of skills." I cannot respond better to this criticism than the authors of this approach:

> Our experience has been that individuals may sometimes begin in an artificial, deliberate manner. However, once attending has been initiated, the person to whom one is listening tends to become more animated and this in turn reinforces the attender, who very quickly forgets about attending deliberately and soon attends naturally.[30]

In other words, just as we are awkward at first when speaking a foreign language we learned in the artificial situation of a classroom, quite soon in the country in the company of indigenous speakers, content quickly takes precedence over our deliberate efforts to find the right verbs and nouns. We start to "think in the language," which is exactly what happens to the counselor as he gains practice and experience.

Many beginners have difficulties with silences, or the hiatuses that do occur in every interview. Actually silences are a natural part of all two-way communication, for if one listens closely or watches a videotape of an interview one notices that *islands* of dialogue alternate with periods of silence. The beginning counselor must learn to become comfortable with these, and not let his own need to keep the flow going to intrude. Silences give important opportunities to both listener and speaker to reflect on what has been said and learned to that moment. It also gives the practitioner a chance to notice carefully the non-verbal aspect or silent language of the speaker. Although we will never meet the patient in Fig. 13.2, just by looking we already know a great deal about her.

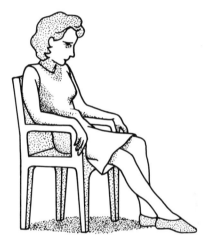

Fig. 13.2
Non-Verbal Communication[31]

In general, the interviewer must learn to take note of his patient's non-verbal language. Here are some common examples:[32]

- A frown, grimace or startled look can reflect lack of understanding, or amazement at you and your idea.
- A stare can mean "I care," "Something about you is pleasant or unpleasant," "I question that."
- A very rigid posture can be indicative of a physical or emotional discomfort, lack of receptivity, a defensive attitude.
- Blushes, perspiration or paleness of face can show how the individual is responding to the dialogue: with embarrassment, anxiety or shock.
- A smile can depict warmth, joy or sincerity; or, if incongruent with the speaker's words, it can be a way of saying, "Yes, but I mean no."

When carried out with genuine caring, respect, interest and true regard for the other, the beginning skills of following the speaker's verbal and non-verbal behaviors are the essence of *empathy*, the heart of every helping relationship. Empathy may be thought of as the ability of the listener/practitioner to put himself, temporarily, in the shoes of the speaker/patient. To do that one has to be able in the first place to listen to the other. Empathy is commonly confused with sympathy, but the contrasting responses in Table 13.3 emphasize their differences.

Empathy	Sympathy
From what you've said about having to work late and then coming home tired and exhausted, I can see how difficult it's been for you to keep to the healthy eating program we established.	It's a real shame you weren't able to keep to the new diet while you were working late.
I sense your strong desire to establish a new and healthy diet, and your frustration too just now that it seems so difficult to maintain it.	I'm very sorry you are having such a tough time getting into the new eating program because of your work schedule.

Table 13.3 Empathy versus Sympathy as Expressed by the Clinician

Of course, there are times when sympathy can be most helpful, but too often it has the subtle connotation of reinforcing powerlessness and confirming victim consciousness. On the other hand, accurate empathy is always empowering, since it represents an understanding and acceptance of the speaker's feelings. Thus the elementary attending skills illustrated in Tables 13.2 and 13.3 represent effective listening and thus serve as the foundation of accurate, elementary empathy.

Yet there is a deeper empathy that goes beyond listening. Apparently, empathy is experienced at its most profound when the practitioner is able to disclose parts of himself, both in sharing his own feelings that arise in the dialogue, but also in offering interpretations and actually striving to assist the patient to find ways to solve the problems that are revealed. In other words, the practitioner's ability to reveal himself as a person, combined with his desire to assist another with his therapeutics, touches the patient and deepens the therapeutic relationship.[33]

One important contribution to empathy is the counselor's ability to radiate warmth and *positive regard*. How does a listener do this? Crucial to the concept is the therapist's ability to assist the patient in bringing out her own positive resources, problem-solving capabilities and interpersonal skills. In other words, the practitioner has to learn to see the positive side of a patient, and to feed back what he hears and sees to the patient. This, in part, is what we mean in holistic medicine by helping the patient find the healer within.

In behavioral terms it means paying selective attention to positive statements and reinforcing them. This explicit policy of giving positive appreciation has also been called giving *strokes*, which are units of human recognition.[34] In fact, it is always possible to find something positive in every individual and to highlight that dimension in the reflection of feelings. The professional can do this by operating on the assumption that people can be helped, and holding fast to a faith and trust that everyone has the ability to change in such a way as to turn an illness, however grim on the surface, into a healing experience.

Some more intermediate and advanced microcounseling skills used in interviews include (1) expediting clarity and *concreteness*, (2) helpful *confrontations*, and (3) suggesting *interpretations*. Many of us have a tendency to talk in vague, general terms. When a patient says, "I drink a few cups of coffee every day," it is helpful if the practitioner does not leave that statement vague, but asks for the exact number of cups. A few could be a dozen, as it turned out in one of my consults. But similarly, in describing interpersonal relationships, difficulties at home or at work, and so forth, the practitioner must press for sufficiently concrete details in order to make the diagnosis, which is the prerequisite for treatment.

Confrontation must be helpful, i.e., non-judgmental. "If you keep on smoking two packs a day you'll probably get lung cancer" is reasonably unhelpful. The patient knows the statistics as well as we do. Helpful confrontations are often possible when the practitioner can objectively see contradictions, incongruities and discrepancies in the patient's values or needs, and then point these out in a caring way. Because our cultural tendency is to blame others for our difficulties, confronting a patient with the degree to which she is playing a role in attracting the events of her life is useful for inviting increased self-responsibility. Helping patients to understand how feelings depend upon beliefs is another kind of important confrontation that the counselor may profitably undertake.

Although interpretations tend to conjure up images of psychoanalysis, those are actually only a particular class of interpretation. In general, an interpretation is the introduction of a new, alternate frame of reference in which to view a set of observations, feelings or behaviors. When interviewers make interpretations they present their clients with a fresh, perhaps more general or all-embracing way of seeing a problem. The interpretation is a kind of expanded paraphrase that brings a group of statements together in a different framework. Often a metaphor that catches the sense of a cluster of comments can serve this purpose too, and has the added advantage that the patient can flesh out the ambiguities and potentials of the image, thereby discovering for herself its healing power. As mentioned, interpretations that go too far beyond the client's own framework often fall flat, not because they are wrong, but because, proposed before the patient herself has reached the point where they can be accepted, they do not produce the emotional effect of a new insight. Wherever possible, the counselor endeavors to lead the patient to make her own interpretations, for then their impact and durability is ensured.

Aside from the communication skills described, the practitioner/interviewer would do well to consider how to arrange the interview setting. Fig. 13.3 shows three seating positions at a desk, each of which subtly affects the communication process.[35] AB1 is the typical seating position suitable for the authoritative/dependent, practitioner/patient relationship mode. Position AB2 actually produces six times more interaction than AB1 and three times more than AB3. The absence of a desk altogether will normally reduce the perceived authority of the practitioner unless he compensates in some other way, such as wearing a white coat.[36]

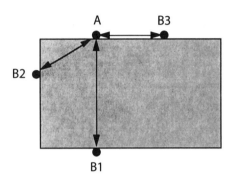

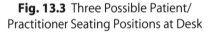

Fig. 13.3 Three Possible Patient/Practitioner Seating Positions at Desk

Finding the Healer Within

Is the power of the patient/practitioner relationship to heal no less magical and mysterious than the dance of the shaman, the charms of the witch doctor, the waters of Lourdes? Somehow the therapeutic alliance established between patient and practitioner provides a force impelling towards wholeness. Yet it is not the practitioner who heals, it is the relationship. True, the practitioner may succeed in curing the physical pathology of disease with any of a variety of natural or allopathic medicines or treatments. Such cures may or may not heal the illness.

Throughout this text I have stressed the discovery of the causes of illness, emphasizing that these can be found scattered widely throughout the entire biopsychosocial field. Discovering the causes of an illness is the first step in establishing an effective treatment protocol. Moreover, the Balints' empowering concept of the patient examining herself suggests that although the practitioner can suggest, interpret and advise, it is the patient who finally must see these causes and make the changes that illness is demanding.

Yet an ill patient, frightened and confused, is often not in a state to start this work. So the holistic physician must begin with support and with the overall viewpoint that the patient will be able to engage her own spiritual and personal resources—strength, courage, determination, the will to live, the ability to see and find meaning in crisis, the grit to convert problems to challenges. Out of the relationship that develops, the practitioner must be able to create a vision of the patient as whole, healed. This vision may or may not mean that the disease is cured. Like the photographic artist who takes many shots of her subject to get the one that best captures the deepest and truest essence, according to her vision of these qualities, so too the physician must learn to see and ally himself with the healthy part of every patient, according to his vision of health. This requires the skills and orienting attitudes of listening, empathy, caring and authenticity, along with knowledge of the body and an effective therapeutics. But in addition the practitioner must clarify his own views on life and living before he can assist another with the deep transformations that chronic or terminal illness may demand. Truly the practitioner must be a man of knowledge, one who, himself scarred and wounded, can boldly walk with another along a stretch of their journey.

In some way yet to be identified, natural medicines and therapies *work with the patient working on herself*. Used allopathically to treat symptoms, neither herbs, chemicals, acupuncture needles nor operations possess the ability to heal. In the context of the healing alliance with practitioner and patient committed to finding and addressing the causes of imbalance, the message of the placebo is that a myriad of diverse agents and procedures can speed the healing process. Yet ultimately healing is the result of the force that resides in us all, the healing power of nature. The practitioner's job is in part to clear away the obstacles to its efficient operation, and in part to be there for, and to attend the patient during the time that the restorative force operates. In the eloquent words of Nobel Prize winner Dr. Albert Schweitzer:

> Each patient carries his own doctor within. They come to us not knowing that truth. We are at our best when we give the doctor who resides within each patient a chance to go to work.[37]

He who can succeed in that task need not worry about the narrow boundaries of particular therapeutics or current medical fashions. Aligned with the greatest tradition in medicine, unbroken since time immemorial—the art of healing—he may in truth be called physician.

Project 13

Conducting a Biopsychosocial Medical Interview

Every effective practitioner finds a way of interacting with his or her patients so as both to foster a caring, helping relationship and to discover the biopsychosocial nexus in which the presenting problem is located. Questions such as

- How would you describe yourself emotionally and mentally?
- How do you feel about your ability to remember and focus your attention?
- Tell me about your relational life?
- What is your libido like? Strong, weak, medium?
- Do you have or think you have a history of abuse—psychological, physical, sexual, emotional?
- Do you have a spiritual life?
- Is there anything I haven't asked you?

can go a long way toward inviting the patient to explore relevant issues that go beyond the somatic presenting complaint, yet may bear critically on it.[38]

The Society for Research and Education in Primary Care Internal Medicine has drawn up extensive guidelines to assist medical students in carrying out a medical interview that not only forms the basis for a physical diagnosis, but also serves as the ground of a humanistic patient/physician relationship.[39]

This patient-centered interview approaches the patient as a unique person with a personal story to tell, and is intended to promote trust and confidence, and to lay the foundations for a strong patient/practitioner relationship. It clarifies the patient's symptoms and concerns, generates and tests many hypotheses that include the full biopsychosocial range of illness dimensions, and creates the basis for an ongoing relationship.

Many of the skills utilized are those described in Chapters 8 and 13. But many other orienting attitudes and areas of knowledge are also included in a series of tables which progressively explicate the principal objectives of the interview, shown here somewhat modified and abbreviated in a form suitable for the practitioner of natural medicine. The tabulated guidelines include:

- Elaborating the elements and structure of a patient-centered interview
- Integrated (physical and psychological medicine) approach to clinical reasoning and patient care
- Physician development of humanistic values.

Project 13 invites the practitioner or student of natural medicine, employing his or her own therapeutic modality, to apply the guidelines set out in the table below to conduct an interview with a patient (or simulated patient), endeavoring to cover as many of the points as practical.

Knowledge

- Recognize open-ended versus closed-ended questions.
- Understand the various stages of an interview:

   opening, characterization of principal complaint, life setting, searching the entire biopsychosocial etiologic field for potential causes and predispositions, appropriate review of body systems, closing.

- Understand the multi-functional objectives of the interview:

   basis for both physical and psychosocial diagnosis, to establish rapport, platform for negotiating treatment contract, vehicle for honest "I-thou" communication, forum for modeling the skills that positively influence health and well-being, classroom for teaching patient about health and disease.

- Be aware of non-verbal behavior of both self and patient.
- Define the characteristics of a helping relationship and unconditional positive regard.
- Understand the three physician/patient relationship modes, and demonstrate awareness of which of the three roles you are currently playing.

Skills

- Assist patients in telling story of illness, which includes detailed symptomatology, at the same time pursuing the broader life setting in which symptoms occur.

- Express interest in and commitment to patient via verbal and non-verbal facilitative communication:

    Verbal: allow patient to tell story of illness, use balance of open- and closed-ended questions, reflect feelings, paraphrase content, seek clarification, maintain empathy, give positive regard.

    Non-verbal: arrange space comfortably for patient and self to minimize power differentials, nod, show affect, communicate interest with body language, echo patient's non-verbal behavior, use quiet attention and silence skillfully.

- Avoid communication-hindering behavior:

    Verbal: over-technical language, false or premature reassurance and advice, frequent interruptions, "there's nothing wrong, it's all in your head."

    Non-verbal: disinterested posture, poor eye contact, excessive note-taking, closed posture.

- Calibrate potential communication barriers and compensate as required: deafness, language or cultural differences, high anxiety, possible hidden agenda.

- Define patient's strengths and use them. Seek out and integrate patient's experience in treatment.

- Negotiate contract that maximizes patient's autonomy, self-responsibility and ability to act as an equal partner. Establish treatment plan with patient, and verify patient's understanding and full agreement. Remain sensitive to patient's non-verbal cues of agreement or disagreement. Don't bulldoze patient into treatment plan.

Attitudes

- Approach patient respectfully and non-judgmentally.

- Respect patient autonomy and individuality.

- Display willingness to join patient as partner, to share diagnostic findings, treatment processes and decisions.

- Display willingness to work with and learn from patients with diverse backgrounds and personal styles.

Table 13.4 Patient-Centered Interview Guidelines

In conducting the interview within the framework of the guidelines of Table 13.4, by modeling the various facilitative attitudes and skills enumerated, you are actually teaching these values to the patient through role-modeling. The ability to establish rapport with patients from a wide diversity of personal and sociocultural backgrounds means applying these guidelines in your own style. Genuineness is essential to achieving strong rapport with the patient. The practitioner's own personal development of humanistic attitudes and his or her own inner work also takes place within the framework of the patient-centered interview. Some of the dimensions where the practitioner may explore personal growth potential are described below:

- Recognition and acceptance of one's own personal strengths and weaknesses, openness and curiosity about one's own attitudes, beliefs and expectations that constitute assets and limitations, value judgments and feelings in working with patients. Learn to feel such feelings, but not necessarily act on them.
- Awareness of one's own stress responses and insecurities. Seek recognition of one's own signs and symptoms of distress, and explore methods of stress reduction.
- Noticing one's personal reactions to patients that include transference and counter-transference. Recognizing when one's own feelings are actually part of the patient's illness.
- Ability to allow patient participation in the treatment process, and to develop patience when patients decline to accept parts of a treatment plan, or fail to carry out agreed assignments involving lifestyle changes.
- Awareness of the nature of suffering and the goals of medicine.

In assisting another we truly help ourselves. The practice of medicine is a spiritual path for those who wish to make it so. The wise practitioner, by maintaining an open, curious, tentative, experimental attitude towards the work, learns from mistakes as well as successes, taking it all in stride. It is the scarred and wounded healer who is indeed best placed to attend another on their journey. Illness is the vehicle, and the practitioner's caring attention and presence are the catalysts for healing, the power of which ultimately lies within each individual.

Annotated Bibliography

Balint, Michael. *The Doctor, His Patient and the Illness*. New York: International Universities Press, 1964; **Michael Balint** and **Enid Balint**, *Psychotherapeutic Techniques in Medicine*. Springfield, IL: C.C. Thomas, 1961. Although written over 30 years ago by two British analysts, these two volumes remain a treasure trove of case histories in psychological medicine. Remarkably free from jargon, psychotherapy—carefully distinguished from "common sense" reassurance and advice—is shown to be an essential therapeutic skill that every physician can learn and use in daily practice.

Cassell, Eric J. *The Healer's Art*. Philadelphia: J. B. Lippincott, 1976. An eminent internist examines in detail what it would mean for the doctor to "treat the whole person." For Cassell, medicine always has been and always will be in part a *moral* discipline, concerned inextricably with values, thus setting limits to the usefulness of science and technology in patient care.

Ivey, Allan E. and **Jerry Authier.** *Microcounseling.* 2nd ed. Springfield, IL: C.C. Thomas, 1978. Notable for its innovative and systematic approach to the teaching of elementary empathic and communication skills—attending, listening, reflecting feelings, paraphrasing content, self-disclosure, interpretation—necessary for psychosocial interviewing. A valuable primer for the practitioner wishing to know exactly what to do to begin to practice basic psychological medicine.

Needleman, Joseph. *The Way of the Physician.* Harmondsworth, Middlesex: Penguin, 1985. Philosophy of medicine as a transcendent art in which the doctor, dealing with life and death, must combine knowledge and technology with a broader vision of meaning and purpose, if he wishes to go beyond "cure" to the archetypal role of assisting healing.

Preston, Thomas A. *The Clay Pedestal.* Seattle: Madrona, 1986. An examination of the roots of Western medical practice, both from the cultural perspective of the past 2500 years, but also as it develops for each one of us from our first encounters with the "omnipotent" doctor in our childhood. The limitations of the biomedical model are related to necessary changes that must come about in the doctor/patient relationship.

Remen, Naomi. *The Human Patient.* Garden City, NY: Anchor/Doubleday, 1980. A pediatrician and eminent practitioner of "mind/body medicine" argues that health is not merely the absence of disease, but is an *ability* to deal creatively with physical and psychosocial change. For Dr. Remen the practice of medicine can never be divorced from the practitioner's view of human nature, and health can never be guaranteed by interventions into human physiology intended to correct body pathology.

14

Case Studies in Psychological Medicine

Here we encounter an important difference between psychological and physical medicine. In physical medicine the examination is done almost entirely by the doctor; what is required from the patient is to agree to it and in a very minor way to co-operate with the doctor. True, in psychological medicine too, it is the doctor who examines the symptom, but the examination is conducted together with the patient with the aim of having the symptoms examined by the patient.

—MICHAEL AND ENID BALINT[1]

Introduction

WHILE THE PRINCIPLES of psychological medicine can be acquired through the study of books, putting these principles into practice with a flesh and blood patient is something else. There is no substitute for hands-on experience, ideally at first supervised by a skilled and seasoned mentor.

Yet practitioners must often begin in less than ideal situations. The patient may be there, complaining of somatic complaints for which the organic basis appears obscure or non-existent, or presenting symptomatology bearing a clear association to stress or personality variables. The clinician is obliged to jump in, knowing that a caring, concerned attitude of non-judgmental listening in the interview can itself be therapeutic, and secure in the knowledge that *vis medicatrix naturae* will operate at the mental as well as the physical level once the impediments to healing have been loosened.

Case histories illustrate how the techniques and orienting attitudes of therapy are applied by masters of the art, and so are useful to the practitioner wondering how to do it. I have selected several—reprinted from their original sources—for this final chapter to illustrate how key ideas can be put into practice. I would have liked to have presented cases from the practices of alternative and complementary practitioners to illustrate important themes of psychological medicine, but a search of the published literature turned up little or nothing where the presenting complaint was somatic and the treatment and analysis were psychological. Thus, I was obliged to take cases from the literatures of mainstream medicine and psychology. Five of the cases (two by Dr. Naomi Remen, two by Dr. Martin Rossman and one by Dr. Larry Dossey) are personal narratives by their authors; one (by Dr. Julian Slowinski) is a detailed description of the multimodal approach to a post-traumatic stress disorder, and yet another case (by Dr. Michael Balint) is developed from clinical seminar discussions with the doctor and his medical colleagues that took place over the course of a two-year period. A final case (by Dr. Melvyn Werbach) illustrates the very important principle that not every syndrome that seems predominately mental is necessarily psychogenic in origin.

Case histories, where the presenting complaint is somatic and the principal therapeutic modality is psychological, are actually rather sparse in the recent literatures of psychology and psychiatry. Many such cases were presented during the heyday of psychoanalytically-oriented psychosomatics, but because those older cases are described in the language of classical psychoanalysis, they are of limited use to the average practitioner of natural medicine, who will be unlikely to operate from that theoretical basis.

Reading the old cases from the vantage point of nearly half a century is an eerie experience. They illustrate an attempt to emulate objective physical diagnosis with psychoanalytic categories of psychopathology, and in so doing invariably cast the patient as a kind of object. Their principal thrust is to explain and interpret symptoms in abstract theoretical terms, many of which are little more than name tags (which quickly acquired a moral judgment) for the dysfunctional or problem behavior to be explained. No doubt this emphasis on theory was in part a consequence of the lack of powerful interventions for changing behavior, coupled with little agreement at the time of the necessary and sufficient conditions for growth and emotional health. In contrast, the more recent humanistic, transpersonal, existential and behavioral approaches employ plain-language descriptions of behavior and experience. In their more person-centered narratives, interpretation and theory have been replaced with pragmatic techniques and the special climate of acceptance that has been found helpful in inducing constructive change and growth. At the same time one cannot but wonder how these cases will read forty years from today. Will they and their conceptual frameworks too come to be seen as so "loaded" with preconceptions and theory, and evincing such a myopic viewpoint so as to be all but unrecognizable and of little more than historical value to the twenty-first century mind?

Case 1

Truck or Motorcycle (by Dr. Naomi Remen—1980)[2]

My first impression of Harold was that he seemed scarcely human, barely alive. Thirteen years old, 5 feet 3, and 253 pounds, he was massive and inert, allowing himself to be brought into my office in a wheelchair by the nurses without the slightest effort to help himself. He sat staring into his lap and did not look up as I took a history from his mother.

Harold had spent an ordinary childhood on his parents' ranch in Northern California, and had been completely well until puberty. In the next year and a half, he had gained 150 pounds. He had been evaluated thoroughly and all his studies were normal. Several physicians had tried to place him on a diet and failed. He was bedridden and totally isolated from his peers.

After getting the information from his mother, I turned to Harold, who had neither spoken nor moved for a full twenty minutes, and asked, "Why did you permit yourself to be brought here?" Harold looked up. His face, like his body, was passive and heavy, but his eyes were alive with anger. As we stared at each other, I felt the force of his anger with respect and relief. Here was energy that could be used.

After a minute or so, in which Harold and I measured each other, he said, "I want you to make me lose weight." His voice was deep and strong—not the voice of his body, but the voice of his eyes. His tone was challenging. Somehow I needed to contact the part that was so strong and angry in this boy and see if it could be turned from an opponent to any plan or diet I had, to a collaborator in resolving the problem.

I decided on a Gestalt technique. Taking a straight chair, I placed it in front of Harold and said, "Imagine that your fat is piled in a heap on this chair." He looked startled and, for the first time, not angry. Hoping that he was close enough to childhood to be able to fantasize, I said, "Can you see your fat here?" He nodded. "Good. Now, talk to it." Harold began to laugh. "What do I say?" "Tell it what you don't like about it."

After a small silence, he began to talk. Resentment after resentment poured out. His fat kept him from having friends, from going to school. It made him ugly. It made it hard for him to walk and even to breathe. When he fell silent, I asked him to tell his fat what he appreciated about it. Harold was shocked. "Appreciate?" This time the silence was longer. Then slowly he said that his fat excused him from chores. "And . . . ?" "And I don't have to do anything I don't want to." "And . . . ?" "And I don't have to try, and maybe if I tried, I couldn't."

"Harold," I said, "who has been talking?" "Why, I have." "Is this 'I' who has been talking fat or thin?" "I don't know . . . no, wait . . . my fat is over there. This 'I' is thin." "Good." And I moved my chair next to his, so that we sat, shoulder to shoulder, facing the empty chair on which he had imagined his fat. "What shall thin-you and I do about this fat?" He laughed delightedly—"Let's make a plan!"

We began to discuss choice. Like many adolescents, he discovered that he was accustomed to having adults make important decisions for him, rather than considering alternatives, seeking advice and choosing for himself. The decision he was making about his fat might be the first of many such decisions he would make in his life. He looked intrigued. I added that adult decisions took careful thought and suggested that he go home and begin a notebook, that he write down all the advantages and disadvantages of being fat and of being thin . . . and then write down everything he ate so he would know for himself. During the two weeks until his next appointment, I asked him to consider these things and to decide if he wanted to lose weight now and let me know when we met again.

Harold stood up and shook my hand. I felt once again a respect for the Angry Man I could still see in his eyes. I sat for a while in the examining room finishing my notes. As I stood up to leave, my eye fell on the empty wheelchair in which Harold had been brought in—and I realized he had left under his own power. It had happened so simply that I wondered if he even noticed.

In two weeks, Harold was back with his notebook and his decision. Yes, he wanted to lose weight. I told him I would call in a dietician to consult with him so that he could begin.

Over the next twelve months, Harold lost 110 pounds. He became interested in nutrition and turned into a creditable cook. He kept careful records of his intake and the dietician and I assessed his decisions and helped him discriminate about which were the wise ones. He wrote in his notebook daily about the inner dialogue between his "fat self" and his "thin self." On occasion, I pointed out how cleverly his fat self had outwitted his thin self, or how resourceful his thin self had been at a family dinner. He came to see that cleverness and resourcefulness were two of his major characteristics.

Then, halfway through the year, Harold stopped losing weight. As the weeks passed I became more and more concerned. In the stress of the situation Harold became silent and withdrawn, and I began to slip into an old pattern of success and failure and feel guilty about "failing" to make Harold lose weight. Now I began to dread his visits, although previously I had always looked forward to them.

On the morning of one of Harold's appointments, I drove to work thinking about him. Never having been fat, I realized that I didn't know what it would mean to me. What would it feel like to have my physical boundaries farther out than they were now? I decided to deliberately experience this. So as I drove, I slowly let my sense of my boundaries expand until I was the size and shape of my car. As I continued down the street in this new shape I experienced an immediate sense of false strength—big is strong— confusing my physical size with a psychological state.

I also remembered a cartoon I'd seen some twenty years ago in which a little Caspar Milquetoast of a man got behind the wheel of his car and was transformed into an aggressive, decisive, forceful driver. Then, as he left his car, he became a little Caspar Milquetoast of a man again. I wondered whether this transformation occurred because the little man suddenly felt his physical boundaries expand. Do fat people do this? Could Harold's fat have this meaning for him?

Harold was on time for his appointment; angry, sullen, and uncommunicative. He was wearing a new pair of jeans, and when I commented on them he replied in a shaking voice that he had needed to buy them recently and they were four sizes smaller than the last pair. For the first time I heard his fear. At the point he stopped losing weight, his weight loss had really begun to become obvious. Perhaps size was strength to him.

I began to tell him of my experience that morning. I talked about Caspar Milquetoast and about the illusion that size is strength, and gave him several similar circumstances where a person could confuse a physical state with a psychological state (i.e., being unable to conceive a child with being unable to mother a child). I said, "I wonder if somewhere inside you there is a driver part who is used to driving a three-axle truck, who would become uneasy if his truck became smaller. The truck is becoming smaller and smaller. Soon it will be the size of"—I hesitated, looking for an image, and my intuition gave me one— "a motorcycle." And that was it.

Harold suddenly got an inward look and with a great deal of intensity said, "Have you ever been on Route 1 on a Sunday when all those big cars are bumper to bumper and no one can move, and there is some dude on a 'cycle' going forty miles an hour right down the white line and thumbing his nose at all of them? Isn't that it? Being strong isn't being big. That's it! Being strong is being able to move." I said, "And?" Harold said, "And being able to decide where you want to go and to go there." And then he smiled. I was deeply touched. "Harold," I said, "who has been eating lately?" He said, "The driver of the truck." "Why?" "Because he didn't understand about motorcycles."

Harold returned in two weeks having lost five pounds. His opening words were, "Here—I have brought a picture of me to show you." He put on my desk a snapshot of an abandoned, rusted–out motor lying on its side in a field. Next to it, he put another snapshot of the motor. This time it had been set up on blocks. It appeared to be in working order, and had been painted a bright light blue.

I looked at him in confusion, and he said, "There, that's what I really look like—I change things—the change is me."

At present Harold is in school and visits me once a year. Recently, he sent me a picture of himself on his new motorcycle.

Dr. Remen's Discussion

The classic treatment of obesity of this sort in an adolescent is prolonged hospitalization and enforced diet. Effective though it may be in weight loss, this method is costly, both in terms of money and in terms of human time and energy. Harold lost weight. Helping him to get in touch with his strengths and personal resources, and to learn to assume responsibility, enabled him to gain something as well: a sense of his own ability to shape the quality and richness of his life through his choices.

Case 2

Whose Asthma? (by Dr. Larry Dossey—1984)[3]

Ted Frank was at the peak of his profession, a forty-eight-year-old attorney with a prestigious law firm. His office was where respectable attorneys in Dallas are supposed to have offices, in a downtown high rise—the prestige of the practice being proportionate to the height of the floor one occupied. Ted was a star in his firm, but he was unhappy with his work— bored with tasks, little gratified even when things went his way, and, worst of all, disgruntled with the way his associates directed the firm. He implemented his "grin and bear it" philosophy with quiet boredom and silent hostility for years, functioning with clear competence professionally, yet becoming increasingly disenchanted with his lot.

Then he developed asthma for the first time in his life—totally unexpected, without any history in childhood of asthma or allergies of any kind, and without any family history of such. At first he tried to ignore the problem. But the wheezing and shortness of breath grew worse, and he began to limit his activity. He could not talk to clients without wheezing audibly, and daytime wheezing gradually turned into nighttime wheezing. When he found himself unable to sleep, he gave in. For one of the few times in his life he went to a doctor.

His physician could find nothing wrong. Indeed, he seemed in peak physical condition aside from the asthma. He was put on a variety of asthma medications and was referred to an allergy specialist, where he underwent testing for a battery of offending agents or allergens that are known to trigger asthma. The tests proved to be of no help; and, although his medications were juggled, the asthma persisted, albeit at a lesser intensity. For six months various medications were started, then stopped when they failed to work. As each medication dosage was adjusted upward to tolerance, all he experienced was the noxious side effects—nervousness, anxiety, insomnia—without any obvious benefit. Finally, when he found himself taking sizeable doses of a hydrocortisone-like drug, he decided to take another direction.

He had learned of a specially designed hospital which focused on allergy problems. Patients were hospitalized for extensive periods, sometimes for months, and were painstakingly isolated from all environmental chemicals such as those in water and foods. Even bed sheets and clothing were scrutinized (no synthetic fibers allowed), as well as the wall coverings, floors, and ceilings, for fear that organic solvents used in the manufacturing process were the asthma-causing culprits. Special organic foods were used, all chemical-free. Nurses were not allowed to wear cosmetics or perfume while working in the isolation area, and even the air entering the rooms was filtered through great charcoal canisters to remove impurities. The goal of the program was to achieve "complete ecological control and environmental isolation." Then, when the asthma had faded, various known common substances would be introduced, one at a time. When the asthma flared following the introduction of a specific food, soap, or clothing of a particular type, it could be concluded that this was the offending agent. If this substance or article was then eliminated from one's exposure, it was expected that the asthma would not return.

The entire logic and rationale of the program infatuated Ted Frank, and he enthusiastically checked himself into the hospital-based unit. He followed every instruction the way he practiced law—attending to every detail—and was delighted when the physicians in charge predicted total success.

There was only one problem: it didn't work. A month later Ted was discharged from the hospital back into the real world of impure air, tainted food, and chemically treated water—several thousand dollars poorer and still wheezing. The compelling logic of the isolation program now seemed spurious, and he felt as if he had been misled. He had begun to develop a logic of his own about why this approach had failed, an idea that he shared with no one, not even the well-intended physicians who had attempted to cure him. Ted began to conclude that the approach of the ecological and environmental program was naive because it conceived of "ecology" and "environment" as something physical, something external, something "out there." No attention was paid to inner states, to emotions, attitudes, feelings—the world of consciousness. He had reluctantly concluded that there were two environments, an inward and an outer one—and that in his own case it was the ecology of his inner environment, his consciousness, that was of greater importance than the outer world in affecting his asthma. His proof? Mainly an intuition, but a string of failures, as well, of approaches that focused on his asthma as the result of an assault from the external world. Ted felt deeply that this approach was wrong.

He saw it as no accident that his official diagnosis, "adult-onset asthma," had befallen him at a time of emotional turmoil related to his increasing disaffection with his work and peers. He simply could not agree with the conclusions of his various physicians that the total origin of his ailment was some external source. Perhaps, he reasoned, there was some validity to an objectively caused illness, but this was not, for him, the whole story. He felt his anxiety and inner chaos were factors also—maybe not a total explanation, but important nonetheless. It seemed simplistic to do what the various approaches had attempted—to treat his body, or to isolate him physically from some offending agent. He was astonished that at no time had any physician, nurse, or respiratory therapist inquired as to the state of his psyche.

Ted Frank sensed a relatedness of body and mind to which his physicians had been oblivious. He felt that if this relatedness had been sundered, and if it were not repaired, his efforts at controlling his asthma would continue to be fruitless. He set out in his usual analytical, logical way in his own investigation of this ineluctable connection, and began to read various books dealing with psychosomatic concepts and the mindbody relationships in various forms of disease.

By the time he appeared in my office he had become a lay authority on his own illness. He even brought a reading list demonstrating the sincerity of his pursuit and the depth of his beliefs. His compendium was far more extensive than what could be found on required reading lists in medical school courses dealing with psychosomatic medicine. His intensity and sincerity convinced me that this man was extraordinarily committed to becoming well, and was willing to expend an enormous personal energy in the process.

From that time forward he always appeared in my office with a new book or two which he brought along to peruse in the waiting room. I found myself wondering what he would bring next, and what I could learn from his latest selections.

He had resigned from his firm, and had hung out his shingle in a small town thirty miles from the metropolis. Resolving to come to terms with the emotional upheavals caused by his work, he saw the move as necessary and as therapeutic as the drugs he was still taking for his asthma. He specified in our initial visit that he wanted to learn biofeedback, a decision he had arrived at after probing several books on the subject. He was infatuated with the possibility of learning to control or abort his asthmatic attacks willfully and consciously. With his characteristic energy and enthusiasm he seemed completely convinced he could do so.

I reveled in our conversations. He had no inflexible belief system to break through, no "Doctor, you make me well" philosophy to deal with. He felt convinced he had a hand in the appearance of his asthma, and was even surer he could have a hand in its control. Furthermore, his grasp of psychophysiological principles was basic and accurate. There was an instant rapport and cohesion between us, the felt magic that lends an experiential wonder to the doctor-patient relationship.

Following a thorough history and physical examination we reviewed his current medications and made some modifications. Then we talked about his reason for wanting to enroll as a subject in my biofeedback laboratory. I reminded him what he already knew: the record of biofeedback in the treatment of asthma is not uniform, the results are mixed, and the most rigorous sorts of studies have yet to be done. Yes, anecdotal and uncontrolled series of cases abound wherein success has been seen, but across-the-board proof of efficacy is lacking. True, we have known for years that emotions can play a key role in asthma, and we know too that asthma is not a homogeneous disease. There are surely several sub-types of asthma, some of which are undoubtedly influenced by emotions in varying degrees. I felt a full disclosure of the present state of the art was important to dispel any illusions and false hopes he might have about the effectiveness of biofeedback. He had been given plenty of inaccurate expectations about treatments in the past, and didn't need more.

We both decided that he was a fit candidate to begin biofeedback training. The biofeedback therapist with whom he worked, interestingly, was also a registered respiratory therapist, and knew well the physiological processes underlying his disease. She was marvelously adept at evoking in her patients an awareness of mind-body relatedness. They were a good match, and he learned the rudiments of biofeedback training quickly.

He learned to recognize inner tension, what emotional stress felt like in his body, and developed a surer conviction that his psychological state affected his asthmatic wheezing. His asthma began to abate.

But not completely. Although his skills at learning to deeply relax his body were enviable in the lab, he, like almost all biofeedback subjects early in their training, had difficulty in maintaining this state outside the laboratory environment in the "real world." Ted's asthma would still flare at predictable times, usually associated with emotional tension.

But his improvement was unmistakable, and he felt he was on the correct path. He affirmed time and again his belief in the body-mind connection that propelled him toward biofeedback in the first place.

He continued to practice his skills at home and in the lab with an admirable discipline. His reading list, which he continued to share with me, became increasingly sophisticated. He gradually developed a calm which reflected an underlying wisdom about his illness. Ted's logical-intellectual probes and his experiential excursions into bodymind domains via his adventures in biofeedback combined in some unfathomable way to emerge as what only can be described as a spiritual approach to the problem.

Illness for him came to take on a new meaning. "My asthma is part of me," he said, and he and I talked frequently about the approaches to his problem that had led him to this formulation. His early ventures in treatment emphasized disease as a malevolent external intruder, a thief in the night who catches one unaware. These views fit poorly with his own inner observations about how his emotions affected his symptoms. He simply could not affirm the notion that disease was "out there." Indeed, the therapeutic approaches that had totally emphasized this philosophy had failed. His statement, "I can't force it out" reflected an understanding that illness can never be vengefully exterminated by any technique, for the reason that it is part of oneself. To hate one's illness is to disdain oneself, he knew. Because of the interrelatedness of body and mind, one cannot focus merely on the physiology without evoking simultaneous repercussions of the psyche; and it was this connectedness that had been ignored by the purely physical approaches he had originally elected. His understanding that he was not different from his asthma led him to a new therapeutic strategy: "I' m taking a more playful attitude toward it." In recognizing the relationship between self and illness, he transcended the grim imperative to "conquer" his problem, to drive it into oblivion, to purge himself of it. Finally a new ontologic understanding emerged: "I'm attempting to integrate myself with the world."

Dr. Dossey's Analysis: Body-Mind Oneness—Beyond Metaphor

Ted Frank's awareness grew from a confrontation with illness. His experience epitomizes the fact that adversity, even dreadful physical diseases, can culminate in breakthroughs in awareness. This is an ancient observation, but one we forget in our blind categorization of illness as enemy. We do not often realize that disease can represent real opportunity for growth and transcendence, and that if we do categorically war against disease there is an element of ourselves that we also combat.

These observations go beyond metaphor. The understanding of inner connection, of body-mind unity, are demonstrable events whose reality can be demonstrated in the physiologist's laboratory. In particular, asthma is an illness that vividly demonstrates the inaccuracy of regarding a disease as if it were some disembodied entity, as if it had no connection with the psyche. The very name of the illness is derived from the Greek word *azein,* meaning "breathe hard." The word implies a smothering, an apt description of the experience of acute asthma. Hinshaw, an authority on diseases of the chest, expressed the interconnectedness of psyche and soma in asthma:

> Fear is both a cause and consequence of asthma. Treatment that serves to quiet fear, be it pharmacologic or psychologic, is good treatment.[4]

Not only is fear capable of triggering asthma, a simple belief can do the same. Several experiments in adults and children have shown that the mere suggestion to an asthmatic subject that he is inhaling an allergic agent (although not, in fact, true) can provoke an attack.

The unity of body and mind illustrated in cases of asthma such as Ted Frank's is not some mystical fabrication, as statements of "oneness" are frequently regarded in medicine. Although much of the mechanism undoubtedly remains to be worked out, it has been suggested that emotions, acting via the autonomic nervous system, cause changes in the lining of the bronchial tubes that make them more sensitive to both infectious and allergic agents.[5] In addition to the effects of the emotions on the lungs, emotions in turn are affected by the asthmatic process once it begins—a vicious cycle. Fear and apprehension, as Hinshaw points out, are part of asthma.

Ted Frank had learned empirically these associations, and set out to change them. He had reasoned, in the footsteps of many researchers, that since so many physiological variables can be modified significantly with a variety of relaxation techniques (e.g., blood pressure, heart rate, galvanic skin response, muscle tension, and certain aspects of the respiratory cycle), it only made sense to try to apply relaxation techniques to the treatment of asthma. The result? Ted himself had begun to replicate the results of many experimenters: both with and without biofeedback, the use of relaxation training in asthmatic persons can result in both immediate and long-term improvement of lung function. In his attempts to voluntarily improve his asthma, Ted was on firm ground.

Ted Frank's asthma illustrates the folly of attempting to understand disease in terms of simple cause-and-effect. The more we learn about the intricate interplay of mind and body, how a psychological event may follow or precede a cascade of physiological events, the more we become mired in an endless reverberating chain of happenings in human illness. Because of this complexity, simple causal explanations for most human diseases have lost much of the authority they once had. Only by considering illness as part of the whole world, including the inner as well as the outer landscapes, will we be able to accommodate the clinical complexities involved in problems such as asthma.

Ted Frank had served as his own body-mind research laboratory. His insight, "My asthma is part of me," seemed an understated expression of the unity of psyche and soma that pervades not just asthma, but all the major diseases of our day.

Case 3

Post-Traumatic Stress (by Dr. Julian Slowinski—1985)[6]

Sally D was a 30-year-old unmarried woman executive who was the victim of an unprovoked attack while walking along a city street. Her assailant repeatedly punched her and stabbed Sally in the face, the weapon piercing her cheek and tongue. The man fled the scene but was later apprehended by the police. Sally received emergency hospital treatment and eventually required plastic surgery and follow-up treatment with a neurologist as a facial nerve was severed in the incident.

The procedure surrounding the trial of the assailant took over a year and was quite stressful. Sally was required to testify a number of times and had to confront her assailant at the court appearances. She also was harassed by people who were suspected to be friends of the assailant.

Sally was referred for therapy more than two years following the stabbing incident chiefly because of labile affect that alarmed friends and colleagues. She had never seen a therapist before. Sally presented as an anxious, sad, and tired-looking woman. Sally wore no make-up, dressed plainly, and wore her hair in a short style that contributed to her overall timid appearance.

Sally complained of difficulty sleeping and of recurrent nightmares about her past attack. During the two years since the incident, she had developed avoidance behaviors that severely limited her freedom. She was frightened of being alone and as a result was escorted by friends or family whenever she was in public. She was taken to and picked up from her job. Sally would not leave her office alone and would not take her lunch hour if she could not be in the company of a colleague. Well-intentioned family, friends, and colleagues were maintaining the avoidant behavior by their solicitude. Sally reported that no one ever told her *not* to be afraid. She avoided crowds and had cut herself off from previously enjoyed activities. Sally described a 50-pound weight loss since the incident. Her interpersonal relationships were characterized by tension, anxiety, and passive behavior that was followed by outbursts of temper. She had become extremely dependent upon her boyfriend, who was supportive, as were solicitous family members and friends. Sally reported that her personality and behavior before the incident were directly at variance with her current state. Sally completed a Life History Questionnaire and Assertiveness Inventory. Her Multimodal Profile (Table 14.1) revealed her chief complaint as well as additional concerns that also were to become the target of therapeutic intervention.

Modality	Problem	Proposed Treatment
Behavior	Fear of being alone	Desensitization via imagery
	Avoidance of crowds and strangers	and *in vivo* experience
	Generally unassertive	Assertive training, bibliotherapy
	Angry outbursts	
Affect	Fear, panic, anxiety	Reassurance, anxiety management training
	Depression	Discuss with Sally possible use of medication
		Proper use of reinforcers
	Fears rejection	Corrective self-talk
	Negative feelings about self & others	Rational disputation
		Role playing

Modality	Problem	Proposed Treatment
	Anger	Rational disputation,
	Guilt about "everything"	bibliotherapy
	Lonely	Relationship building
	Unresolved guilt over death of father	Empty-chair dialogue
Sensation	Somatic complaints: stomach upset, bowel disturbance, headache	Relaxation training
		Abdominal breathing exercise
		Consultation with Sally's physician
	Decreased interest in sex	
	Tension	Relaxation and prescribed exercise
	Fatigue	
Imagery	Nightmares of attack (frequent) and images of being attacked	Desensitization
	Negative self-image as unattractive	Corrective self-talk
	Hypersensitive about facial scar	Positive imagery
	Disturbing image of father's death	Desensitization
		Empty-chair technique
Cognition	Negative statements about self-worth	Cognitive restructuring
		Coping imagery
	Needs approval of others	Assertive training
	Sees self in stereotyped role of passive and compliant daughter and female ("doormat")	Vocational counseling
	Unfulfilled wishes for further professional advancement and education	Relationship building
	Fears not finding a spouse	Rational emotive therapy
	Perfectionistic beliefs about performance	Desensitization
	Thoughts of people harming her	Rational emotive therapy
Interpersonal relationships	Passive and compliant at expense of self-esteem	Assertive training
	Avoidance of men and strangers	Desensitization
		Positive imagery rehearsal
	Frequent volatile encounters with colleagues	Role playing, assertive training
	Unassertive with family members	Assertive training
	Secondary gain from concerned persons	Explain reinforcement principles and elicit cooperation
Drugs/ biology	Sleep disturbance	Referral to physician for checkup
	Weight loss/poor appetite	
	Cigarette smoking	Smoke-stopping program
	Frequent colds	
	Lack of exercise	Exercise program

Table 14.1 Sally D's Multimodal Profile

Sally's Multimodal Profile revealed much more than the diagnosis of post-traumatic stress disorder would imply. While her symptoms reflected the classic aspects of the delayed stress syndrome, Sally's assessment also disclosed a basically shy, unassertive woman with negative feelings about herself. She carried with her a host of cognitive imperatives that were the result and residue of a strict, traditional ethnic upbringing that severely hampered her behavior and interpersonal relations. Her family history revealed that as a child at home her role was to nurse a sickly father and be protected by siblings. Her father's death a decade before treatment had left her with unresolved feelings that brought immediate resistance and tears when it was discussed in therapy. In addition, Sally was locked in a long-term relationship that was not meeting her needs or goals for the future. While she was respected and successful in her career, Sally felt frustrated by not being able to advance further without more formal education.

Treatment. While Sally recognized both the chronicity and seriousness of the symptoms of the delayed stress syndrome, she requested that initial therapeutic intervention be directed at her interpersonal difficulties on the job. Sally's volatile affect irritated her colleagues to the point that she received several severe admonitions from her boss.

From the viewpoint of the therapist, the initial intervention was one that served several purposes: rapid rapport was established, results were easily measurable, and the techniques employed could and would be used to deal with many of the same symptoms seen in the delayed stress syndrome.

In fact, treatment was directed in several areas simultaneously. Relaxation training was begun with immediate positive results reported. Evaluation showed that Sally was adept at visual imagery, and appropriate behavior rehearsal was begun in this modality using day-to-day scenes of coping appropriately on the job. This laid the foundation for the transition to using images to cope with the avoidance behavior and fears she had developed. Behavioral rehearsal and rational discussion of dealing with problematic people at the office yielded rapid, positive results and built Sally's confidence in tackling her greater fears. Consultation with her physician gave assurance that her condition and physical complaints were being monitored, and no medical intervention was required at the time therapy began.

Detailed second-order BASIC I.D. tracking of Sally's response to fear, and her subsequent avoidance behavior, yielded valuable clinical information.[7] For example, Sally's first awareness of becoming anxious when she was with strangers or in public places was the feeling of tension in her stomach. The sensation triggered thoughts that people were going to harm her. She then would begin to walk rapidly and engage in various avoidance behaviors. Once Sally was safely back at home or in the office, she would become angry with herself for having behaved in such a way. She then engaged in generating negative self-statements and feelings. Eventually, Sally became angry at others and believed that she then behaved by displacing her anger on colleagues. Specific treatment was prescribed to assist Sally to cope through each step along her own "firing order."[8] Relaxation, corrective self-talk, and self-monitoring were recommended. Graded desensitization exercises were begun, which exposed Sally to public places and strangers.

As Sally progressed, a series of graded *in vivo* exercises were also conducted, accompanied by the therapist in the crowded downtown areas. Sally eventually walked at noon down busy streets that she had avoided for two years. Graded tasks involving decreasing dependency on friends and family also met with continued success. Selected "bibliotherapy" readings paralleled treatment and helped deal with cognitive distortions and irrational interpretations of events. As Sally gained more mastery of her fears of people and public places, *in vivo* desensitization sessions with the therapist included visits to the day hospital, psychiatric unit, and retardation services at the hospital where the therapist was on staff.

Imagery was repeatedly employed in sessions to deal effectively with the painful images of the traumatic event. The fact that she was finally able to talk freely about the episode was a breakthrough for Sally. During this time there was a noticeable decrease in the frequency of nightmares. Sally continued to master her fears through daily practice using both *in vivo* exposure and imagery rehearsal. She became increasingly more adept at discriminating both internal and environmental stimuli that had previously been associated with maladaptive responses. As Sally's confidence grew she reported improvement across the BASIC I.D. modalities. Earlier somatic complaints were no longer a concern. Associated vegetative signs and symptoms of depression decreased and eventually were absent. Interpersonal relations improved as Sally's new assertive skills were supported and reinforced by her friends and colleagues. A significant event occurred when Sally witnessed a mugging of a woman on a city street and came to the victim's aid after the attacker fled. Rather than becoming fearful and upset over the incident, Sally used the opportunity in therapy to deal constructively with her anger over her own attack. Also by chance, and well along in therapy, Sally reported seeing her attacker standing on a street corner one day. She reported that she was not upset at seeing him and only "felt sorry for him."

By her own admission, Sally recognized that she had become extremely self-conscious about the residual scar on her cheek and had developed defensive behaviors and negative cognitions that interfered with her interpersonal functioning. Through the use in the sessions of behavioral rehearsal, shame-risk exercises, rational disputation, and flooding techniques,[9] Sally's hypersensitivity about her facial scar was dramatically reduced.

Once Sally's chief complaints involving the sequelae of the trauma had responded to treatment, attention was turned to additional problems presented in her modality profile.

Sally overcame her initial resistance, and managed to face the conflicts connected to the memory of her father's illness and death. The empty-chair technique and imagery exercises allowed for therapeutic gains in assisting Sally to experience and put to rest a host of negative experiences and affective associations she had previously avoided.

Sally turned her attention to the interpersonal area. After thoughtful consideration she terminated a long-standing relationship that was not meeting her needs and, in her mind, did not predict a future that she wanted. Similarly, Sally dealt assertively and more appropriately with family members with whom her previously unassertive behaviors had locked her into dependent relationships.

As a better sense of self emerged, Sally concentrated on her physical and personal appearance. She began wearing make-up, changed her hair style and bought fashionable clothes. Her appearance was significantly improved, and Sally was determined to enjoy socializing and expanding her network of friends. Plans were also made for career advancement by exploring appropriate ongoing education programs.

Dr. Slowinski's Discussion

The case of Sally reports her progress in 30 sessions of multimodal therapy spanning over six months. Initial sessions were scheduled twice weekly to allow for assessment and initial intervention in Sally's stressful psychological state.

A multimodal analysis of Sally's status allowed the therapist to simultaneously intervene across several modalities. Flexibility was essential, for not only was Sally suffering from the ongoing results of the traumatic stress disorder, but also from situational difficulties in her professional and personal life. Sally was a very cooperative patient who readily followed specific suggestions and assignments between sessions. While Sally's cooperation might have reflected her basically compliant personality style, her commitment to treatment worked in her favor as gains were rapidly achieved. It is a shame to think that Sally had not come to treatment for two years despite the severity of her problems. It appeared that as long as Sally remained passive and dependent, her supportive network maintained her. However, the system could not cope with her eventual anger and depression, and she was urged to seek treatment.

As mentioned, Sally responded quickly to initial therapeutic interventions, especially relaxation training and anxiety management. The techniques provided her with coping skills as "ammunition" to deal with her daily stress. Imagery techniques were extremely helpful for Sally. They were used as a form of behavior rehearsal in helping her to successfully cope with her fears of being in public places. Imagery was also important in dealing effectively with memories of her trauma flowing from the event itself right through to the discomfort caused by the protracted process of the trial of Sally's assailant. *In vivo* desensitization exercises proved to be a valuable adjunct to imagery and relaxation training in overcoming the variety of avoidance behaviors she had developed. Attention was paid at the same time to the contributing cognitions that maintained Sally's maladaptive behaviors. Much of therapy centered around examinations of her faulty beliefs and the use of cognitive and rational-emotive techniques.

Once Sally began making progress with her chief causes of anxiety, rapid progress was seen across other modalities. The signs and symptoms associated with depression lessened, the frequency of nightmares diminished, and general interpersonal functioning improved. Somatic complaints all but disappeared. Sally's new confidence allowed her to be less resistant in dealing with issues surrounding her father's death. The Gestalt therapy technique (the empty chair) gave Sally an avenue to deal with her affect appropriately and helped to resolve long-standing painful memories.

Sally's therapy is still ongoing. We are emphasizing future planning and continued adjustment to the changes in daily events and relationships that flow from her improved behavior and openness. Attention will also be paid to periodically reviewing events that may recall the initial traumatic incident so that Sally will be prepared to cope with future anxiety-producing situations. This allows for a type of "emotional fire drill" that supports appropriate behavior patterns and emotional responses.

While Sally's case is certainly not unique in terms of presenting with a cluster of symptoms following a trauma, it serves to demonstrate the effectiveness of multimodal therapy for a specific diagnostic category. Multimodal assessment and therapy provided a specific and systematic set of interventions that met both her clinical needs and her own expectations.

Case 4

The Inner Advisor (by Dr. Martin Rossman—1984)[10]

A technique we have found extremely valuable is the dialogue with what we term an "inner advisor," a figure of wisdom and caring evoked in imagery. Catholics learn in catechism that they have a guardian angel available to them in times of need. Spirits and spirit guides are a part of the belief system of a surprising number of people in this culture. As the two cases below illustrate, the advisor can be a helpful source of not only psychological and spiritual, but also physical guidance. Jung used a variant of this approach which he described in *Mysterium Conjunctionis* as internal talk to another who is invisible.[11]

It is important to evoke the patient's reaction to and interpretation of the advisor to make best use of it. If the aura of the spiritual is bothersome to someone, a neurological model is stressed, and the advisor is presented as a way of evoking right-brain activity that may provide new pertinent information. In *Healing Yourself*[12] a non-dogmatic model of this phenomenon that accommodates most belief systems is described. If, however, the patient has specific spiritual beliefs about the advisor, these beliefs must be respected, since we really do not know exactly what this phenomenon represents.

Whatever the mechanism of the inner advisor, it has proven to be a useful introduction to imagery. Once people can relax with some confidence and imagine themselves in a quiet place, they are encouraged to invite into their awareness an image which represents the qualities of great wisdom and caring. This figure may be someone familiar or unfamiliar to the person, an old man or woman, a religious figure, a child, an animal, plant, ball of light, or just a sense of a wise presence. The image need not be visual, though it usually is. When the advisor appears, the individuals should invite it to be comfortable and should talk with it and ask it questions about their problem or illness. They should allow themselves to be receptive to the answers they receive in response, whether through thoughts, auditory imagery, or in mime or symbolism. Further dialogue is encouraged until it seems that some clear contact or resolution of at least some aspect of the problem is reached. Individuals are asked to record in their journal these experiences with the advisor, noting insights, feelings, and questions that seem relevant to the problem.

Case 4.A: A twenty-nine-year-old woman, who worked as a secretary, complained of severe tension headaches which had been occurring several times a week for ten years. Relaxation training helped somewhat, but her headaches continued at a reduced frequency and intensity for several weeks. One day she came in with a severe, generalized headache she had developed the night before. I asked her to relax and ask her inner mind for an inner advisor, a figure that could help her understand the headache and what she could do about it. Immediately the image of a mynah bird came to her mind. She said it was like one she had had when she was nine years old and had died because she did not know how to nurture it. The imaginary mynah was friendly, however, and when she asked it about her headache it began to peck her all over her head. The message she received was that she let people pick on her too much. Specifically, the day before she had heard that a fellow employee, a man whom she had helped obtain a job in her office, had been slandering her behind her back to her boss and other office staff. She became infuriated, but instead of expressing her anger, began to feel sick and went home with a headache. She then asked the mynah what to do—it told her to assert herself, to tell the man to his face to stop slandering her, and to apologize. She visualized herself doing that (it was a very frightening idea for her) and was surprised to see the man sheepishly apologize and shrink in size. She laughed as she saw this, and to her surprise, she found that her headache was gone. The next day she confronted this man in real life and found to her amazement that he acted very much as she had seen him act in her imagery. In a later talk with the mynah, it told her that she should not have been surprised at that man's reaction because she had known all along that he was this type of person, and she had recommended him for a job because of what she thought others thought of him. She recognized that often her personal assessment of people was accurate, yet she had ignored it and had related to people according to the opinions of others. Consequently, she had been consistently disappointed in relationships and work situations. The continuing process of inner dialogue, leading to growing self-respect and assertiveness, resulted in far fewer and less severe headaches and in an ability to respond effectively when a headache did occur.

Case 4.B: A thirty-year-old woman lawyer with multiple severe allergies complained of constant fatigue, abdominal bloating and cramping, skin rashes, and sinus congestion. Allergy testing had revealed her to be sensitive to almost every inhalant and food product tested. Several years of environmental manipulation, rotary elimination diets, hyposensitization, and psychotherapy had helped little, if at all. A course of acupuncture treatments was only somewhat helpful. Her advisor was a thin, willowy young woman who called herself Laura. When asked if she knew anything about this patient's allergies, Laura answered, "You have light compression." Neither the patient nor I understood this enigmatic answer and we asked Laura for more information. She refused, however, to say more, but offered in her outstretched hand a prism, which was refracting a beam of white light into the seven colors of the spectrum. She gave this to the patient and then disappeared. The patient was instructed to meet with Laura again and ask her for more guidance and also to be aware of possible meanings in this image that might occur to her over the next few days. Three days later she called, excitedly saying she was browsing through some old books and found one which cited evidence of the adverse effect of less than full spectrum lighting on the immune system. The author emphasized the possible role this might play in allergies, among other illnesses. The patient consulted with her advisor who confirmed the meaning of the imagery. She advised the patient to spend one hour a day in the sun when possible and to replace all her light bulbs at home and in the office with full-spectrum bulbs. After three weeks the patient reported that she was "95 percent" better, and follow-up a year-and-a-half later revealed that she had stayed well.

Dr. Rossman's Conclusions

Information received from the inner advisor needs to be evaluated before it is put into action. We do not advocate that people abandon their responsibility to their inner advisors any more than we encourage them to abandon it to anyone else. In fact, we tell people that they need not do whatever the advisor recommends, but to consider it carefully. If the advice seems reasonable and the risk is acceptable, we encourage people to act on it and see how it works.

The relationship with the advisor is an ongoing one, and in time, a person may develop several advisors, each with a different area of expertise. I encourage people who have reached this point to think of the entire unconscious mind as an advisor, which can appear in different forms to deliver different messages. Thus people attain a conscious attitude which, as Jung said, "allows the unconscious to cooperate instead of being driven into opposition."[13]

Case 5

Advice and Reassurance (by Dr. Michael Balint—1964)[14]

It is generally agreed that at least one-quarter to one-third of the work of the general practitioner consists of psychotherapy, pure and simple. Some investigators put the figure at one-half, or even more, but, whatever the figure may be, the fact remains that present medical training does not properly equip the practitioner for at least a quarter of the work he has to do.

Although the need for a better understanding of psychological problems and for more therapeutic skill is keenly felt by many practitioners, they are reluctant to accept professional responsibility in this respect. The reason most frequently advanced is that they have too much to do as it is, and it is impossible for them to sit down and spend an hour with a single patient at a time, week after week. This argument, impressive as it sounds, is not, in fact, firmly based. It is true that establishing and maintaining a proper psychotherapeutic relationship takes much more time than prescribing a bottle of medicine. In the long run, however, it can lead in many cases to a considerable saving of time for the doctor and for his patient.

What happens in practice in most so-called psychological cases is an almost mechanical prescribing of sedatives if the patient is not depressed, and of some "tonic" if he is. When this fails, various specialists are consulted, usually resulting in "reassuring" reports that nothing organically wrong has been found.

Thrown back on his own resources, the doctor, often shamefacedly prescribes some placebo, and gives advice or a "reassuring" pep talk. (It is a common joke to ask: "Reassuring—but to whom?") Then there are the advocates of "common-sense" psychology who advise the patient to take a holiday, to change his job, to pull himself together, not to take things too seriously, to leave home, to get married, to have a child, or not to have any more children but to use some contraceptive, etc. None of these recommendations is necessarily wrong, but the fallacy behind them is the belief that an experienced doctor has acquired enough well-proved "common-sense" psychology to enable him to deal with his patient's psychological or personality problems even without attempting a proper diagnosis. But minor surgery, for instance, does not mean that a doctor can pick up a well-proved carving-knife or a common-sense carpentry tool and perform minor operations. On the contrary, he has to observe carefully the rules of antisepsis and asepsis, he must know in considerable detail the techniques of local and general anesthesia and must have acquired skill in using scalpel, forceps, and needle, the tools of the professional surgeon. Exactly the same is true of psychotherapy in general practice. The uses of empirical methods acquired from everyday life are as limited in professional psychotherapy as are carving-knife and screwdriver in surgery.

To demonstrate the limited usefulness of "common-sense" advice and reassurance, I wish to quote a case in which this method, and nothing else, was used. Dr. S., in spite of the severe criticisms of the seminar,[15] did not go beyond the traditional limits of medicine: taking a history, carrying out a physical examination when he thought it necessary, "reassuring" his patient, and giving her common-sense advice in an avuncular way as his nature is. In this way Mrs. B. never had any psychotherapy and was not even examined psychologically. The many well-observed details of her history, however, enabled the seminar to get good glimpses into the mechanisms and the problems of her case. Thus we were able to follow the ups and downs of the history of her illness, criticize her doctor for his technique, and appreciate with understanding the limited success he achieved. In May Dr. S. [the treating physician] mentioned

> Mrs. B., aged 24, whom I had known since she was 17, when she had an appendicostomy for colitis. She is the only daughter of a very neurotic woman who had kept her under strict control. Some years ago I advised the patient to get out more, go to dances, etc. She took my advice, and met her husband at a dance. They live now with her mother, who does not get on too well with her son-in-law. The couple tried to emigrate, but it was discovered that the husband had a shadow on his lung. The T.B. clinic could find nothing wrong at first, but one of the many samples taken was positive, and he was sent to a sanitarium. After four months he came home, and husband and wife came to see me a fortnight ago, together. She has nervous symptoms, palpitations, insomnia, and sometimes diarrhea. She asked me whether it would be advisable to have a child, and I said it would, but the husband said he did not want a child, as he was not in a secure enough position, not having a house and not knowing whether they would

be going to emigrate, as is their intention as soon as his health permits. This morning the girl's mother rang up to say her daughter was very ill with nerves. The patient then came to see me, and told me she was obsessed with the idea of being changed from a female into a male and has to pray all the time that such a thing will not happen. She had read of such a case in the papers. Sexual relations with her husband are very infrequent. I examined her, and assured her that her genitals were quite normal and there was nothing for her to worry about. She felt happy at being told this, and said she would think no more about it. Her husband is rather a peculiar man, has no friends, is lazy. He wants to wait six months to make sure his chest is all right and they will then try to emigrate. They have been married two years and he insists on having no children; contraceptives are used.

Dr. S. was criticized on two counts in the seminar. It was pointed out to him that "reassuring" the patient by telling her that there was "nothing wrong" with her would have only a short-lived effect. Admittedly his prompt examination eased the patient's anxieties, but this was not necessarily a desirable result. He intervened therapeutically before establishing the correct diagnosis. He allayed Mrs. B.'s anxieties, probably only temporarily, but certainly missed an opportunity for finding out more about her problems and the causes of her anxieties. Dr. S. produced the ever-ready excuse of not having enough time just now, but promised to be more thorough when he saw the patient again. A week later he reported:

I was called to see the girl, who was in bed with colitis. She told me that after the examination she thought she was convinced that she was not changing her sex, but since then she had changed her mind again, and she was not sure now. The patient's mother told me that her daughter is always wanting to compare her genitals with her mother's to make sure she is normal, but the mother will not allow this. Apparently my examination had not been sufficient to reassure the girl as I had hoped.

The seminar, and its psychiatrist leader in particular, triumphantly pointed out to Dr. S. how short-lived had been the effects of his reassurance, that exploding one "offer"[16] by the patient by a physical examination had resulted only in her producing another "offer" in the form of colitis, and lastly that it would be advisable for him either to do a psychological examination himself or to refer Mrs. B. to a psychiatrist. A further week later we heard from Dr. S.—

Mrs. B. came to see me last Thursday, when she said she was feeling very much better, but she still thinks sometimes there is a possibility of her changing into a man. She is very depressed, her husband never takes her out. It was arranged that she should call to see me the following Monday. She is now training to be a shorthand typist and goes to school. She came on Monday with her husband, said she was very depressed, but she was very changeable—sometimes she is deeply depressed and then she feels very exhilarated. She even threatens suicide, but neither mother nor husband takes her seriously. She blames her de-pression on lack of friends and lack of entertainment. As the patient felt better, and I was very busy, she was asked to come again in a fortnight.

The "offer" of colitis apparently not having been accepted, Mrs. B. produced a third "offer," depression and some slight threats of suicide. This third offer did not make much impression either. Mother, husband, and doctor alike refused to take it seriously. Dr. S. then admitted to the seminar that he was trying to mark time. As the couple intended to emigrate, it would be inadvisable to start probing into Mrs. B.'s problems, this might create highly emotional reactions, which could not be dealt with in the time available. As there was some truth in this argument it had to be accepted, but Dr. S. was again warned that unexpected things might happen.

> The next report came at the beginning of July, about seven weeks after the first:
>
> Although she believes me when I say she cannot change her sex, yet she cannot help feeling sometimes that it might happen, and she has to pray to God. If the change happens, she feels perhaps it will be a kind of punishment because she was not nice to her parents when she was young. She said that when she was five she played with another girl, and they touched each other's genitals. She felt later on that it was wrong, and told her mother. Before she tells me anything she always discusses it first with mother, who usually says things are not important and there is no need to tell me about them. Mother is still very strict with her. Patient said she would like to go overseas to get away from her, but it is a little too far and she would rather go somewhere where she could visit her mother if she wanted to. Her general depression has been much less lately but she has attacks of disbelief about the impossibility of changing her sex. She was told to come back in a week. She says she likes to come and see me as when she leaves me she feels cheered up, because I listen to her.

Dr. S. then added:

> Patient does not talk about father much. He once had a slipped disc and was in bed for two weeks, and in January he was suffering from melaena, from which he soon recovered. He is a traveler, and often away. His wife domineers him and tells him what to do.

At long last, Dr. S. found time "to listen"[17] to his patient. Apart from repeating her doubts about changing her sex, some important material was produced. We got an idea of the closeness and tenseness of a mother-daughter relationship which went so far that a married woman of twenty-four had to report to her mother all the details of her sexual life, and even had to ask her advice about what to discuss and what not to discuss with her doctor. That this relationship was not exclusively one-sided—i.e., caused only by the domineering mother—was shown by the daughter's wish to compare her genitals with her mother's for the sake of the reassurance which that might give her. This, taken in conjunction with the sexual play with another girl at the age of five, plainly indicated a strongly ambivalent attachment to the mother. The obsessional idea and fear of changing her sex thus became intelligible as a fantastic method of escaping from the conflict of ambivalence, and also explained why it was felt as a punishment. If this train of thought is roughly correct, we can understand why a "common-sense reassurance"—which failed even to touch on her real problems—could not have much effect on her.

> A week later a dramatic denouement started. Dr. S. told us:
>
> A couple of days ago I received an urgent telephone call from the girl's mother that the girl had had a row with her husband and had taken poison. She had really only taken six aspirins and one sleeping tablet. When I called, mother, father and daughter were in a room together, and they all started talking about the row. A few minutes later the girl's husband came in and said the matter should not be discussed in public, so the mother and father went out. The daughter then blamed her husband for not giving her a child, and threatened divorce. I told the husband that it was the primitive right of a

woman to have a child, and that if his wife divorced him it would be his own fault. This morning the patient came in much happier. She said they had had intercourse three nights running, which she had enjoyed because no preventive measures were taken. However, after intercourse the husband said that if they had a child as a consequence, he would not like it, as it would be in the way and an unwanted expense; now she is worried about that. In spite of this, she still has fleeting ideas about changing her sex, and asked what she should do when she has these ideas, which question I did not answer.

Nearly all the doctors turned against Dr. S. for again giving premature advice before finding out what the real situation was. Dr. S. retorted that in an emergency such as this a general practitioner was entitled to use his personality; he simply could not sit and wait for results, he had to do something, and whether it was to the advantage of his patient or not remained to be seen. The urgency was admitted, but it was pointed out that the urgency had been partly created by Dr. S.'s procrastinating policy, which always found good reasons for not probing deeper at any particular moment.

In mid-August, Dr. S. reported:

Since last reporting on the case I saw her twice. She and her husband are now getting on very well, they have regular, satisfactory intercourse, and are looking forward to having a child. Patient has taken a job as a secretary and has passed her typing examination. She is feeling very much better and very pleased with everything, though I had not been able to reassure her completely that she would not change her sex. She asked me several times whether it was not possible that she had changed since I examined her, but I refused to make further examinations as it would mean loss of prestige for me, and the girl would think I was uncertain about it too.

Reluctantly the seminar had to admit that the advice to the husband to accept his wife's right to have children had not been so bad after all. Dr. S. had certainly succeeded to a certain extent, but how and why nobody knew. Still less was known about what the price of his success would be and who would pay it. So Dr. S. was advised not to rest too contentedly on his laurels, but to watch for further developments.

In October we learned that the young couple had found a flat several miles away from mother's and that they had come to say goodbye to Dr. S. Sexual relations were satisfactory, but the girl "still had silly ideas occasionally about changing her sex, but she was able to reject them straight away."

In May of the following year we heard again about Mrs. B.:

Her mother came yesterday, and she was very nervy and full of aches and pains. She said her daughter was not happy in her first flat and she had moved to another place, where she was quite happy. Moreover, she is working and she is pregnant, but does not want to see her mother at all. Mother is very sad about it, the more so as Mrs. B. threatens that she does not want her mother to see the child either. Perhaps there is no need now for the girl to feel she is not a proper woman.

Now I wonder whether all this was due to the overwhelming mother, who talked for the daughter all the time and who had to be told all about the sexual affairs between the daughter and her husband? Was it this that made the girl so inconclusive about her own state? Now, not only has she become pregnant, which proves she is a woman, but she has become independent of mother.

Six months later Dr. S. received a letter from Mr. B. announcing that a baby had arrived without any trouble, and that Mrs. B. had never looked better. They had given up the idea of emigrating, and in a few weeks were moving to a house which was being built for them in the country. Dr. S. then rang up the mother and

> congratulated her, and she was very surprised that I knew about the baby. They did not let her know about it at all, she heard from someone else in a roundabout way that her daughter was having a baby. She went to see her the day before yesterday and spent an hour with her. The daughter and her husband say they will not have anything to do with her, and they will not allow her to touch the baby. The mother offered to have the daughter with her for a week when she comes out of the home, but they refused point-blank. They made a complete break with the mother.

The neurotic conflicts had not been resolved, but only adjusted. But the adjustment was definitely there, and it was undeniable that Dr. S. had played a great part in it. This case history shows that "common-sense" methods may have successes, but not because they are "common-sense." They represent shots in the dark in a possibly correct direction. It may even happen that they get near the target.

We asked who would pay the price for the doctor's success. Recent events seemed to suggest that it would be Mrs. B.'s mother, but more was to come. Three months later we heard from Dr. S.:

> The mother of this girl sprained her ankle soon after her daughter left her, and now she has broken her wrist. I think that is very interesting. She broke the wrist of the right hand, which ought to have hit her daughter. She was full of hate; she is a nervous wreck now.

Dr. Balint's Analysis and Discussion of the Case

One partner of the intense and richly ambivalent relationship had escaped into femininity and motherhood, the other had broken her wrist and become an overt neurotic. What were the chances of the young woman remaining as healthy as she appeared to be, and of the older woman recovering from the severe trauma that befell her? No one knew, and now it might be impossible for any one doctor to assess these chances in their mutual relation, as the two women were separated and under two different doctors. Was the present situation more favorable for therapy than that in which Dr. S. did a physical examination and "reassured" Mrs. B., or otherwise? Was it the right decision in the early stages not "to go deeper"? So far as we can tell, Dr. S. and his advice helped the young woman to free herself at her mother's expense. Was it a fair price, or could a better bargain have been struck if Dr. S., instead of carrying out a physical examination and "reassuring" his patient, had embarked there and then on "going deeper"?

In spite of our almost pathetic lack of knowledge about the dynamisms and possible consequences of "reassurance" and "advice," these two are perhaps the most often used forms of medical treatment. In other words, they are the most frequent forms in which the drug "doctor" is administered. It will be easy to accuse me of being a trouble-maker, who sees untold dangers in something perfectly simple and human. What, after all, can be more natural than to sympathize with a patient in distress, and to try to show him that much of his distress has no physical cause? Moreover, the patient is often relieved by our sincere "reassurance," and afterwards things develop in a favorable direction. As everyday practice shows, these two statements are true—in a way.

If we take the beginning and the end of the story, we cannot but be deeply impressed by what happened. Here was a young woman, unhappy, under the thumb of a domineering mother, receiving hardly any help and support, or even normal sexual affection, from her husband, thinking of divorce and suicide in her despair, and eventually developing a fixed idea, not knowing whether she was really a man or a woman. At the end of the story we hear about her as a happy mother, who has had an easy confinement, has freed herself from her mother, and is looking forward to settling down as mistress of her own home and of her own life. Undoubtedly Dr. S.'s therapy of reassurance and advice contributed considerably to these impressive changes, i.e., was both helpful and effective. That is my opponents' argument, and I readily concede that it is valid as far as it goes.

But it is only a superficial picture, which does not tell us anything about what really happened or why it happened. When we take into consideration the other details which Dr. S.'s frank reports enable us to follow closely, the convincing argument based on this case history dissolves into a haze of what, for the time being, are unanswerable problems, and Dr. S.'s simple and straightforward therapy appears to have been a lucky shot in the dark. Indeed, unless a detached observer made himself disagreeable by drawing attention to it, it would be easy to forget that one shot—the physical examination and ensuing reassurance—was a complete failure. On the other hand, the other shot—the advice to the couple to have a child—was a resounding success.

That too is typical of this situation. Failures are suppressed and forgotten while successes are proudly paraded. I should like to remind the reader that both therapeutic measures—the reassurance about the woman's sex and the advice that she should have a child—were "common sense." One had no effect, while the effect of the other was excellent. *So the question is not how much common sense is required but how better to aim it.* The answer must come from more research, the only way by which reliable information about these most important problems can be obtained. I wish to reiterate, though it is pretty obvious, that this research can be conducted only by general practitioners; no one else, certainly no specialist, has access to the patient material. The answers to questions of this kind can be obtained only in a close and constant relationship with the patient, which is the essence of general practice.

Case 6

Dedicated Doctor (by Dr. Naomi Remen—1980)[18]

In the following case, a man is identified with a part of himself that he later came to call the Dedicated Doctor, whose values, priorities, and goals conflicted with the needs of his body. The technique used by his internist to help him get past the limitation of his identification is quite new and will be discussed further.

Dr. Paul R.'s secretary called to say that he would be a few minutes late for his appointment with me. As I put the receiver down, I realized that I had not been looking forward to Paul's visit this afternoon. A crisis was developing and some decisions would be needed.

Paul had been coming to see me for eight months. As I waited for him I thought back to his first visit and re-experienced my dismay at hearing his story: five weeks of intense stomach pain with weight loss and vomiting. His physical examination, laboratory findings, and X-rays had led to a clear diagnosis of gastric ulcer—on the wall of the stomach close to where it joins the small intestine.

Together we had reviewed the standard ulcer diet and the importance of rest and drug therapy. It was, all in all, a very gratifying first visit. Paul, being a physician, had understood his physical situation and the needed treatment more thoroughly than the average person. We had good communication, the main points had been covered, and I anticipated prompt results.

At first Paul seemed to be an excellent patient. He followed the diet, took his medications faithfully, and rested a bit more than was his habit. Unfortunately, his cooperation with his treatment proved short-lived. He was extremely active professionally, and very devoted to his patients. I had not realized how difficult it would be for him to take adequate periods of rest, to remember both his medications and his diet.

He said that he "did his best" but it just was not always possible. His patient load was enormous—he worked long hard days, his reputation was excellent, and he seemed unable to say "no" and refuse a new patient his care. Despite his workload, he spent a great deal of time battling the house staff and the nursing service in order to drive them to even greater efforts in behalf of those in his care. "The hospital administration . . . bureaucracy . . . inefficiency . . . burdensome forms . . . it's all designed to harass sick people and consume my valuable time," he would exclaim with aggravation.

After the first month he started missing appointments, and I became concerned because he was not staying in touch with me. I asked my secretary to remind him of his appointments but this did not help. The few times that he did come in, he seemed to understand perfectly the importance of medication, diet, rest, and avoidance of emotional stress and strain. Yet he did not act from this understanding.

Despite many hours of talking, I had not gotten through to Paul, even though at one point I had actually begged him to take care of himself. I think that he appreciated my efforts and he tried to placate me by promising that he would change, though I suspect both of us knew that he wouldn't. Yesterday the not unexpected crisis occurred and Paul had his first episode of overt bleeding from his stomach. Unsurprisingly, a new set of X-rays showed that despite months of therapy, the ulcer crater had not changed. I'd done everything I knew. Perhaps now that he had experienced one of the serious consequences of his behavior, he might be willing to act differently. I considered the idea of hospitalization and complete rest. Looking at the evidence before me, I was forced to face the fact that Paul had a refractory ulcer and surgery was quite possibly the next step.

My thoughts about his condition were interrupted when Paul arrived, apologizing for being late. I showed him the films. He looked at his X-ray in silence and didn't seem surprised. His face showed no expression. I suggested that he go into the hospital for several days; perhaps with the strictest medical management, surgery might yet be avoided. Paul rejected that almost out of hand, saying that he could not take time off just now, his practice was very busy and his patients needed him. I was shocked. How could he afford not to take the time, given the consequences? It was the only sensible thing to do, the only available alternative to major surgery. Surely as a physician he must know this.

Suddenly it became clear to me that my colleague, so responsible in caring for the health problems of others, did not seem to be capable of acting responsibly with regard to his own problem. It seemed to me that he had lost sight of the seriousness of his physical problem; he was responding to his patients' needs and not to his own.

Paul seemed to be locked into a certain way of being, a certain role, a certain attitude toward his body and its needs, and even his medical knowledge of the consequences of his actions was not sufficient to change the pattern of his behavior. I decided to try a novel approach to increase his sensitivity to his body's needs.

"Paul," I said, "the reason your ulcer hasn't healed is that you have not actively participated in your own care."

"I don't understand that," Paul said with feeling, "I'm doing my best."

"Well," I continued, "perhaps there's a part of you that has not been involved, that's not doing its best. A part that says to your stomach, 'Yes, I want to be well but not on your terms.'"

Paul's skepticism and impatience with this philosophical and introspective turn of events was obvious in his face. However, it seemed important to continue. How unfortunate that the only voice Paul's stomach had, its only mode of expression, was pain. Eloquent as this was, it was not clear enough for Paul to hear and act on. If only his stomach could talk to Paul directly. I asked him if he was willing to try something to clarify matters. When he agreed, I asked him to tell his stomach how he felt about its behavior.

He looked incredulous, but seeing my determination, sighed, and said, "Well, stomach, I'm upset about your behavior; you're getting in my way and I resent it." "Say it again, Paul," I said. He repeated his sentence, this time speaking with strong feeling.

"Now close your eyes and in your imagination become your stomach. Lend it your voice and allow it to answer you." He sat back in his chair and closed his eyes. After a few minutes of silence he said, "Well, I'm upset too. Paul complains about the pain, but I'm the one who is suffering. Paul, I want you to take care of me."

Paul opened his eyes and said, "I do the best I can."

The dialogue continued with Paul alternately closing his eyes and speaking from his stomach's perspective, and opening his eyes and speaking from his own. The conversation went something like this:

STOMACH: "That's not true, Paul. You haven't paid attention to my needs."

PAUL: "What! Didn't I almost stop smoking? Don't I chew Maalox when you hurt? I even drink decaffeinated coffee and I hate it."

STOMACH: "You call that caring because you take care of me when I hurt you? If I didn't hurt you, you'd never take care of me. Half the time you even forget to feed me."

PAUL: (with his usual intensity): "Well, I hate you for getting in my way. You really cramp my style. My patients need me, and I can't work well with all this pain."

STOMACH: "Your style! Well, I have my style too and I want to live by it! I've hurt you for eight months and I'll keep hurting you until you notice me and take care of me."

A period of prolonged silence ensued.

DOCTOR: "Sounds like a standoff."

STOMACH: "No, I'm ahead."

DOCTOR: "What do you mean?"

STOMACH: "Well, I can force the issue and bleed. Then I'll get to go into the hospital and there I'll get some real attention. Someone there will really care about me even though Paul doesn't."

I couldn't help but smile at the triumphant tone in the stomach's voice. "Paul," I said, "why don't you find out what the stomach means by his statement that you don't care about him?"

PAUL: "What do you mean by that, stomach?"

STOMACH: "I mean that you don't care about me. You're so busy being a dedicated doctor. You care about your patients, their babies, the interns, the nurses, the administrators. But, Paul, all the time we've been sitting here, talking about me, you've been thinking about Sally Thompson's cesarean section. Don't you understand? I'm bleeding. I'm in pain. I want you to care about my pain."

At this point I spoke to Paul's stomach directly. "What do you need, stomach?"

STOMACH: "I need Paul to care for me in the way he cares for his patients. Paul, I want you to understand my needs. I need you to stop getting irritated about every unimportant little thing; that just forces me to pour out acid. I want you to stop avoiding me. I need some rest and I need peace. I need relaxation. I need some consideration and compassion. I'm sick and I deserve it, Paul."

PAUL: "I hear him. He wants rest. He wants me to be aware of his needs. He wants me to take care of him."

DOCTOR: "Is that right, stomach?"

STOMACH: "Yes, I want you to take care of me, Paul. You give me Maalox not because you care about me but because you want me to get out of your way so you can take care of other people."

PAUL: "Yes, I can understand that."

DOCTOR: "Can you, Paul?"

PAUL: "Yes, I see what he means. I've been very unfair to him. I haven't been considering him. I've been so busy that I haven't been taking care of his needs."

DOCTOR: "Say that again, but this time say, 'I haven't been considering me. I haven't been taking care of my needs.'"

PAUL: "I haven't been taking care of me. I need all those things too. I deserve all those things too."

I said, "Paul, you need to take care of yourself." Paul looked at me with tears in his eyes and said simply that he did need help and would accept my advice for immediate hospitalization. Arrangements were easily made. Paul's partners willingly stepped in to help and took over his patient responsibility. I felt gratified that I had been able to help Paul to see his danger and take a course of action that might yet avert it.

Dr. Remen's Discussion

Through his illness, Paul began a re-examination of his priorities and lifestyle which ultimately led him to make wiser choices about certain of his needs and to find ways to consider them in the course of his busy day. Health professionals are frequently called on to suggest such reexamination to their patients. The illness, of course, often makes the suggestion first, and the professional acts to help the patient hear it and act on it. Despite his medical knowledge, Paul was identified with the Dedicated Doctor and could not respond to his own needs. Identification, even briefly, with his stomach made his body's needs clear to him. By *identifying* with the painful part, *Paul disidentified from the Dedicated Doctor for the first time* and could see this aspect of his personality from the outside, from the point of view of his stomach, a part of himself which was suffering at his hands. He was then freed to make choices and set priorities on the basis of a more inclusive set of values than those of the Dedicated Doctor with whom he had been so strongly identified. From this broader perspective, he could find ways to achieve the goals of the Dedicated Doctor and care for others as well as making a plan to care for his stomach so that he could continue to serve his patients.

Disease, by causing pain or weakness, tends to naturally direct an individual's attention to a certain body part and its needs. Some people initially resist paying attention and act much as if they have disowned the part of themselves which is ill. Behind this resistance may lie fear of what will be seen if one looks, or simply anger that one's body is no longer obeying one's every command. Asking people to deliberately focus their attention on the painful part, even to the extent of becoming it in their imagination, may overcome this resistance. This technique not only explicates the needs of the part but may, in some cases, clarify larger issues of attitude and lifestyle.

Occasionally the needs of the part and certain unmet needs of the individual may coincide. When this occurs, an understanding of the needs of the disowned part may provide insight about larger areas of need which too have been disowned. By this means, some people may gain useful information about what is missing in their lives and can then take the steps to provide it.

Recognizing the multiplicity of human personality is useful in being a physician, a nurse, a brother, friend, or wife to someone who persists in ignoring their illness and in behaving in ways that will harm them. Such people are most commonly seen as rejecting help, being stubborn or even irrational. Often we may lose patience and withdraw. If we see the person, not as unreasonable, but struggling to maintain their accustomed sense of identity at the expense of their well-being, we can often take an attitude which is more helpful and productive. One physician finds it useful in such circumstances to directly say, "You know, there is some part of you which seems to be working to defeat you, working against your best interests. How can I be of help to you?"

Any aspect of the personality may have specific goals, values, and priorities which conflict with a person's physical needs. Often the effect of identifying with such a part is to prevent the person from coming into relationship with their disease or their symptoms and thereby taking the necessary steps to help themselves.

The first case in this chapter is an example of this. Harold's Fat Self did not wish to lose weight and did not have the qualities and strengths that his more inclusive identity possessed. It was necessary for him to disidentify from his fat and come into *relationship* with it—rather than *being* it—before he could mobilize his full strength and take effective action.

Unless this step is taken, people may persist in damaging themselves through ignoring their physical condition or become unable to learn useful information from what is happening. Quite often, focusing attention on this lack of relationship between the person and their problem and not on the identification which may be behind it is the most effective way to help a person out of this situation. Simply working with people to clarify their relationship to their disease may enable them to better integrate it into their old lifestyle or adopt a new and more mutually satisfying way of living. In the course of improving a person's relationship with their disease or problem, the part of themselves which is avoiding relationship may become obvious and apparent to the professional. Although it is not usually necessary to point to this, some people may spontaneously become aware of it, as did Paul.

The relationship of a person to a disease commonly passes through stages. At first, the disease may be denied and the person avoids relating to it. The body part which is affected is ignored and its needs not considered, almost as if it has been cast out. Usually this sort of relationship does not last very long; due to the nature of subsequent events, illness is almost impossible to ignore indefinitely.

Denial may then give way to an acceptance with conflict. The attitude of the person toward their body part or their condition might be characterized by the statement, "I see you but I won't give you any quarter." Paul's initial relationship to his ulcer was much like this. People in this stage often will do things that hurt themselves, such as lifting a heavy load when they have a bad back or forgetting to take their medications. Feelings of resentment and anger toward the body are prominent at this time although perhaps not fully conscious until examined through various psychological techniques.

After some time in conflictual relationship, many may spontaneously move into a relationship of acceptance with harmony. At this point, a disease may be seen almost as a partner and the person's attitude toward it might be characterized as, "I take you wherever I go. I consult with you about your needs as I do my activities. Sometimes I respect your needs and leave a party early or take a day of rest. Sometimes I expect you to respect mine as I commit a dietary indiscretion on an important occasion like an anniversary."

Ultimately this partnership may disappear and the disease become incorporated fully into the lifestyle of the individual. The needs of the body are no longer consciously considered but unconsciously considered, just as a tall man will instinctively stoop as he passes through a low doorway. Needed treatment becomes just another part of life, and a person will take an insulin shot or put on a leg brace much in the same way they brush their teeth or shave.

Paul was helped on his way to such a relationship with his ulcer through the use of imagination, a relatively unused human resource. At present, a sick person's imagination is not an asset, often causing unnecessary fears, anxiety, and worry. They may envision what is happening in some unrealistic and frightening way, imagine painful outcomes which never materialize, or the rejection of others, which never occurs. Yet, under purposeful direction, the imagination may be a means of resolving inner conflict and of coming into a better relationship with what is, indeed, real.

Case 7

Mental Symptoms Do Not Always Mean Psychogenic
(by Dr. Melvyn Werbach—1986)[19]

Linda's illness began without warning one morning when, upon awakening, she suddenly experienced a strange, cool sensation over part of her face which was mildly painful. The sensation soon left her but returned another day and gradually increased in its frequency, severity and area of distribution. She eventually sought the aid of her internist. He referred her to a neurologist who found nothing on his initial exam to explain her symptoms. He then ordered a full battery of studies including skull X-rays, an EEG (brain wave tracing) and a brain scan, all of which failed to reveal any abnormalities. Since she also had a history of headaches which seemed to be migrainous, he decided to start her on cyproheptadine, a histamine and serotonin antagonist. The drug helped her headaches but had no effect on her facial pain.

In taking Linda's history, the neurologist found that she had been going through a period of considerable stress. Her daughter not only had headaches like hers, but had also had a recent episode during which she lost consciousness and had a seizure. After her daughter's seizure, Linda's facial pains were worse, and she also lost her appetite. The neurologist concluded that her facial pains were 'a conversion problem'; i.e., that she was unconsciously expressing her feelings through imagined sensory changes in her face.

Linda was not satisfied with his diagnosis, so she sought the services of another physician. He thought that her sensation of coolness might be due to spasm of the blood vessels and prescribed niacin. Unfortunately, the niacin was ineffective. Yet another physician was consulted, and again he failed to suggest anything which brought her relief. After four years of searching, she began a program of acupuncture. At first she felt considerable improvement but, after fifty acupuncture sessions, she found she was back to where she had started.

After six years, Linda went to see another neurologist who, once again, could find no evidence of an organic cause for her facial pain. He felt that he had nothing to offer her, since he was convinced that she did not have organic disease, and suggested that she see me for a consultation.

I found Linda to be a pleasant and intelligent woman of menopausal age who appeared neither anxious nor depressed, but was clearly frustrated over the failure of her doctors to find an effective treatment for what had become an increasingly severe pain syndrome. By now, her pain was becoming almost unbearable. On a scale of one to ten, where one represents a slight discomfort and ten represents unbearable pain, she stated that her pain was reaching nine. It was a constant pain over most of her face as well as her ears and part of her neck. The episodes would occur anytime without warning, from daily to as rarely as a few times a month. They were unrelated to heat, cold, emotional or physical distress or the season of the year. She continued to have occasional migraine headaches, but these were much less frequent since she was placed on propanol.

I probed her for a possible psychological cause to explain her symptom. She was most cooperative, but we could find no clues from her history other than the fact that her husband had had a heart attack three years earlier which had made her worry about his health. She noted that she often had an attack of facial pain not long after he left for work, a fact which she thought might indicate that her worry over his health bore some relationship to the syndrome, even though the onset of the pain seemed to be unrelated to what she was thinking at the moment.

Despite this information, I was not convinced that her pain was psychogenic. Linda seemed to be too healthy psychologically to have developed such a severe pain syndrome because of inability to cope with her husband's heart condition. I gave her a psychological test (MMPI) which confirmed my impression. Her psychological profile was essentially normal and her ego strength, or general coping abilities, was much above average.

I then questioned whether her pain could be due to some type of hyperactivation syndrome wherein normal structures might become overactivated from some unidentified stimulus to produce pain. To assess this possibility, I attached her to physiologic monitoring instruments and found her to display no evidence of hyperactivation. Since the physiologic readings were taken when she had no pain, I asked her to call me during an episode and arrange to see me immediately so that I could see if she showed a hyperactivation pattern at that time. She did so, and once again she showed no evidence of excessive physiologic activity which could explain her severe level of pain.

I then performed a brief trial of electrical acupuncture. These succeeded in decreasing the area of pain, but had no effect on its frequency or intensity. I was convinced that I was missing something, but what? Earlier I had reviewed her allergic history, which was negative. Now, however, as we searched for additional historical clues, Linda revealed that two years ago her skin had broken out in an itchy rash which cleared up as soon as she stopped her multivitamin.

Perhaps Linda was food sensitive! She noted that her syndrome worsened soon after her husband's heart attack. While earlier she thought that perhaps it had worsened because of the stress, she now recalled that, after his heart attack, they stopped eating eggs each morning to cut down on cholesterol. Instead they began to eat a daily bowl of raisin bran. Could something in the cereal be causing the pain?

We decided to try a five-day fast during which she drank only spring water. By 10 A.M. on the first morning of the fast she began to note facial pain which gradually worsened until it became severe and she became nauseated. Later in the day she developed what she described as the worst migraine in her life, which persisted until the fourth day. On the second day she noted muscular pains in her thighs and calves which gradually faded away. On the fourth day she had a second attack of facial pain which was much milder, but persisted all day. By the fifth day she was feeling fine except for hunger. Linda had been through the classical withdrawal syndrome described for masked food sensitivities!

We began to slowly return foods to her diet. She had no symptoms until a few hours after adding wheat, when she had a typical episode of facial pain. We removed wheat from her diet and gradually added back all other foods without incurring any further episodes of pain.

Since then, Linda has usually been free of all facial pain. Occasionally, between thirty minutes and four hours after ingesting a food, she develops her pain syndrome. When this occurs, she attempts to discover the exact ingredients of that food. Invariably, she finds that one of those ingredients was wheat.

Dr. Werbach's Discussion

Linda's case illustrates the folly of assuming that symptoms which cannot be shown to be accompanied by physical changes are necessarily psychological in origin when, in fact, they may have a physical cause which routine procedures are unable to demonstrate. Even worse, the statement that a symptom is psychogenic carries such negative connotations in our society that it often justifies a dismissal of treatment efforts as well as of third-party insurance coverage to pay for those efforts.

Summary and Conclusions

The eight cases reprinted above illustrate a variety of techniques and orienting attitudes towards psychological medicine. In Dr. Remen's two cases, gestalt dialogues and imagery play an important part, as does the climate of self-acceptance that the therapist (as teacher) plays. Dr. Slowinski's case illustrates the comprehensive nature of a meticulous behavioral analysis along many dimensions which encompass virtually every pertinent aspect of the patient's life. Once the behavioral deficits or emotional insecurities are described, then precise techniques can be applied to assist the patient in remedying that deficit or insecurity. In Dr. Rossman's two cases, the "inner advisor" imagery technique revealed crucial diagnostic information that led to successful resolutions. Evidently, patients often know more about their illnesses than they are aware. Dr. Dossey's case illustrates the very profound changes in life attitudes and orientations that can result when an individual comes to the conclusion that their illness can be a teacher, or even a spiritual path. Evidently, the practitioner can play midwife to this process when appropriate. Dr. Balint's narrative, and the accompanying discussion of Dr. S.'s case by his peers, is notable for revealing the hit-and-miss characteristics of a casual rendering of advice and reassurance, those two standbys of those practitioners who have not yet come to realize the subtleties of psychological medicine, and the degree to which a clinician practices it willy-nilly, whether or not he or she is aware of it.

Like any other treatment modality, psychological medicine requires skill, sensitivity, knowledge and flair. Many professionals who ought to know better imagine that psychological medicine is only a matter of common sense. Would that it were so easy! The final case by Dr. Werbach is an important antidote to the over-psychologization of medicine. Just because symptomatology has a strong emotional or mental content is no guarantee that a case necessarily is principally psychogenic or will require primarily psychological medicine. As every effective holistic practitioner is aware, until the causes of a problem are unraveled, treatment must be conservative and the diagnosis tentative. In general, psychological medicine is merely one dimension of a case, one skill in the holistic practitioner's repertoire of treatment modalities. Often neglected, sometimes taken for granted, both underused and overused, attention to the emotional plane in disease and illness must always remain in the practitioner's awareness as one dimension of every case that may—or may not—need attention. I hope that the principles elaborated in this text will go some way towards giving the practitioner of natural medicine the confidence to make the necessary assessments, and to incorporate in the full treatment protocol whatever elements of psychological medicine seem appropriate.

Chapter Notes

Chapter 1

1. W. R. Houston, "The Doctor Himself as a Therapeutic Agent," *Annals of Internal Medicine* 11 (1938): 1416-25.
2. From J. Calnan, *Talking with Patients* (London: William Heinemann, 1983), with the kind permission of the author.
3. The term "holism" was introduced by Jan Smuts in 1926 as an antidote to reductionism in science. See J. C. Smuts, *Holism and Evolution* (London: Macmillian & Co., 1926).
4. A. F. Tredgold, *Psychological Medicine* (Baltimore: Williams and Wilkins, 1945).
5. This usage is not without precedent. See, e.g., M. Balint and E. Balint, *Psychotherapeutic Techniques in Medicine* (Springfield, IL: C. C. Thomas, 1961); J. J. Strain, *Psychological Interventions in Medical Practice* (New York: Appleton-Century-Crofts, 1978).
6. See, e.g., D. Ullman, *Discovering Homeopathy* (Berkeley: North Atlantic, 1991); M. Werbach, *Nutritional Influences on Illness: A Sourcebook of Clinical Research*, 2d ed. (Tarzana, CA: Third Line Press, 1993); D. Hoffman, *Successful Stress Control: The Natural Way* (Rochester, VT: Inner Traditions International, 1987); L. Hammer, *Dragon Rises, Red Bird Flies* (Barrytown, NY: Station Hills Press, 1991); H. Beinfield and E. Korngold, *Between Heaven and Earth* (New York: Ballantine Books, 1991).

Chapter 2

1. M. Werbach, *Third Line Medicine: Modern Treatment for Persistent Symptoms* (Tarzana, CA: Third Line Press, 1986).
2. The word *paradigm* is used here to refer to world views that encompass broad areas of theory and practice. For instance, the view that the earth is a flat surface about which all the planets and stars revolve was the geo-ethnocentric paradigm,

and influenced religion, science, agriculture and philosophy. Eventually it was replaced by the Copernican paradigm in which the earth and planets are spherical bodies circling the sun, which itself is only one of trillions of stars in the Milky Way galaxy. It was this new paradigm which gave impetus to the various modern sciences as we know them today, and even forced religion to take a new view of man. More on paradigms in science can be found in the classical work by T. Kuhn, *The Structure of Scientific Revolutions* (Chicago: University of Chicago Press, 1962).

3. Without diminishing the value of chemical medicine, it should be noted that a number of these common infections had already begun to decline in incidence to a low level before the introduction of antibiotics and immunization. This decline in infectious disease was due at least as much to improved public health measures, which eliminated malnutrition, provided effective sewage disposal and corrected overcrowded living conditions.

4. Iatrogenic: medically generated, or what are usually called unwanted side effects of medicines and medical procedures.

5. The Eastern medicines in particular have always incorporated mental states into both diagnosis and treatment. As the focus of the present text is the Western medical tradition, a detailed exposition of these systems would take us too far afield.

6. J. M. F. Camp, *The Healer's Art: The Doctor through History* (New York: Taplinger, 1977).

7. The terms we use for Galen's four temperaments—"choleric," "sanguine," "melancholic" and "phlegmatic"—were introduced in the ninth century by the Arab physician Johannitius.

8. Reproduced in G. C. Davison and J. M. Neale, *Abnormal Psychology*, 3rd ed. (New York: John Wiley & Sons, 1982), courtesy of The New York Public Library.

9. As shown, e.g., in the etymology of the word therapeutics, from the Greek *therapeuin*, to attend. This emphasizes the ancient physician's role as an attendant or assistant to the natural healing process, which Hippocrates called *vis medicatrix naturae*.

10. Pronounced *batch*.

11. E. Bach, *Heal Thyself* (Saffron Walden, England: C. W. Daniels, 1931), 10.

12. To attempt to minimize sexist terminology, in even-numbered chapters of this book the practitioner is female and the patient male; vice versa for odd-numbered chapters. For similar considerations I also use *they*, *their* and *them* when referring to individuals who could be of either gender, a practice which will occasionally produce ungrammatical usage.

13. Bach, *Heal Thyself*, chapters 1 & 2.

14. As fundamental to our understanding of illness as it is, we must not elevate Bach's doctrine to a panacea: illness is a multi-determined event. Bach was merely drawing our attention to a crucial, long-neglected factor, one that must always be considered, and the one that is central to psychological medicine.

15. R. S. Blacklow, *MacBryde's Signs and Symptoms,* 6th ed. (London: J. B. Lippincott, 1983), 277.
16. Ibid., 284.
17. Ironically, Selye was himself trained as a medical doctor.
18. After G. L. Engel, "The Clinical Application of the Biopsychosocial Model," *American Journal of Psychiatry* 137 (1980): 535-44, and used with the kind permission of the publishers. For more details about the systems view as applied to psychology and medicine, see G. E. Schwartz, "Testing the Biopsychosocial Model: The Ultimate Challenge Facing Behavioral Medicine?" *Journal of Consulting and Clinical Psychology* 50 (1982), 1040-53; and W. T. Powers, "A Systems Approach to Consciousness," in *Psychobiology of Consciousness,* eds. R. J. Davidson and J. M. Davidson (New York: Plenum Press, 1980).
19. F. Capra, *The Turning Point* (New York: Simon & Schuster, 1982), 266-7.
20. See G. L. Engel, "Towards a New Medical Model: A Challenge for Biomedicine," *Science* 196 (1977): 129-36; and Engel, "Clinical Application of Biopsychosocial Model."
21. I have intentionally used the masculine form for the doctor in this section to emphasize that 80 percent of medical doctors in the Western world are men.
22. Hopefully this mechanistic view will increasingly become a caricature of allopathic medicine. More and more doctors are fostering patient autonomy and responsibility in lieu of the older paternalistic view. Indeed, many allopathic physicians these days see illness as inseparable from the context in which it exists. See, e.g., E. Cassell, *The Healer's Art* (Philadelphia: J. B. Lippincott, 1976); J. Needleman, *The Way of the Physician* (Harmondsworth, Middlesex: Penguin, 1985); L. Dossey, *Meaning and Medicine* (New York: Bantam, 1991); and many of the other references in later chapters.
23. Samuel Hahnemann, *The Organon of Medicine,* 6th ed., trans. W. Boericke (1852; reprint, Calcutta: Bhattacharya, 1960).
24. H. Coulter, "Homeopathic Medicine," in *Ways of Health,* ed. D. S. Sobel (London: Harcourt Brace, 1979), 296.
25. The word doctor has its roots in the Latin word *docere,* meaning teacher.
26. A psychological game is a technical concept popularized by psychoanalyst Eric Berne in his book, *Games People Play* (New York: Grove Press, 1964), to refer to transactions between individuals that are based on hidden, unconscious motives.

Chapter 3

1. I. Shah, *The Subtleties of the Inimitable Mulla Nasrudin* (Harmondsworth, Middlesex: Penguin, 1987).
2. This paragraph is a free paraphrase from G. Ryle, *The Concept of Mind* (Harmondsworth, Middlesex: Penguin, 1949).
3. One revealing hint of that is the ease with which we can, without any change in

meaning, substitute simpler equivalents for the word "mind" in a sentence. For example, "She has a scientific mind" = she approaches problems scientifically; "It came to my mind" = the thought came to me; "I put my mind to it" = I put my attention on it; "When they make up their minds" = when they decide; "Our minds can't grasp" = we can't grasp, etc.

4. Hysteria: physical symptoms such as paralysis, sensory deficits and motor dysfunctions lacking any demonstrable organic pathological basis. Nowadays such symptomatology is termed *somatization*.

5. The id was a kind of underground sewer system through which rushed dank, pent-up forces restrained from exploding out into the world by the leaky pipes and sewer caps of an imperfect superego. Meanwhile the ego acted as a kind of overworked and flawed sewage treatment plant whose job it was to sanitize this prurient effluent before allowing it to flow out into the world.

6. Often mistakenly called *behaviorism*. I avoid the word behaviorism because it is rarely used by behavior theorists themselves, but by detractors who are generally not conversant with the technical concepts and subtleties of the theory.

7. And as it does so the machine is gradually going to resemble us in its behavioral and perceptual skills. There's no fear, however, that it will overtake us, since after all we its creator remain logically always one leap ahead of our prodigy's development.

8. In that emphasis, cognitive psychology is an antidote to both the extreme environmentalism of behavior theory and the extreme determinism of classical psychoanalysis.

9. A. Ellis, *Inside Rational-Emotive Therapy* (San Diego: Academic Press, 1989).

10. A. H. Maslow, *Motivation and Personality*, 2nd ed. (New York: Harper and Row, 1970).

11. From S. R. Wilson, "The 'Real Self' Controversy," *Journal of Humanistic Psychology* 28 (1988): 39-65.

12. A. H. Maslow, cited in M. Daniels, "The Myth of Self-actualization," *Journal of Humanistic Psychology* 28 (1988): 7-38.

13. B. Schwartz, *The Battle for Human Nature* (London: W. W. Norton, 1986).

14. Reprinted with kind permission of Brilliant Enterprises, 117 W. Valerio St., Santa Barbara, CA 93101.

Chapter 4

1. G. R. Elliott and C. Eisdorfer, *Stress and Human Health* (Berlin: Springer-Verlag, 1982).

2. The value to an organism of a stimulus can be described as its *valence*, a quantity denoting how desirable (+) or undesirable (-) it may be. Valence can be measured by appropriate behavioral and possibly neurophysiological procedures. See E. Rolls, "A Theory of Emotion and Consciousness, and Its Application to Understanding the Neural Basis of Emotion," in *The Cognitive Neurosciences*, ed. M. S.

Gazzinaga (Cambridge, MA: MIT Press, 1995), 1091-1106.

3. R. S. Lazarus and S. Folkman, *Stress, Appraisal, and Coping* (New York: Springer, 1984).

4. See S. E. Hobfoll, "Conservation of Resources: A New Attempt at Conceptualizing Stress," *American Psychologist* 44 (1989): 413-524.

5. Many thanks to Jonas Roth for these illustrations.

6. G. F. Mahl, "Relationship Between Acute and Chronic Fear and the Gastric Acidity and Blood Sugar Levels in *Macaca mulatto* Monkeys," *Psychosomatic Medicine* 14 (1952): 982-90.

7. J. W. Mason, "A Historical View of the Stress Field," *Journal of Human Stress* 1 (1975): 6-12 (Part I), 22-36 (Part II).

8. Levels of metabolic breakdown products of various hormones were measured either in plasma obtained from blood drawn at various intervals, or from urine samples.

9. J. W. Mason, "Emotions as Reflected in Patterns of Endocrine Integration," in *Emotions—Their Parameters and Measurement,* ed. L. Levi (New York: Raven Press, 1975), 143-81.

10. G. Everly, *A Clinical Guide to the Treatment of the Human Stress Response* (New York: Plenum Press, 1989), 34-9.

11. S. A. Corson, "Pavlovian and Operant Conditioning Techniques in the Study of Psychosocial and Biological Relationships," in *Society, Stress and Disease,* vol. 1, ed. L. Levi (London: Oxford University, 1971), 7-21.

12. J. W. Mason et al., "Selectivity of Corticosteroid and Catecholamine Response to Various Natural Stimuli," in *Psychopathology of Human Adaptation,* ed. G. Servan (New York: Plenum Press, 1976), 147-71.

13. J. R. Millenson, *Principles of Behavioral Analysis* (New York: Macmillan, 1967), 451-5.

14. Mason, "Emotions Reflected in Patterns"; Corson, "Pavlovian and Operant Conditioning Techniques."

15. Mason, "Historical View of Stress," 24.

16. It should be noted in this connection that unconscious animals and patients do not show the endocrine changes of the General Adaptation Syndrome. See J. C. Norton, *Introduction to Medical Psychology* (New York: Macmillan, 1982), 203.

17. This section and its evidence are derived from D. Oken, "Musculoskeletal Disorders," in *American Handbook of Psychiatry,* vol. 4, ed. M. F. Reiser (New York: Basic Books, 1981), 726-66, to which the reader is referred for specific citations to the literature.

18. J. I. Lacey, "Somatic Response Patterns and Stress," in *Psychological Stress,* ed. M. H. Appley and R. Trumbull (New York: Appleton Century Crofts, 1967), 14-37; I. Goldstein Balshan et al., "Study in Psychophysiology of Muscle Tension, I: Response Specificity," *Archives of General Psychiatry* 11 (1964): 322-30.

19. I. D. Balshan, "Muscle Tension and Personality in Women," *Archives of General*

Psychiatry 7 (1962): 436-48.

20. A. C. Guyton, *Human Physiology and Mechanisms of Diseases,* 5th ed. (Philadelphia: W. B. Saunders, 1992) provides a readable account.

21. See the review by R. Ader and N. Cohen, "Conditioning and Stress," *Annual Review of Psychology* 44 (1993): 53-85.

22. M. Stein and A. H. Miller, "Stress, the Immune System, and Health and Illness," in *Handbook of Stress,* eds. L. Goldberger and S. Breznitz (New York: Macmillan, 1993), 127-41.

23. For the relevant literature, see S. Maier, L. R. Watkins, and M. Flesler, "Psychoneuroimmunology: The Interface between Behavior, Brain and Immunity," *American Psychologist* 49 (1994): 1004-17.

24. Specific citations can be found in J. K. Kiecolt-Glaser and R. Glaser, "Psychoneuroimmunology: Can Psychological Interventions Modulate Immunity?" *Journal of Consulting and Clinical Psychology* 60 (1992): 569-75; R. Ader and N. Cohen, "Psychoneuroimmunology: Conditioning and Stress," *Annual Review of Psychology* 44 (1993): 53-85; R. Glaser and J. K. Kiecolt-Glaser, *Handbook of Human Stress and Immunity* (San Diego: Academic Press, 1994).

25. R. J. Booth and K. R. Ashbridge, "A Fresh Look at the Relationships between the Psyche and Immune System: Teleological Coherence and Harmony of Purpose," *Advances* 9, no. 2 (1993): 4-23.

26. J. K. Kiecolt-Glaser and R. Glaser, "Stress and Immune Function in Humans," in *Psychoneuroimmunology,* 2nd ed., eds. R. Ader, D. L. Felton, and N. Cohen (San Diego: Academic Press, 1991), 849-67.

27. Mitogens are plant proteins that can nonspecifically trigger lymphocytes to respond in the way they do to their specific antigen. A mitogen is thus a kind of immunological skeleton key.

28. Maier, Watkins, and Flesler, "Psychoneuroimmunology."

29. Ibid.

30. R. Glaser et al., "Stress-related Immune Suppression: Health Implications," *Brain, Behavior and Immunity* 1 (1987): 7-20.

31. Mason, "Historical View of Stress Field."

32. This questionnaire is adopted from the original source, and reproduced by kind permission of *Nursing Times* where it first appeared in the November 1991 issue.

Chapter 5

1. The original report by T. H. Holmes and R. H. Rahe is to be found in the *Journal of Psychosomatic Research* 11 (1967): 213-18.

2. Recent research, however, indicates that when the "undesirable" aspects of adjusting to a positive event are partialed out there is no relationship between these events and the usual deleterious outcomes of stress. See S. E. Hobfoll, "Conservation of Resources: A New Attempt at Conceptualizing Stress,"

American Psychologist 44 (1989): 513-24.

3. See B. S. Dohrenwend and B. P. Dohrenwend, eds., *Stressful Life Events: Their Nature and Effects* (New York: Wiley, 1974).

4. G. Brown, "Meaning, Measurement and the Stress of Life Events," in B. S. Dohrenwend and B. P. Dohrenwend, *Stressful Life Events,* 217-43.

5. See chapter 1 of J. P. Henry and P. M. Stephens, *Stress, Health, and the Social Environment* (Berlin: Springer-Verlag, 1977).

6. Ibid.

7. See Chapter 9 for a discussion of the concept of stress hardiness.

8. A. D. Kanner et al., "Comparison of Two Modes of Stress Measurement: Daily Hassles and Uplifts Versus Major Life Events," *Journal of Behavior Medicine* 4 (1981): 1-39.

9. See S. E. Taylor, *Health Psychology* (New York: McGraw-Hill, 1991), 224.

10. See S. Cobb, "Social Support as a Moderator of Life Stress," *Psychosomatic Medicine* 38 (1976): 300-14.

11. See chapter 18 in G. S. Everly, Jr., *A Clinical Guide to the Treatment of the Human Stress Response* (New York: Plenum Press, 1989).

12. M. Frankenhauser, "Experimental Approaches to the Study of Catecholamines and Emotion," in *Emotions: Their Parameters and Measurement,* ed. L. Levi (New York: Raven Press, 1975), 22-35.

13. R. Karasek et al., "Job Decision Latitude, Job Demands, and Cardiovascular Disease," *American Journal of Public Health* 71 (1981): 694-705.

14. Many retrospective studies are also reported in D. O'Neill, *Doctor and Patient* (Philadelphia: J. B. Lippincott, 1955).

15. Ibid., 101.

16. Ibid., 117.

17. Ibid., 132.

18. Ibid., 133.

19. R. Freidman and L. K. Dahl, "The Effect of Chronic Conflict on the Blood Pressure of Rats with a Genetic Susceptibility to Experimental Hypertension," *Psychosomatic Medicine* 37 (1975): 412-16; R. Freidman and L. K. Dahl, "Psychic and Genetic Factors in the Etiology of Hypertension," in *Stress and the Heart,* ed. D. Wheatley (New York: Raven, 1977), 137-56.

20. From Freidman and Dahl, "Psychic and Genetic Factors," reproduced with the kind permission of the publishers.

21. Two other groups (not shown in Fig. 5.1), one of each genetic strain, were treated identically for 13 weeks but did not receive shock, and did not develop hypertension.

22. S. Cohen and G. M. Williamson, "Stress and Infectious Disease in Humans," *Psychological Bulletin* 109 (1991): 5-24.

23. R. S. Lazarus and S. Folkman, *Stress, Appraisal, and Coping* (New York: Springer, 1984).

24. E. L. Diamond, "The Role of Anger and Hostility in Essential Hypertension and Coronary Heart Disease," *Psychological Bulletin* 92 (1982): 410-33; H. Weiner, *Psychobiology and Human Disease* (Amsterdam: Elsevier, 1977); J. Sommers-Flanagan and R. P. Greenberg, "Psychosocial Variables and Hypertension," *Journal of Nervous & Mental Diseases* 177 (1989): 14-24.

25. N. Cousins, *Anatomy of an Illness* (London: W. W. Norton, 1979). It should be pointed out that Cousins' treatment also included megadoses of intravenous vitamin C.

26. J. Borysenko, *Minding the Body, Mending the Mind* (New York: Bantam, 1987).

27. E. Light and B. Lebowitz, eds., *Alzheimer's Disease Treatment and Family Stress: Directions for Research* (Washington, D.C.: Government Printing Office, 1988).

28. J. I. Kiecolt-Glaser et al., "Spousal Caregivers of Dementia Victims: Longitudinal Changes in Immunity and Health," *Psychosomatic Medicine* 53 (1991): 345-62.

29. See Cohen and Williamson, "Stress and Infectious Disease," for citations to specific studies discussed in this paragraph.

30. See Kiecolt-Glaser, "Spousal Caregivers of Dementia Victims," for a survey of the literature supporting the conclusions reached in this paragraph.

31. Ibid.

32. S. V. Kasl, A. S. Evans, and J. C. Niederman, "Psychosocial Risk Factors in the Development of Infectious Mononucleosis," *Psychosomatic Medicine* 41 (1979): 445-66.

33. Cohen and Williamson, "Stress and Infectious Disease."

34. The ideas in this section are drawn from chapter 3 of K. R. Pelletier, *Mind as Healer, Mind as Slayer* (New York: Dell, 1977), to which the reader is referred for citations to the original sources.

35. More detailed information may be found in G. T. Lewith and D. Aldridge, eds., *Clinical Research Methodology for Complementary Therapies* (London: Hodder & Stoughton, 1993); and D. H. Barlow and M. Herson, *Single Case Experimental Designs* (New York: Pergamon, 1984).

36. Copyright 1976 by Thomas H. Holmes, M.D., Dept. of Psychiatry and Behavioral Sciences, University of Washington School of Medicine, Seattle, WA 98195. Reproduced with permission of University of Washington Press.

Chapter 6

1. From K. R. Gaarder and P. S. Montgomery, *Clinical Biofeedback: A Procedural Manual for Behavioral Medicine* (Baltimore: Williams & Wilkins, 1977). Reproduced with the kind permission of the publisher.

2. This table has been compiled from data reported in F. Adrasik, D. Coleman, and L. H. Epstein, "Biofeedback: Clinical and Research Considerations," in *Behavioral Medicine: Assessment and Treatment Strategies,* eds., D. M. Doleys, R. L. Meredith, and A. R. Ciminero (London: Plenum Press, 1982); D. Shapiro and R.

S. Surwitt, "Biofeedback," in *Behavioral Medicine: Theory and Practice*, ed. O. F. Pomerleau and J. P. Brady (London: Plenum Press, 1979); D. I. Mostofsky and Y. Loyning, eds., "The Neurobehavioral Treatment of Epilepsy" (Hillsdale, NJ: Erlbaum Associates, 1993).

3. J. Achterberg, *Imagery in Healing: Shamanism and Modern Medicine* (Boston: Shambhala, 1985).

4. Ibid.

5. See, e.g., A. Hannay, *Mental Images: A Defence* (London: George Allen & Unwin, 1971).

6. O. C. Simonton, S. Simonton, and J. Creighton, *Getting Well Again* (Los Angeles: Tarcher, 1978); O. C. Simonton, S. Matthews-Simonton, and T. F. Sparks, "Psychological Intervention in the Treatment of Cancer," *Psychosomatics* 21 (1980): 226-7, 231-3.

7. For details see M. Rossman, "Imagine Health! Imagery in Medical Self-Care," in *Imagination and Healing*, ed. A. A. Sheikh (Farmingdale, NY: Baywood, 1984), 231-58. More illustrations are presented in Chapter 14 of our book.

8. J. R. Cautela and L. McCullough, "Covert Conditioning," in *The Power of Human Imagination*, eds. J. L. Singer and K. S. Pope (New York: Plenum Press, 1978), 227-54.

9. R. S. Hall, J. A. Anderson, and M. P. O'Grady, "Stress and Immunity in Humans: Modifying Variables," in *Handbook of Human Stress and Immunity*, eds. R. Glaser and J. Kiecolt-Glaser (San Diego: Academic Press, 1994), 183-215. In some cases patients have used other metaphors, including the visualization of cancer as weeds in a flower garden that are being removed.

10. Simonton, Matthews-Simonton, and Sparks, "Psychological Intervention in the Treatment of Cancer."

11. Hall, Anderson, and O'Grady, "Stress and Immunity in Humans."

12. J. Schneider et al., "Guided Imagery and Immune System Function in Normal Subjects: A Summary of Research Findings," in *Mental Imagery*, ed. R. G. Kunzendorf (New York, Plenum Press, 1991), 179-91. In injury, damaged cells emit a chemical which causes circulating neutrophils to become sticky and then adhere to blood vessel walls. They then squeeze themselves through the pores of these walls and migrate to the site of the injury where they voraciously phagocytose bacteria and debris.

13. Hall, Anderson, and O'Grady, "Stress and Immunity in Humans." What we do know is that NK cell activity affects artificial tumor growth in mice.

14. D. Meichenbaum, "Why Does Using Imagery in Psychotherapy Lead to Change?" in *Power of Human Imagination*, eds. J. L. Singer and K. S. Pope (New York: Plenum Press, 1978), 388.

15. Hall, Anderson, and O'Grady, "Stress and Immunity in Humans," 191.

16. R. B. Stuart, "Behavioral Control of Overeating," *Behavioral Research and Therapy* 5 (1967): 357-65.

17. This section is derived in large part from M. L. Russell, *Behavioral Counseling in Medicine* (New York: Oxford University Press, 1986).

18. After Russell, ibid.

19. Defined as rhythmic, vigorous activity capable of being sustained for at least 30 minutes, and that elevates the heart rate to 65-75 percent of its age-related maximum.

20. After Russell, *Behavioral Counseling in Medicine.*

21. Ibid.

22. D. C. Turk, P. Salovey, and M. D. Litt, "Adherence: A Cognitive-Behavioral Perspective," in *Compliance: The Dilemma of the Chronically Ill,* eds. K. E. Gerber and A. M. Nehemkis (New York: Springer, 1988).

23. M. Weintraub, "Intelligent Non-compliance and Capricious Compliance," in *Patient Compliance,* vol. 10, ed. L. Lasagne (Mt. Kisco, NY.: Futura, 1976).

24. R. W. Hanson, "Physician-patient Communication and Compliance," in *Compliance: The Dilemma of the Chronically Ill,* eds. K. E. Gerber and A. M. Nehemkis (New York: Springer, 1988).

25. L. H. Epstein and B. J. Masek, "Behavioral Control of Medicine Compliance," *Journal of Applied Behavioral Analysis* 11 (1978): 1-9.

Chapter 7

1. Slightly modified from M. Feurerstein, E. E. Labbe, and A. R. Kuczmierczyk, *Health Psychology* (London: Plenum Press, 1986), 247.

2. For more details about this third coping mechanism, see P. Carrington, *Releasing: The New Behavioral Science Method for Dealing with Pressure Situations* (New York: Morrow, 1984).

3. Figs. 7.1, 7.2 and 7.3 are adapted from A. P. Chesney and W. D. Gentry, "Psychosocial Factors Mediating Health Risk: A Balanced Perspective," *Preventative Medicine* 11 (1982): 612-17. Reproduced here with the kind permission of the publisher and authors.

4. The practitioner interested in more than the sketch of the rationale and methodology provided in this section should consult one of the available relaxation training manuals, e.g., D. A. Bernstein and T. D. Borkovec, *Progressive Relaxation Training* (Champaign, IL: Research Press, 1973).

5. D. A. Bernstein and B. A. Given, "Progessive Relaxation: Abbreviated Methods," in *Principles and Practice of Stress Management,* 2d ed., eds. R. L. Woolfolk and P. M. Lehrer (New York: Guilford, 1993).

6. P. Charrington, "Modern Forms of Meditation," in *Principles and Practice of Stress Management,* Woolfolk and Lehrer.

7. The TM mantra is assigned by a certified TM instructor.

8. Paul Brunton's *In Search of Sacred India* (New York: Dutton & Co., 1935) is a useful book to recommend to patients whose skepticism borders on close-mindedness.

9. C. Patel, "Yogic Therapy," in *Principles and Practice of Stress Management*, Woolfolk and Lehrer.

10. M. Lee, E. Lee, and J. Johnstone, *Ride the Tiger to the Mountain* (New York: Addison-Wesley, 1989).

11. From D. C. Turk, D. Meichenbaum, and M. Genest, *Pain and Behavioural Medicine* (London: Guilford Press, 1983), 332-3. Reprinted with the kind permission of the publisher.

12. Personal communication from Dan Bensky.

13. R. Melzack and P. Wall, "Pain Mechanisms: A New Theory," *Science* 150 (1965): 971-9.

14. After R. L. Karol et al., "A Therapist Manual for the Cognitive-Behavioral Treatment of Chronic Pain," JSAS *Catalog of Selected Documents in Psychology* 11 (1981): 15-16.

15. F. O. Schmitt, "Molecular Regulators of Brain Function: A New View," *Neuroscience* 13 (1984): 991-1001; C. B. Pert et al., "Neuropeptides and Their Receptors: A Psychosomatic Network," *Journal of Immunology* 135 (1985): 820-6; C. B. Pert, "The Wisdom of the Receptors: Neuropeptides, the Emotions, and Bodymind," *Advances* 3 (1986): 8-16.

16. R. Melzack, "The McGill Pain Questionnaire," *Pain* 1 (1975): 277-99. Reproduced here with the kind permission of the publisher and author.

17. P. D. Wall and R. Melzack, eds., *Textbook of Pain*, 2nd ed. (London: Churchill Livingstone, 1989).

18. T. X. Barber, "Hypnosis, Deep Relaxation, and Active Relaxation," in *Principles and Practice of Stress Management*, Woolfolk and Lehrer. The ellipses do not refer to material left out, but to deliberate pauses by the therapist which serve to slow down the mental and bodily processes of the patient.

19. Although introduced here in the context of pain control, hypnotherapy has potential value in alleviating stress-related problems generally for those patients able to enter the trance state.

20. A. Antonovsky, *Health, Stress, and Coping* (London: Jossey-Bass, 1979), 10. See also A. Antonovsky, "Pathways Leading to Successful Coping and Health," in *Learned Resourcefulness*, ed. M. Rosenbaum (New York: Springer, 1990), 31-63; and A. Antonovsky, "The Structural Sources of Salutogenic Strengths," in *Personality and Stress: Individual Differences in the Stress Process*, eds. C. I. Cooper and R. Payne (New York: Wiley, 1991).

21. Barber, "Hypnosis, Deep Relaxation, and Active Relaxation," 162.

Chapter 8

1. Practitioners of Eastern medicine are also trained to take emotional and psychological factors into account in both their diagnosis and treatment. Depending on their orientation, they may or may not find the Western principles of psychological

medicine enunciated here to be of value in supplementing their own distinctive ways of working within their energetic frameworks.

2. Carl Simonton quoted in F. Capra, *Uncommon Wisdom* (New York: Simon & Schuster, 1988), 201.

3. Although the West dissociated general medicine from psychological medicine some time ago, most traditional medical systems, e.g., Tibetan, Ayurvedic and Chinese, never made this distinction.

4. From E. F. Borgatta and W. W. Lambert, eds., *Handbook of Personality Theory and Research* (Chicago: Rand-McNally, 1968).

5. T. Gordon, *Leader Effectiveness Training* (New York: Wyden Books, 1977).

6. M. Balint, *The Doctor, His Patient and the Illness* (New York: International Universities Press, 1964).

7. Rogers replaced the term "patient" with "client" to emphasize the non-hierarchical nature of person-centered counseling.

8. C. R. Rogers and J. K. Wood, "Client-centered Theory: Carl R. Rogers," in *Operational Theories of Personality*, ed. A. Burton (New York: Brunner/Mazel, 1974), 227.

9. Ibid., 234-5. This case is reprinted with the kind permission of the publisher. I have added the running commentary.

10. W. Glasser, *Reality Therapy* (New York: Harper and Row, 1965).

11. Glasser selected the verbal forms rather than the more familiar adjectival ones in order to stress that these emotions are actually chosen by the person, not something imposed on him from outside. Recall cognitive psychology's explanation of how, once certain beliefs are chosen, our emotional gun is then cocked for predictable emotions to be fired by external events.

12. Unless of course we have the power and are prepared to coerce through superior physical force; or to control others' survival needs. These methods are known respectively as oppression and manipulation, and although both are sadly still in common use by some parents, teachers, industries and oppressive governments, control by force is always temporary and invariably destructive of human relationships.

13. Behavioral therapy includes *systematic desensitization* (i.e., counter-conditioning of relaxation responses to anxiety-producing stimuli), *skills learning* through behavioral rehearsal and modeling, *reinforcement contingency contracting* that strengthens the patient's adaptive and self-fulfilling behaviors, and *assertive training*.

14. The exact instructions to the patient are similar to the therapist's question guidelines given in the text, but in somewhat less technical language. They can be found in A. A. Lazarus, *The Practice of Multimodal Therapy* (London: McGraw Hill, 1981), 17-18, 76. Illustrative cases (of which Table 8.2 is a modified example) of BASIC I.D. assessment and treatment plans can be found in A. A. Lazarus, ed.,

Casebook of Multimodal Therapy (London: Guilford Press, 1985), and A. A. Lazarus, ed., *Multimodal Behavior Therapy* (New York: Springer, 1976).

15. R. May and I. Yalom, "Existential Psychotherapy," in *Current Psychotherapies*, eds. R. Corsini and D. Wedding (Itasca, IL: Peacock, 1989), 364-5.
16. Ibid., 377.
17. E. van Deurzen-Smith, *Existential Counselling in Practice* (London: Sage, 1988).
18. After M. Rosenberg, *From Now On: Without Blame* (St. Louis: Community Psychological Consultants, 1977).

Chapter 9

1. See, e.g., E. H. Ackerknecht, "The History of Psychosomatic Medicine," *Psychological Medicine* 12 (1982): 17-24; Z. J. Lipowski, "Psychosomatic Concepts in Historical Perspective," in *Proceedings of the 15th European Conference on Psychosomatic Research*, eds. J. H. Lacey and D. A. Sturgeon (London: John Libbey, 1986).
2. These became known, somewhat facetiously, as the "holy seven" psychosomatic illnesses. In fact, as this chapter goes on to describe, there are *no* psychosomatic illnesses in the sense of an illness being purely psychogenic in origin. On the other hand, *all* illness is psychosomatic to the degree that psychosocial influences are a part of the holistic, multicausal matrix of every disease.
3. Z. J. Lipowski, "The Holistic Approach to Medicine," in *Psychosomatic Medicine and Liaison Psychiatry*, ed. Z. J. Lipowski (New York: Plenum, 1985).
4. Lipowski, "Psychosomatic Concepts in Historical Perspective."
5. Or the opposite, as in the less-used term "somatopsychic," which denotes the emotional and behavioral effects of bodily dysfunction.
6. Lipowski, "Holistic Approach to Medicine."
7. The letters A, C, N, E and O stand for five fundamental dimensions of personality: **A**greeable vs. Antagonistic, **C**onscientious vs. Undependable, **N**eurotic vs. Self-secure, **E**xtroversion vs. Introversion, **O**penness vs. Closed to Experience. In principle, any personality trait whatsoever can be located as a particular combination of these five.
8. The student wishing to pursue the conceptual development of psychosomatics further may consult the following: J. J. Groen, "Emotional Factors in the Etiology of Internal Diseases," especially chapters 1, 2 and 21, in *Psychosomatic Research*, ed. J. J. Groen (New York: Pergamon, 1964); Z. J. Lipowski, "Psychosomatic Medicine: An Overview," in *Modern Trends in Psychosomatic Medicine*, 3rd ed., ed. O. Hill (Boston: Butterworths, 1976); Lipowski, "Holistic Approach to Medicine"; B. Lask and A. Fosson, *Childhood Illness: The Psychosomatic Approach* (Chichester: Wiley, 1989); M. Christie, ed., *Foundations of Psychosomatics* (Chichester: Wiley, 1981); J. W. Todd, "The Psychosomatic Concept in Medicine," in *Modern Trends in Psychosomatic Medicine*, ed. D. O'Neil (London: Butterworths, 1955).

9. F. Alexander, T. M. French, and G. H. Pollock, *Psychosomatic Specificity,* vol. 1 (Chicago: University of Chicago Press, 1968), 9.

10. The information for this section is drawn from various reviews and original research reports. The following references will lead the interested reader to the original sources: R. Totman, *Mind, Stress and Health* (London: Souvenir, 1990); G. Davison and J. M. Neale, *Abnormal Psychology,* 5th ed., chapter 8 (London: John Wiley, 1990); C. E. Thoresen and L. H. Powell, "Type A Behavior Pattern: New Perspectives on Theory, Assessment, and Intervention," *Journal of Consulting and Clinical Psychology* 60 (1992): 595-604; J. J. Ray, "If A-B Does not Predict Heart Disease, Why Bother with It?" *British Journal of Medical Psychology* 64 (1991): 85-90; J. Rodin and P. Salovey, "Health Psychology," *Annual Review of Psychology* 40 (1989): 533-79.

11. Davison and Neale, *Abnormal Psychology,* 208.

12. Friedman and Rosenman called type A an "action-emotion complex" and assiduously avoided referring to it as a personality trait, perhaps because they did not wish their work to be identified with Alexander's earlier psychoanalytic psychosomatic hypotheses. Nevertheless, no one has ever shown how type A differs operationally from a cluster of personality traits. See J. Suls and J. D. Rittenhouse, "Personality and Physical Health: An Introduction," *Journal of Personality* 55 (1987): 155-67.

13. Thoresen and Powell, "Type A Behavior Pattern," 597.

14. After V. A. Price and M. Friedman, "Modifying Type A Behavior and Reducing Coronary Recurrence Rates," in *Proceedings of the 15th European Conference on Psychosomatic Research,* eds. J. H. Lacey and D. A. Sturgeon (London: Libbey, 1986).

15. Thoresen and Powell, "Type A Behavior Pattern," 597.

16. R. Totman, *Mind, Stress and Health* (London: Souvenir, 1990), 84.

17. T. W. Smith and P. G. Williams, "Personality and Health: Advantages and Limitations of the Five-factor Model," *Journal of Personality* 60 (1992): 395-423.

18. R. R. McCrae and O. P. John, "An Introduction to the Five-factor Model and its Applications," in R. R. McCrae, ed., "The Five-factor Model: Issues and Applications" [special issue], *Journal of Personality* 60 (1992): 175-215.

19. As suggested, e.g., in M. Angell, "Disease as a Reflection of the Psyche," *New England Journal of Medicine* 312 (1985): 1570-72.

20. H. S. Friedman and S. Booth-Kewley, "The 'Disease-prone Personality': A Meta-analytic View of the Construct," *American Psychologist* 42 (1987): 539-55.

21. S. C. Kobasa, "The Hardy Personality: Toward a Social Psychology of Stress and Health," in *Social Psychology of Health and Illness,* eds. G. S. Sanders and J. Suls (Hillsdale, NJ: Erlbaum, 1982), 3-32; J. G. Hull, R. R. Van Treuren, and S. Virnelli, "Hardiness and Health: A Critique and Alternative Approach," *Journal of Personality and Social Psychology* 53 (1987): 518-30; S. C. Ouellette, "Inquiries into Hardiness," in *Handbook of Stress,* vol. 2, eds. L. Goldberger and S. Breznitz (New York: Macmillan, 1993), 77-96.

22. A. Antonovsky, "Pathways Leading to Successful Coping and Health," in *Learned Resourcefulness,* ed. M. Rosenbaum (New York: Springer, 1990), 31-63.

23. E. Orr and M. Westman, "Does Hardiness Moderate Stress, and How? A Review," in Rosenbaum, *Learned Resourcefulness,* 64-94.

24. Smith and Williams, "Personality and Health," 395-423; M. F. Scheier and C. S. Carver, "Dispositional Optimism and Physical Well-being," *Journal of Personality* 55 (1987): 169-210.

25. Scheier and Carver, "Dispositional Optimism and Physical Well-being."

26. A complex of traits called "unstressed affiliation motive." See Smith and Williams, "Personality and Health."

Chapter 10

1. See C. G. Stephens, "Reflections of a Post-Flexnerian Physician," in *The Task of Medicine,* ed. K. L. White (Menlo Park, CA: Kaiser Foundation, 1988), 177.

2. See S. Sontag, *Illness as Metaphor* (New York: Farrar, Straus, Giroux, 1977); M. Angell, "Disease as a Reflection of the Psyche," *New England Journal of Medicine* 312 (1985): 1570-72.

3. P. R. Williamson, "Support Groups: An Important Aspect of Physician Education," *Journal of General Internal Medicine* 6 (1991): 179-80.

4. The information in this section is drawn from reviews by S. Thornton, "Irritable Bowel Syndrome," in *Practice of Behavioural Medicine,* eds. S. Pearce and J. Wardle (Oxford: BPS Books, 1989); W. E. Whitehead and M. M. Schuster, "The Treatment of Functional Gastrointestinal Disorders," in *The Psychosomatic Approach to Illness,* ed. R. L. Gallon (Oxford: Elsevier, 1982); B. Lask and A. Fosson, *Childhood Illness: Psychosomatic Approach* (New York: John Wiley, 1989); W. E. Whitehead, "Behavioral Medicine Approaches to Gastrointestinal Disorders," *Journal of Consulting and Clinical Psychology* 60 (1992): 605-12.

5. More exact criteria for IBS are provided in Whitehead, "Behavioral Medicine Approaches to Gastrointestinal Disorders."

6. I generally prefer to avoid this pejorative term and use the more neutral equivalent, "negative-affect" (the "N" personality dimension described in Chapter 9), but the dimension does include low self-esteem, negative self-image, ambivalence in action, dependency on others' judgments, pessimistic outlook, feelings of helplessness and hopelessness.

7. J. Svedlund and I. Sjödin, "A Psychosomatic Approach to Treatment in the Irritable Bowel Syndrome," in *Proceedings of the 15th European Conference on Psychosomatic Research,* eds. J. H. Lacey and D. A. Sturgeon (London: Libbey, 1986).

8. Whitehead and Schuster, "Treatment of Functional Gastrointestinal Disorders," 206-7.

9. For further details, see Thornton, "Irritable Bowel Syndrome."

10. This section has been abstracted from reviews by J. Bastiaans and J. Groen, "Psychogenesis and Psychotherapy of Bronchial Asthma," in *Modern Trends in Psychosomatic Medicine,* ed. D. O'Neill (London: Butterworths, 1955); A. Steptoe, "Psychological Aspects of Bronchial Asthma," in *Contributions to Medical Psychology,* vol. 3, ed. S. Rachman (Oxford: Pergamon, 1984); A. B. Alexander, "Behavioral Medicine in Asthma," in *Adherence, Compliance and Generalization in Behavioral Medicine,* ed. R. B. Stuart (New York: Brunner-Mazel, 1982); F. M. Lehrer, D. Sargunaraj, and S. Hochron, "Psychological Approaches to the Treatment of Asthma," *Journal of Consulting and Clinical Psychology* 60 (1992): 639-43.

11. Alexander, "Behavioral Medicine in Asthma," 38.

12. K. Purcell et al., "The Effect on Asthma of Children of Experimental Separation from Family," *Psychosomatic Medicine* 31 (1969): 144-64.

13. Bastiaans and Groen, "Psychogenesis and Psychotherapy of Bronchial Asthma," 236.

14. The information presented in this section is abstracted from A. A. Kaptein, "Skin Disorders," in *Behavioural Medicine: Psychological Treatment of Behaviour Disorders,* eds. A. A. Kaptein et al. (London: John Wiley, 1990); D. G. Folks and F. C. Kinney, "Role of Psychological Factors in Dermatologic Conditions," *Psychosomatics* 33 (1992): 45-54; S. C. Wessely, "Dermatological Complaints," in *Somatization: Physical Symptoms and Psychological Illness,* ed. C. Bass (Oxford: Blackwell, 1990); H. Musaph, "Psychodermatology," in *Modern Trends in Psychosomatic Medicine,* vol. 3, ed. O. Hill (London: Butterworths, 1976); M. A. Gupta, A. K. Gupta, and H. F. Haberman, "Psoriasis and Psychiatry: An Update," *General Hospital Psychiatry* 9 (1987): 157-66.

15. K. W. van der Schaar and M. Couperus, "A Psychosomatic Study of Skin Disease in Ten Adolescent Girls," in *Proceedings of 15th European Conference on Psychosomatic Research,* Lacey and Sturgeon.

16. Ibid.

17. M. Bremer-Schulte et al., "Group Therapy of Psoriasis. Duo Famila Group Treatment as an Example," *Journal of the American Academy of Dermatology* 12 (1985): 61-6.

18. The information presented in this section is derived from reviews by L. D. Young, "Psychological Factors in Rheumatoid Arthritis," *Journal of Consulting and Clinical Psychology* 60 (1992): 619-27; K. A. Anderson et al., "Rheumatoid Arthritis: Review of Psychological Factors Related to Etiology, Effects, and Treatment," *Psychological Bulletin* 98 (1985): 358-87; G. F. Solomon, "Psychophysiological Aspects of Rheumatoid Arthritis and Autoimmune Disease," in *Modern Trends in Psychosomatic Medicine,* Hill.

19. R. Rimon, "Psychosomatic Aspects of Rheumatoid Arthritis," *Psychiatrica Fennica Supplement* (1981): 97-101.

20. Solomon, "Psychophysiological Aspects of Rheumatoid Arthritis," 196.

22. Ibid.; H. Weiner, *Psychobiology and Human Disease* (New York: Elsevier, 1977).

22. A. O'Leary et al., "A Cognitive-behavior Treatment for Rheumatoid Arthritis," *Health Psychology* 7 (1986): 527-44.

Chapter 11

1. This section draws on information from reviews by H. E. Adams, M. Fuerstein, and J. L. Fowler, "Migraine Headache: Review of Parameters, Etiology, and Intervention," *Psychological Bulletin* 87 (1980): 217-37; E. B. Blanchard, "Psychological Treatment of Benign Headache Disorders," *Journal of Consulting and Clinical Psychology* 60 (1992): 537-51; H. van der Helm-Hylkema, "Headache," in *Psychological Treatment of Somatic Disorders,* eds. A. A. Kaptein et al. (New York: John Wiley, 1990); R. C. Packard, "Life Stress, Personality Factors and Reactions to Headache," in *Wolff's Headache and Other Head Pain,* 5th ed., ed. D. J. Dalesio (New York: Oxford University Press, 1987).
2. A. van Boxtel and P. Goudswaard, "Absolute and Proportional Resting EMG Levels in Chronic Headache Patients in Relation to the State of Headache," *Headache* 24 (1984): 259-65.
3. Blanchard, "Psychological Treatment of Benign Headache Disorders."
4. Biofeedback for migraine was discovered serendipitously in unrelated experiments in 1970 at the Menninger Foundation. One subject, a woman regularly suffering from migraine, discovered that an approaching attack disappeared when she succeeded in raising her finger temperature.
5. From van der Helm-Hylkama, "Headache," 75. Reproduced with the kind permission of the publisher.
6. J. Klapper, J. Stanton, and M. Seawell, "The Development of a Support Group for Headache Sufferers," *Headache* 32 (1992): 193-6.
7. G. P. Holmes, "Defining the Chronic Fatigue Syndrome," *Review of Infectious Diseases* 13 (1991): 53-5; E. G. Dowsett et al., "It's Called Myalgic Encephalomylitis—A Persistent Enteroviral Infection," *Postgraduate Medical Journal* 66 (1990): 326-30.
8. Dowsett, "It's Called Myalgic Encephalomylitis."
9. J. Hooge, "Chronic Fatigue Syndrome: Cause, Controversy, and Care," *British Journal of Nursing* 1 (1992): 440-6.
10. Ibid.
11. C. Shepherd, *Living with ME: A Self-help Guide* (London: Heinemann, 1989); A. MacIntyre, *M.E. Postviral Fatigue Syndrome: How to Live with It* (London: Unwin, 1989); J. Millenson, "M.E.: An Alternative View," *ME Action Campaign Interaction* (Jan./Feb., 1992).
12. D. B. Greenberg, "Neurasthenia in the 1980s: Chronic Mononucleosis, Chronic Fatigue Syndrome and Anxiety and Depressive Disorders," *Psychosomatics* 31 (1990): 129-37; S. Wessely, "Old Wine in New Bottles: Neurasthenia and 'ME'," *Psychological Medicine* 20 (1990): 35-53.

13. G. F. Drinka, *The Birth of Neurosis : Myth, Malady, and the Victorians* (New York : Simon and Schuster, 1984).

14. C. Ray, "Chronic Fatigue Syndrome and Depression: Conceptual and Methodological Ambiguities," *Psychological Medicine* 21 (1991): 1-9; Hooge, "Chronic Fatigue Syndrome."

15. M. Craig, *Psychological Medicine* (London: J. & A. Churchill, 1912).

16. Ray, "Chronic Fatigue Syndrome and Depression."

17. Wessely, "Old Wine in New Bottles."

18. S. Butler et al., "Cognitive Behavior Therapy in CFS," *Journal of Neurology and Neurosurgery in Psychiatry* 54 (1991): 153-8.

19. Z. J. Lipowski, "Somatization and Its Clinical Application," *American Journal of Psychiatry* 145 (1988): 1358-68; H. Fabrega, "The Concept of Somatization as a Cultural and Historical Product of Western Medicine," *Psychosomatic Medicine* 52 (1990): 653-72.

20. M. Hersen and D. H. Barlow, *Single Case Experimental Design Strategies for Studying Behavioral Change* (New York: Pergamon, 1976).

Chapter 12

1. L. Webster, *Dream-work* (London: Dryad, 1987).

2. Summarized, e.g., in H. Lindlaur, *Philosophy of Natural Therapeutics* (Maidstone, Kent: Maidstone Osteopathic Clinic, 1975). The nineteenth-century naturopaths meant of course "violating the natural laws of health," for by definition a law of nature is an invariance which admits of no violations.

3. See, e.g., the case histories in K. Duff, *The Alchemy of Illness* (New York: Pantheon, 1993); D. Talman, *Heartsearch* (Berkeley: North Atlantic, 1991); and K. Wilber, *Grace and Grit* (Boston: Shambhala, 1991).

4. The technical meaning of hysteria is a conversion somatization, nothing to do with its popular connotations of easily roused to over-dramatic tears or scenes.

5. G. Groddeck, *The Meaning of Illness* (New York: International Universities Press, 1977), 197.

6. Ibid., chapter 6.

7. D. Jennings, "The Confusion between Disease and Illness in Clinical Medicine," *Canadian Medical Association Journal* 35 (1986): 865-70.

8. The categories listed here (excluding family therapy) are abridged and modified from Wilber, *Grace and Grit*.

9. Ibid., 266.

10. After a suggestion by M. Kidel, "Illness and Meaning," in *The Meaning of Illness*, eds. M. Kidel and S. Rowe-Leete (London: Routledge, 1988), and compiled from interpretations given by L. Hay, *You Can Heal Your Life* (London: Eden Grove, 1984) and by T. Dethlefsen and R. Dahlke, *The Healing Power of Illness*, trans. P. Lemesurier (Shaftsbury, Dorset: Element, 1990).

11. Dethlefsen and Dahlke, *Healing Power of Illness,* 78.
12. N. Shealy and C. Myss, *The Creation of Health* (Walpole, NH: Stillpoint, 1988), 23.
13. Dethlefsen and Dahlke, *Healing Power of Illness,* 83.
14. R. F. Rosenthal and J. S. Gordon, *The Healing Partnership* (Washington, D.C.: Aurora, 1991), 9.
15. Karl Robinson quoted in R. Leviton, "What Does Illness Mean?" *Yoga Journal* (Nov./Dec. 1991): 50.
16. See the autobiographical accounts of Duff, *Alchemy of Illness,* Talman, *Heartsearch,* and Wilber, *Grace and Grit,* for a description of the long and tortuous journeys undertaken to seek out the meaning of chronic illness.
17. R. Moss, *The I that is We* (Berkeley: Celestial Arts, 1981), 105.
18. B. Levine, *Your Body Believes Every Word You Say* (Lower Lake, CA: Aslan, 1991).
19. A. Guggenbühl-Craig and N. Micklem, "No Answer to Job: Reflections on the Limitations of Meaning in Illness," in *Meaning of Illness,* Kidel and Rowe-Leete, 144.
20. S. Sontag, *Illness as Metaphor* (New York: Farrar, Straus and Giroux, 1977).
21. Duff, *Alchemy of Illness;* Talman, *Heartsearch;* Wilber, *Grace and Grit.*
22. Guggenbühl-Craig and Micklem, "No Answer to Job," 150.
23. L. Dossey, *Meaning and Medicine* (New York: Bantam, 1991), 19.
24. The remainder of this section is taken, with minor changes, from a previously unpublished thesis by Susan Holden, "The Pearl of Sensation" (Durham University, 1992), and is reprinted here with her kind permission.
25. A. Mindell, *Dreambody* (New York: Arkana, 1982), 32.
26. J. Goodbread, *The Dreambody Toolkit* (New York: Routledge & Kegan Paul, 1987), 10.
27. Mindell, *Dreambody,* 69.
28. Ibid., 16.
29. Dethlefsen and Dahlke, *Healing Power of Illness,* 89.

Chapter 13

1. J. Needleman, *The Way of the Physician* (Harmondsworth: Penguin, 1985).
2. Although we commonly use the word "physician" to mean one who is certified, authorized or licensed by the state to practice medicine, the primary meaning of the word is "one who is skilled in the art of healing" (*Webster's 3rd International Dictionary*). As this chapter illustrates, it is the relationship that heals; therefore, one who can create a healing relationship is a physician, and that ability cuts across the spectrum of practitioners, orthodox or otherwise.
3. T. A. Preston, *The Clay Pedestal* (Seattle: Madrona, 1986), 67.
4. M. Balint, *The Doctor, His Patient and the Illness* (New York: International Universities Press, 1964); J. Borysenko, "Removing Barriers to the Peaceful Core," in

Healers on Healing, eds. R. Carlson and B. Shield (Los Angeles: J. P. Tarcher, 1989).

5. Adapted from T. S. Szasz and M. H. Hollander, "A Contribution to the Philosophy of Medicine: The Basic Models of the Doctor-patient Relationship," *Archives of Internal Medicine* 97 (1956): 585-92.

6. P. S. Jensen, "The Doctor Patient Relationship: Headed for Impasse or Improvement?" *Annals of Internal Medicine* 95 (1981): 769-71.

7. E. J. Cassell, "Preliminary Explorations of Thinking in Medicine," *Ethics in Science & Medicine* 2 (1981): 1-12; T. Mizrahi, *Getting Rid of Patients* (New Brunswick, NJ: Rutgers Press, 1986); L. Dossey, *Beyond Illness* (Boston: New Science Library, 1984).

8. E. J. Cassell, *The Healer's Art* (Philadelphia: J. P. Lippincott, 1976), 117.

9. The physicians were general practitioners who had a general interest in psychological medicine and met once a week in roundtable discussion with Michael Balint, a psychoanalyst, to discuss their problem cases.

10. J. Needleman, *The Way of the Physician* (Harmondsworth, Middlesex: Penguin, 1985); D. H. Johnson, "Presence," in *Healers on Healing,* Carlson and Shields.

11. A. Weil, *Health and Healing* (Boston: Houghton Mifflin, 1983), chapter 19.

12. Cf. H. Spiro, *Doctors, Patients, and Placebos* (New Haven, CT: Yale University Press, 1986).

13. Weil, *Health and Healing,* 226.

14. Ibid., 109.

15. N. Cousins, *Anatomy of an Illness* (New York: W. W. Norton, 1979), 58.

16. P. Suedfeld, "Subtractive Placebo," *Behavioural Research and Therapy* 22 (1984): 159-64.

17. Cf. Spiro, *Doctors, Patients, and Placebos*; Weil, *Health and Healing.*

18. A. H. Roberts et al., "The Power of Nonspecific Effects in Healing: Implications for Psychosocial and Biological Treatments," *Clinical Psychology Review* 13 (1993): 375-91; J. A. Turner et al., "The Importance of Placebo Effects in Pain Treatment and Research," *Journal of the American Medical Association* 271 (1994): 1609-14.

19. Turner, "Importance of Placebo Effects," 1609.

20. E.g., Spiro, *Doctors, Patients, and Placebos,* 75.

21. M. Sidman, *Tactics of Scientific Research* (New York: Basic Books, 1960).

22. E. J. Cassell, "The Nature of Suffering and Goals of Medicine," *New England Journal of Medicine* 306 (1982): 639-45.

23. Modified from P. Tate, "Doctors Style," in *Doctor/Patient Communication,* eds. D. Pendleton and J. Hasler (New York: Academic Press, 1983), and used with the kind permission of the publisher.

24. Balint, *The Doctor, His Patient and the Illness,* 125.

25. S. Matthews, A. L. Suchman, and W. T. Branch, "Making 'Connexions': Enhancing the Therapeutic Potential of Patient-clinician Relationships," *Annals of Internal Medicine* 118 (1993): 973-7.

26. For more detail and case histories concerning how to do this delicate job, cf. M.

Balint and E. Balint, *Psychotherapeutic Techniques in Medicine* (Springfield, IL: C. C. Thomas, 1961).

27. Closed-ended questions are those that admit of yes/no or very limited response. For instance, "Do you take any exercise?" or "How many brothers and sisters do you have?" Open-ended questions offer a broader range of response: "Were there any other family problems at that time?" or "Could you say a little bit more about that?" or "I'm wondering if you can give me an idea of the type of physical exercise you get in a typical week?"

28. Cf. C. L. Bowden and A. G. Burstein, *Psychosocial Basis of Medical Practice,* 2nd ed. (Baltimore: Williams & Wilkins, 1979), 37.

29. Adapted from M. L. Russell, *Behavioral Counseling in Medicine* (New York: Oxford University Press, 1986), 44.

30. A. E. Ivey and J. Authier, *Microcounseling,* 2nd ed. (Springfield, IL: C. C. Thomas, 1978), 52.

31. From M. J. O'Brien, *Communication and Relationships in Nursing* (St. Louis: C. V. Mosby, 1974), 61, and reproduced with the kind permission of the publisher.

32. Ibid., in abridged form.

33. S. Jourard, *The Transparent Self* (New York: Van Nostrand Reinhold, 1971).

34. E. Berne, *Games People Play* (New York: Grove, 1964).

35. See P. Pietroni, "Non-verbal Communication in the General Practice Surgery," in *Language and Communication in General Practice,* ed. B. Tanner (London: Hodder and Stoughton, 1976).

36. Tate, "Doctor's Style," 75-85.

37. Quoted in Cousins, *Anatomy of an Illness,* 68.

38. These seven questions are used routinely by Dr. Leanna J. Standish in her naturopathic practice, and I am grateful for her permission to reprint them here.

39. M. Lipkin, T. E. Quill, and R. J. Napodano, "The Medical Interview: A Core Curriculum for Residencies in Internal Medicine," *Annals of Internal Medicine* 100 (1984): 277-84.

Chapter 14

1. M. Balint and E. Balint, *Psychotherapeutic Techniques in Medicine* (Springfield, IL: C. C. Thomas, 1961), 49.

2. From N. Remen, *The Human Patient* (Garden City, New York: Anchor/Doubleday, 1980), 1-7. Reprinted here with the kind permission of the author.

3. From L. Dossey, *Beyond Illness* (Boston: Shambhala, 1984), 148-54. Reprinted here, in slightly modified form, with the kind permission of the author.

4. H. C. Hinshaw, *Diseases of the Chest,* 3rd ed. (Philadelphia: W. B. Saunders, 1969), 332.

5. C. W. Moorefield, "The Use of Hypnosis and Behavior Therapy in Asthma," *American Journal of Clinical Hypnosis* 13 (1970): 162-8.

6. From Julian W. Slowinski, "Three Multimodal Case Studies," in *Casebook of Multi-modal Therapy,* ed. A. A. Lazarus (New York: Guilford Press, 1985), 101-7. Reprinted here with the kind permission of the publisher.

7. A second order BASIC I.D. consists of subjecting any item in the profile to a more detailed recursive microanalysis in terms of the seven BASIC I.D. dimensions.

8. "Firing order" refers to the typical sequence of modalities culminating in a problem behavior or emotion. Ascertaining this sequence is important since therapeutic interventions will be directed toward interrupting it.

9. Not all of the techniques used by Dr. Slowinski (listed in Table 14.1) have been discussed in prior chapters. For more details, please consult the original source plus the references provided in Chapter 6, as well as the references to behavioral therapy provided in Chapter 8.

10. From M. Rossman, "Imagine Health! Imagery in Medical Self-care," in *Imagination and Healing,* ed. A. A. Sheikh (Farmingdale, NY: Baywood, 1984), 244-7. Reprinted here with the kind permission of the author and publisher.

11. C. G. Jung, *Mysterium Conjunctionis* (Princeton: Princeton University Press, 1970), 497.

12. A graduated learning program in self-care relaxation and imagery skills developed by Drs. Rossman and Remen. This program (a workbook and set of six cassettes entitled *Healing Yourself: A Step-by-Step Program for Better Health through Imagery)* is available to health professionals and others from the Academy for Guided Imagery, P. O. Box 2070, Mill Valley, CA 94942.

13. C. G. Jung, *Practice of Psychotherapy* (Princeton: Princeton University Press, 1975).

14. From M. Balint, *The Doctor, His Patient and the Illness* (New York: International Universities Press, 1964), 107-17. Reprinted here, in slightly modified form, with the kind permission of the publisher.

15. The seminar consisted of about a dozen family practitioners and two psychiatrists (Dr. Balint being one) that met weekly on a long-term basis. A main purpose of these seminars was to train doctors to make accurate psychogenic diagnoses and to give them the confidence to work on the psychological dimensions of their cases, if they so wished. A second purpose was to provide a basis for conducting research into what is and is not effective psychological medicine.

16. Patients frequently "offer" one symptom after another in an (unconscious) attempt to get the practitioner to listen to the underlying problem(s) of living.

17. That is to say, to *listen actively.*

18. Remen, *The Human Patient,* 59-67. Reprinted here with the kind permission of the author.

19. From M. R. Werbach, *Third Line Medicine* (Tarzana, CA: Third Line Press, 1986), 164-7. Reprinted here with the kind permission of the author. This book is available exclusively from Third Line Press, 4751 Viviana Dr., Tarzana, CA 91356.

Index